BETWEEN THE DEVIL AND THE DRAGON

Books by Eric Hoffer

The True Believer
The Passionate State of Mind
The Ordeal of Change
The Temper of Our Time
Working and Thinking on the Waterfront
First Things, Last Things
Reflections on the Human Condition
In Our Time
Before the Sabbath
Between the Devil and the Dragon

BETWEEN
THE DEVIL AND
THE DRAGON

The Best Essays and Aphorisms of

ERIC HOFFER

HARPER & ROW, PUBLISHERS, New York
Cambridge, Philadelphia, San Francisco, London
Mexico City, São Paulo, Sydney

1817

This collection includes *The True Believer* and substantial selections from *Working and Thinking on the Waterfront; The Passionate State of Mind; The Ordeal of Change; The Temper of Our Time; First Things, Last Things; Reflections on the Human Condition; In Our Time;* and *Before the Sabbath,* all published by Harper & Row, Publishers, Inc. Reprinted by permission.

The aphorisms and essays in this book were selected by the publisher in consultation with the author and edited where necessary to avoid repetition.

BETWEEN THE DEVIL AND THE DRAGON. Copyright 1951, 1952, 1953, 1954, © 1955, 1956, 1958, 1959, 1961, 1962, 1963, 1964, 1965, 1966, 1967, 1968, 1969, 1970, 1971, 1973, 1976, 1979, 1982 by Eric Hoffer. All rights reserved. Printed in the United States of America. No part of this book may be used or reproduced in any manner whatsoever without written permission except in the case of brief quotations embodied in critical articles and reviews. For information address Harper & Row, Publishers, Inc., 10 East 53rd Street, New York, N.Y. 10022. Published simultaneously in Canada by Fitzhenry & Whiteside Limited, Toronto.

FIRST EDITION

Designer: Sidney Feinberg

Library of Congress Cataloging in Publication Data

Hoffer, Eric.
　Between the devil and the dragon.
　　1. Social history—20th century. 2. United States—
Social conditions. 3. United States—Intellectual life.
I. Title.
HN27.H62　　　　303.4′0973　　　81–48040
ISBN 0–06–0149841–1　　　　AACR2

82 83 84 85 86 10 9 8 7 6 5 4 3 2 1

CONTENTS

I

ON NATURE

AND HUMAN NATURE

Man made God in his own image. In whose image did he make the devil? The devil with hoofs, tail, and horns is obviously a beast masquerading as a man. Does he, then, personify nature? Is there a confrontation—God and man on one side, the devil and nature on the other?

It is significant that where men live in awe of nature and see it as inexorable and inscrutable fate, nature is personified not in a devil but in a dragon. The dragon is a composite of the fearsome strengths and uncanny faculties of the animal world. Any piecing together of parts of various animals will result in something like a dragon. Vasari tells how the young Leonardo da Vinci, wanting to paint something that would frighten everybody, brought to his room every sort of living creature he could lay his hands on and set out to paint a composite animal. "He produced an animal so horrible and fearful that it seemed to poison the air with its fiery breath. This he represented coming out of some dark broken rocks, with venom issuing from its jaws, fire from its eyes, and smoke from its nostrils. A monstrous and horrible thing indeed." In the course of time the dragon came to embody the menace and the mystery of the whole nonhuman cosmos. "The dragon," says Kakuzo Akakuro, "unfolds himself in the storm clouds, he washes his mane in the blackness of the seething whirlpool. His claws are in the forks of lightning, and his scales begin to glisten in the bark of rainswept pine trees. His voice is heard in the hurricane." Since societies awed by nature tend to equate power with nature, they will invest omnipotent individuals—emperors, despots, warriors, sorcerers, and so on—with the attributes of the dragon. Thus, unlike the devil, the dragon is a man masquerading as a beast.

The dragon is infinitely more ancient than the devil. The earliest representation of the dragon is the painting of the sorcerer in the cave of Trois Frères, from the Late Paleolithic period. It presents a sorcerer decked out as a composite animal with the horns of a reindeer, the ears of a wolf, the eyes of an owl, the paws of a bear, and the tail of a horse.

The devil is coetaneous with Jehovah, the God who is not nature but its creator. It was the feat of the ancient Hebrews that, though without an advanced technology, they lost their awe of nature and saw it as man's task to "subdue the earth." And once man, backed by Jehovah or a potent technology, assumes a cocky attitude toward nature, the devil comes upon the scene and takes the place of the dragon. The devil personifies not the nature that is around us but the nature that is within us—the infinitely ferocious and cunning prehuman creature that is sealed in the subconscious cellars of the psyche.

Outside the Occident, where nature has the upper hand, the dragon is still supreme; the Occident is the proper domain of the devil.

It is of interest that at his first appearance in the Garden of Eden, before clothes were invented, the devil came undisguised and contrived the fall of man from a paradisiacal existence. Nowadays the devil is decked out in the latest fashion and quotes the latest scriptures.

We of the present are vividly aware that the slaying of the dragon is the opening act in a protracted, desperate contest with the devil. The triumphs of the scientist and the technologist set the stage for the psychiatrist and policeman. We also know that we can cope with the devil only by using the tension between that which is most human and nonhuman in us to stretch souls in a creative effort.

Σ

Has the dread of a nuclear holocaust brought the dragon to the Occident? A generation made aware of a nuclear threat from birth seems to have a superstitious awe of nature. Ecological fervor may be the manifestation of an urge to propitiate nature; so, too, the revival of astrological superstitions and the receptivity to Asian cults.

Σ

Deep probings into man's nature invariably come up with the scandalous evidence of his innate vileness. The historian Friedrich Meinecke was so disconcerted by the dark and impure origins of great cultural values that it seemed to him as though "God needed the devil to realize himself." Yet, considering man's origins, the startling thing is not the evil that is at the root of cherished values, but the alchemy of the soul which transmutes unflagging malice and savagery into charity and love. For the prehuman creature from which man evolved was unlike any living thing in its malicious viciousness toward its own kind. Had it not been for the appearance of a mutation of sociableness, by means of babbling, laughter, and the dance, the species would have perished. Humanization was not a leap upward but a groping toward survival. Original sin has its roots in man's origins: we are descended from a devil. And since it still holds true that man is mankind's deadliest enemy, the survival of the species still depends on further humanization.

Until we become wholly human, we are all to some extent devils—beasts masquerading as men.

Σ

Laughter to begin with was probably glee at the misfortunes of others. The baring of the teeth in laughter hints at its savage ancestry. Animals have no malice, hence also no laughter. They never savor the sudden glory of *Schadenfreude*. It was its infectious quality which made of laughter a medium of mutuality.

Beasts are not beastly. The evil of dehumanization is not that it turns us into animals but that it turns us into the malignant prehuman monstrosity from which man evolved.

Σ

The capacity for transcending the senses—for telepathic transmission and for sensing the unseen—is an animal characteristic. It is doubtful whether the mutation of passionate sociableness, which started the process of humanization, would have been possible without a blunting of the capacity to sense evil intentions. It is still true that a misunderstanding takes place not when people fail to understand each other but when they sense what is going on in each other's mind and do not like it. Pascal feared that if men knew what each thought of the other, there would be no friends in the world.

Σ

How does a vivid awareness of the evil that is in us affect a person's view of the world?

Most of the people who delved deeply into man's nature were not overly disconcerted by the discovery that ill will and hatred are all-pervading ingredients in the compounds and combinations of our inner life. Montaigne, Bacon, La Rochefoucauld, Hume, Renan, and others derived an exquisite delight from tracing and identifying the questionable motives which shape human behavior. Pascal saw it as evidence of divine grace that an impulse of charity is distilled from the evil brew that simmers in men's souls.

In John Calvin the combination of intense self-awareness with a fervent belief in God had outlandish results. Calvin knew beyond doubt that there was no such thing as a genuinely good deed. "No work of pious men ever existed which, if it were examined before the strict judgment of God, did not prove damnable." The jealous, malicious, all-hating "I" thrives on the misfortunes of others, and this "I" is the bedrock on which virtue and piety rest. Calvin had, therefore, to assert categorically that we cannot earn salvation by good deeds. From this it was but a step to the preposterous doctrine of predestination.

Σ

It is not only more sensible but more humane to base social practice on the assumption that all motives are questionable and that in the long run social improvement is attained more readily by a concern with the quality of results than with the purity of motives. The establishment of a desirable pattern of habits is more vital than the implanting of right beliefs and motives. A concern with right and wrong thinking is the manifestation of a primitive, superstitious mentality.

Σ

In the alchemy of man's soul almost all noble attributes—courage, honor, love, hope, faith, duty, loyalty, and so on—can be transmuted into ruthlessness. Compassion alone stands apart from the continuous traffic between good and evil proceeding within us. Compassion is the antitoxin of the soul: where there is compassion, even the most poisonous impulses remain relatively harmless.

Nature has no compassion. It is, in the words of William Blake, "a creation that groans, living on death; where fish and bird and beast and tree and metal and stone live by devouring." Nature accepts no excuses, and the only punishment it knows is death.

Σ

It was not the least part of the uniqueness of the ancient Hebrews that they were the first to enunciate a clear-cut separation between man and nature. In all ancient civilizations there was a feeling of a profound relationship between the things that happen in nature and the course of human affairs. The whole structure of magic was founded on the assumption of an identity between human nature and nature. The ancient Hebrews were the first to reject any close ties of kinship between man and the rest of creation. The one and only God created both nature and man, yet made man in his own image and appointed him his viceroy on earth. Jehovah's injunction to man is unequivocal: Be fruitful and multiply and subdue the earth. Nature lost its divine attributes. Sun, stars, sky, earth, mountains, wells, rivers, sea, plants, and animals were no longer the seat of mysterious powers and the arbiters of man's fate. Since the Hebrews, history rather than cosmic phenomena has been the meaningful drama of the universe.

The writers of the Old Testament picked as the father of the race not Esau, a man of nature whose garments, like Thoreau's ideal man, smelled of grassy fields and flowery meadows, but his twin, Jacob, who was all too human in his anxieties and cunning scheming, and who preferred the inside of a tent to the great outdoors, and the smell of lentil soup to the smell of trees and fields.

Σ

The formidableness of the human species stems from the survival of its weak. Were it not for the compassion that moves us to care for the sick, the crippled, and the old, there probably would have been neither culture nor civilization. The crippled warrior who had to stay behind while the manhood of the tribe went out to war was the first storyteller, teacher, and artisan. The old and the sick had a hand in the development of the arts of healing and of cooking. One thinks of the venerable sage, the unhinged medicine man, the epileptic prophet, the blind bard, and the witty hunchback and dwarf.

Σ

Unlike the pattern which seems to prevail in the rest of life, in the human species the weak not only survive but often triumph over the strong. The self-hatred inherent in the weak unlocks energies far more formidable than those mobilized by an ordinary struggle for existence. The shifts and devices the weak employ to escape an untenable reality are often preposterous, yet they somehow turn out to be generators of power. One thinks of the magic of words which turns thin air into absolute truths, and the alchemy of conviction which transmutes self-contempt into pride, lack of confidence into faith, and a sense of guilt into self-righteousness. Finally, self-hatred endows the weak with an exceptional facility for united action. Flight from the self almost invariably turns into a rush for a compact group. And certainly, this readiness to unite with others is a source of unequaled strength. Thus the soul intensity generated in the weak endows them as it were with a special fitness. There is sober realism in St. Paul's words: "God hath chosen the weak things of the world to confound the things which are mighty."

Σ

The resentment of the weak does not spring from any injustice done to them but from their sense of impotence. They hate not wickedness but weakness. When it is in their power to do so, the weak destroy weakness wherever they find it. Woe to the weak when they are preyed upon by the weak! The self-hatred of the weak is likewise an instance of their hatred of weakness.

Σ

By renouncing the self we are getting out from underneath the only burden that is real. For however much we identify ourselves with a holy cause, our fears on its behalf can never be as real and poignant as our fear and trembling in behalf of a perishable self. The short-lived self, teetering on the edge of extinction, is the only thing that can ever really matter. Thus the renunciation of the self is felt as a liberation and salvation.

Σ

We almost always prove something when we act heroically. We prove to ourselves and others that we are not what we and they thought we were. Our real self is petty, greedy, callous, cowardly, dishonest, and stewing in malice. And now in defying death and spitting in its eye we grasp at the chance of a grand refutation.

Σ

We need not only a purpose in life to give meaning to our existence but also something to give meaning to our suffering. We need as much something to suffer for as something to live for.

Σ

It is not sheer malice that pricks our ears to evil reports about our fellow men. For there are frequent moments when we feel lower than the lowest of mankind, and this opinion of ourselves isolates us. Hence the rumor that all flesh is base comes almost as a message of hope. It breaks down the wall that has kept us apart and we feel one with humanity.

Σ

When we are conscious of our worthlessness, we naturally expect others to be finer and better than we are. If then we discover any similarity between them and us, we see it as irrefutable evidence of their worthlessness and inferiority. It is thus that with some people familiarity breeds contempt.

Σ

Man feels truly at ease only when he pities. His love and admiration for his equals and betters is beset with misgiving. Sometimes, indeed, we convince ourselves of the innate weakness of others for no better reason but that we may love them unreservedly.

Σ

We associate brittleness and vulnerability with those we love, while we endow those we hate with strength and indestructibility. It is perhaps true that the first conception of an almighty God had its origin in the visualization of an implacable enemy rather than a friendly protector. Men loved God the way the Russians loved Stalin. Only by convincing ourselves that we really and truly love an all-powerful and all-seeing enemy can we be sure of never betraying ourselves by a word or gesture. "How are you going to love," said Tertullian, "unless you are afraid not to love!"

Σ

It fares ill with the world when the strong imitate the weak. The shifts and devices by which the weak turn weakness into strength become instruments of oppression and dehumanization when used by the strong. The Stalins and Hitlers act as if they were "a company of poor men."

Σ

Nature attains perfection, but man never does. There is a perfect ant, a perfect bee, but man is perpetually unfinished. He is both an unfinished animal and an unfinished man. It is this incurable unfinishedness which sets man apart from other living things. For, in the attempt to finish himself, man becomes a creator. Moreover, the incurable unfinishedness keeps man perpetually immature, perpetually capable of learning and growing.

There is something unhuman about perfection. The performance of the expert strikes us as instinctual or mechanical. It is a paradox that, although the striving to master a skill is supremely human, the total mastery of a skill approaches the nonhuman. They who would make man perfect end up by dehumanizing him.

Σ

The savior who wants to turn men into angels is as much a hater of human nature as the totalitarian despot who wants to turn them into puppets.

There are similarities between absolute power and absolute faith: a demand for absolute obedience, a readiness to attempt the impossible, a bias for simple solutions—to cut the knot rather than unravel it, the viewing of compromise as surrender, the tendency to manipulate people and "experiment with blood." Both absolute power and absolute faith are instruments of dehumanization. Hence absolute faith corrupts as absolutely as absolute power.

Σ

Anyone aware of the imperfections inherent in human affairs is hardly capable of total commitment. Part of him will inevitably remain uncommitted. It is this perch of uncommitment which makes an act of self-sacrifice sublimely human and distinguishes the man of faith from the fanatic.

Σ

Free men are aware of the imperfections inherent in human affairs, and they are willing to fight and die for that which is not perfect. They know that basic human problems can have no final solutions, that our freedom, justice, equality, and so on are far from absolute, that the good life is compounded of half measures, compromises, lesser evils, and gropings toward the perfect. The rejection of approximations and the insistence on absolutes are the manifestations of a nihilism that loathes freedom, tolerance, and equity.

Σ

In human affairs every solution serves only to sharpen the problem, to show us more clearly what we are up against. There are no final solutions.

Σ

You dehumanize a man as much by returning him to nature—by making him one with rocks, vegetation, and animals—as by turning him into a machine. Both the natural and the mechanical are the opposite of that which is uniquely human. Nature is a self-made machine, more perfectly automated than any automated machine. To create something in the image of nature is to create a machine, and it was by learning the inner working of nature that man became a builder of machines.

When you automate an industry you modernize it; when you automate a life you primitivize it.

Σ

The mindlessness of nature frightens us, particularly when we are made aware of the ingenuity and precision by which it achieves its ends. That chance should accomplish, even over immeasurably long periods and with immeasurable waste, what only the subtlest mind could devise seems to us beyond belief. We find it easier to believe in God than in the purposeful working of blind chance.

Σ

Nature is rational and is ruled by mathematics. Every answer we pry from her is severely logical. It seems paradoxical that that which has no mind should be unfailingly rational. Man is the only spontaneous force in the universe.

Σ

It is significant that in Stalin's Russia not only did Stalin treat the Russians as if they were matter, part of nature, but the Russians saw Stalin as fate and a force of nature. When fate strikes, one has to lie low until the wrath has passed. There can be no sense of humiliation. We do not feel humilated when the sea spits on us or the wind forces us to our knees. Nor does one protest or conspire against a natural calamity.

Σ

Both the scientist and the savage postulate the oneness of man and nature. The difference between them is that the savage tries to influence nature by means which have proved their efficacy in influencing human nature, while the scientist wants to deal with human nature the way he deals with matter and other forms of life. The scientist reads the equation *human nature = nature* from left to right, while the savage reads it from right to left. Yet it is worth noting that Darwin, too, read the equation from right to left when he read cutthroat capitalist competition into the economy of nature.

The remarkable thing is that the fanatic deals with men the way the scientist deals with matter. There is a startling similarity between Bacon's prescription for mastering nature—"Nature, to be commanded, must be obeyed"—and Loyola's formula for manipulating men—"Follow the other man's course to your own goal."

Σ

Unpredictability is an essential ingredient of human uniquencess. Compared with man, all other living things are predictable automata. Yet, paradoxically, man has to be immersed in a predictable universe if his creative unpredictability is to unfold. The creative individual needs not only a predictable natural and social environment but also a predictable body and a more or less routinized everyday life. Thus man, a uniquely unpredictable creature, has a hunger for predictability, and will use whatever power he has to turn variables into constants. Indeed, he measures power by the ability to predict.

Σ

Spiritual stagnation ensues when man's environment becomes unpredictable or when his inner life is made wholly predictable. In Stalin's Russia the social environment was unpredictable: one never knew what might happen between going to bed and getting up. At the same time, terror and indoctrination made Russians as predictable as numerals.

Σ

Man was nature's mistake—she neglected to finish him—and she has never ceased paying for her mistake. For it was in the process of finishing himself that man got out from underneath nature's inexorable laws and became her most formidable adversary.

Σ

The source of man's creativeness is in his deficiencies; he creates to compensate himself for what he lacks. He became Homo faber—a maker of weapons and tools—to compensate for his lack of specialized organs. He became Homo ludens—a player, tinkerer, and artist—to compensate for his lack of inborn skills. He became a speaking animal to compensate for his lack of the telepathic faculty by which animals communicate with each other. He became a thinker to compensate for the ineffectualness of his instincts.

Σ

That man, a deficient lesser animal, became more than an animal was due to his singular talent for turning handicaps into advantages. Man's tools and weapons more than made up for his lack of specialized organs, and his capacity for learning did more for him than inborn skills and organic adaptations. It still holds true that man is most uniquely human when he turns obstacles into opportunities.

Σ

Since man has to finish and "make" himself, there are unavoidably greater differences between individual men than between individual animals. The *Gleichschaltung* of individuals always results in some degree of dehumanization. This is true even when individuality is sacrificed for a declared common good.

One must also expect chance to play a greater role in the lives of men than in the lives of animals. It is true that where sheer survival is concerned accidents are less decisive for man than for other forms of life. Much of the time society shields a person against death by accident. But in the unfolding of the individual's life, chance is everything. In a vigorous society, chance and example have full play, and in such a society the talented are likely to be lucky.

Σ

Language was invented to ask questions. Answers may be given by grunts and gestures, but questions must be spoken. Humanness came of age when man asked the first questions. Social stagnation results not from lack of answers but from the absence of the impulse to ask questions.

Σ

Animals can learn, but it is not by learning that they become dogs, cats, or horses. Only man has to learn to become what he is supposed to be.

Σ

Due to the imperfection of man's instincts, there is a pause of faltering and groping between his perception and action. A shrinking of the pause results in some degree of dehumanization. This is as true of highly trained specialists and dogmatic true believers as of the mentally deficient.

Both iron discipline and blind faith strive to eliminate the pause before action, while the discipline that humanizes and civilizes aims at widening the interval between impulse and execution.

Art humanizes because the artist must grope and feel his way, and he never ceases to learn.

Σ

The most fateful consequence of man's incurable unfinishedness is his chronic immaturity, his inability to grow up, his perpetual youthfulness. By all odds, earliest man, so naked to the elements and to deadly enemies, should have existed in a state of constant shock. We find him instead the only lighthearted being in a deadly serious universe. All around him were living creatures superbly equipped—and driven by grim purposefulness. He alone, with childish carelessness, tinkered and played and exerted himself more in the pursuit of superfluities than of necessities. Yet the tinkering and playing, and the fascination with the nonessential, were a chief source of the inventiveness which enabled man to prevail over better-equipped and more purposeful animals.

Σ

Man is a luxury-loving animal. Take away play, fancies, and luxuries, and you will turn him into a dull, sluggish creature, scarcely energetic enough to obtain a bare subsistence. A society becomes stagnant when its people are too rational or too serious to be tempted by baubles.

Σ

Both the revolutionary and the creative individual are perpetual juveniles. The revolutionary does not grow up because he cannot grow, while the creative individual cannot grow up because he keeps growing.

Σ

Patience is a by-product of growth—we can bide our time when it is the time of our growth. There is no patience in acquisition or in the pursuit of power and fame. Nothing is so impatient as the pursuit of a substitute for growth.

Σ

To some, freedom means the opportunity to do what they want to do; to most it means not to do what they do not want to do. It is perhaps true that those who can grow will feel free under any condition.

Σ

A plant needs roots in order to grow. With man it is the other way around: only when he grows does he have roots and feel at home in the world.

Σ

A sensitive conscience is often a by-product of a decline in vigor. When we are growing, our doings are transitory, mere stepping-stones to be left behind, but when we stop growing we are what we do and think.

Σ

Our achievements speak for themselves. What we have to keep track of are our failures, discouragements, and doubts. We tend to forget the past difficulties, the many false starts, and the painful groping. We see our past achievements as the end result of a clean forward thrust, and our present difficulties as signs of decline and decay.

Σ

There are many who find a good alibi far more attractive than an achievement. For an achievement does not settle anything permanently. We still have to prove our worth anew each day: we have to prove that we are as good today as we were yesterday. But when we have a valid alibi for not achieving anything we are fixed, so to speak, for life. Moreover, when we have an alibi for not writing a book, painting a picture, and so on, we have an alibi for not writing the greatest book and not painting the greatest picture. Small wonder that the effort expended and the punishment endured in obtaining a good alibi often exceed the effort and grief requisite for the attainment of a most marked achievement.

Σ

When people do us good, our exhilaration is due not merely to the good we receive. In addition we feel that we are on the right path, that we have chosen well to be where we are. We see the good that happens to us as a good omen.

Σ

The people we meet are the playwrights and stage managers of our lives: they cast us in a role, and we play it whether we will or not. It is not so much the example of others we imitate as the reflection of ourselves in their eyes and the echo of ourselves in their words.

Σ

Our credulity is greatest concerning the things we know least about; and since we know least about ourselves, we are ready to believe all that is said about us. Hence the power of flattery and calumny.

Σ

Those who are ready to praise others take praise from others with a grain of salt. On the other hand, those who praise reluctantly accept praise from others at its face value. Thus the less magnanimous a soul, the more readily does it succumb to flattery.

Σ

The capacity for identifying ourselves with others seems boundless. No matter how meagerly endowed, we yet find it easy to identify ourselves with persons of exceptional endowments and achievements. Can it be that even in the least of us there are crumbs of all abilities and potentialities so that we can comprehend greatness as if it were part of us?

Σ

That we pursue something passionately does not always mean we really want it or have a special aptitude for it. Often, the thing we pursue most passionately is but a substitute for the one thing we really want and cannot have. It is usually safe to predict that the fulfillment of an excessively cherished desire is not likely to still our nagging anxiety.

In every passionate pursuit, the pursuit counts more than the object pursued.

Σ

So true is it that the path of desire, once trodden, remains frequented that we not only keep wanting what we cannot have but go on wanting what we no longer really want.

Σ

There is perhaps an element of malice in the readiness to overestimate people. We are laying up for ourselves the pleasure of later cutting them down to size.

Σ

It seems that we are most busy when we do not do the one thing we ought to do, most greedy when we cannot have the one thing we really want, most hurried when we can never arrive, most self-righteous when irrevocably in the wrong.
    There is apparently a link between excess and unattainability.

Σ

The feeling of being hurried is not usually the result of living a full life and having no time. It is, on the contrary, born of a vague fear that we are wasting our life. When we do not do the one thing we ought to do, we have no time for anything else—we are the busiest people in the world.

Σ

So long as our capacity to savor a fulfillment is unimpaired, we keep on trying no matter how numerous the misses—we cannot learn from experience. It is only when a fulfillment no longer brings a singular joy that the slightest disappointment can teach us a lesson for good.

Σ

The end comes when we no longer talk with ourselves. It is the end of genuine thinking and the beginning of the final loneliness. The remarkable thing is that the cessation of the inner dialogue marks also the end of our concern with the world around us. It is as if we note the world and think about it only when we have to report to ourselves.

Σ

To grow old is to grow common. Old age equalizes—we are aware that what is happening to us has happened to untold numbers from the beginning of time. When we are young we act as if we were the first young people in the world.

Σ

A man's heart is a grave long before he is buried. Youth dies, and beauty, and hope, and desire. A grave is buried within a grave when a man is buried.

Σ

The remarkable thing is that it is the crowded life that is most easily remembered. A life full of turns, achievements, disappointments, surprises, and crises is a life full of landmarks. The empty life has even its few details blurred, and cannot be remembered with certainty.

Σ

It is the individual only who is timeless. Societies, cultures, and civilizations—past and present—are often incomprehensible to outsiders, but the individual's hungers, anxieties, dreams, and preoccupations have remained unchanged through the millennia. Thus we are up against the paradox that the individual who is more complex, unpredictable, and mysterious than any communal entity is the one nearest to our understanding; so near that even the interval of millennia cannot weaken our feeling of kinship. If in some manner the voice of an individual reaches us from the remotest distance of time, it is a timeless voice speaking about ourselves.

1 THE UNNATURALNESS

OF HUMAN NATURE

In the early days of modern science we find outstanding scientists expressing their wonder and delight that the prodigious variety of nature should be the work of but a few simple laws. Galileo saw it as "a custom and habit of nature" to achieve its ends by means which are "common, simple, and easy." Kepler was convinced that "nature loves simplicity," and Newton wrote feelingly how "nature is pleased with simplicity and affects not the pomp of superfluous causes."

During the same period, the men whose preoccupation was with human nature spoke not of simplicity but of incredible complexity. Montaigne never wearied of expatiating on the inconstancy, lack of uniformity, involuteness, and unpredictability of human manifestations. It seemed to him that every bit in us plays every moment its own game and that "there is as much difference between us and ourselves as between us and others." Pascal, a student of both nature and human nature, contrasted the simplicity of things with man's double and complex nature. He saw man as a mass of contradictions: an angel and a brute, a monster and a prodigy, the crown and scum of created things, the glory and scandal of the universe. Whatever harmony there is in us is "fantastic, changeable, and various." He concluded that "men are of necessity so mad that not to be mad were madness in another

---

This essay is a somewhat shorter version of the essay that appeared under the same title in *The Ordeal of Change*.

form." He thought it quite in order that Plato and Aristotle should have written on politics as though they were laying down rules for a madhouse.

In the study of nature, an explanation must not only be consistent with the facts but also as simple and direct as possible. Where several explanations are advanced, the rule is followed that the one which is most simple is also most nearly correct. To choose a more complex explanation, says a recent writer on the nature of science, would be as sensible "as traveling eastward around the world to reach your neighbor's house which is next door to the west."

In human affairs the sensibleness of the direct, simple approach is by no means self-evident. Here it is often true that the simplest ends are reached only by the most roundabout and extravagant means. Even the predictable comes here to pass in unpredictable ways. To forget that man is a fantastic creature is to ignore his most crucial trait, and when contemplating human nature the wildest guesses and hunches are legitimate.

2

The fantastic quality of human nature is partly the product of man's unfinishedness. Being without specialized organs, man is in a sense a half-animal. He has to finish himself by technology, and in doing so he is a creator—in a sense a half-god. Again, lacking organic adaptations to a particular environment, he must adapt the environment to himself and re-create the world. The never-ending task of finishing himself, of transcending the limits of his physical being, is the powerhouse of man's creativeness and the source of his unnaturalness. For it is in the process of finishing himself that man sloughs off the fixity and boundless submissiveness of nature.

The unnaturalness of human nature should offer a clue to the central meaning of man's ascent through the millennia: it was the result of a striving to break loose from nature and get out from under the iron laws which dominate it. The striving was not conscious, and it did not start from an awareness of strength. The process of reflection—of self-awareness—which fueled man's ascent was to begin with an awareness of helplessness: man the half-animal became poignantly aware of his unfinishedness and imperfection. He worshiped the more favored forms of life; worshiped their specialized organs, their skills and strength. He probably first killed animals, ate their flesh, and put on their skins, not to still his hunger and keep warm but to acquire their strength, speed, and skill and become like them. Naked, unarmed, and unprotected, man clung desperately to an indifferent mother earth and passionately claimed kinship with her more favored children. But the discovery that he could create substitutes for the organs and inborn perfections which he lacked turned worship and imitation into a process of vying—into a striving to overcome and overtake nature and leave it behind. In finishing and making himself man also remade the world, and the man-made world no longer clung to nature but straddled it. Instead of claiming kinship with other forms of life, man now claimed a descent and a line apart and began to see his uniqueness and dignity in that which distinguished him from the rest of creation.

Seen thus, the human uniqueness of an aspiration or an achievement should perhaps be gauged by how much it accentuates the distinction between human affairs and nonhuman nature; and it should be obvious that the aspiration toward freedom is the most essentially human of all human manifestations. Freedom from coercion, from want, from fear, from death are freedom from forces and circumstances which would narrow the gap separating human nature from nature and impose on man the passivity and predictability of matter. By the same token, the manifestation most inimical to human uniqueness is that of absolute power. The corruption inherent in absolute power derives from the fact that such power is never free from the tendency to turn man into a thing and press him back into the matrix of nature from which he has risen. For the impulse of power is to turn every variable into a constant and give to commands the inexorableness and relentlessness of laws of nature. Hence absolute power corrupts even when exercised for humane purposes. The benevolent despot who sees himself as a shepherd of the people still demands from others the submissiveness of sheep. The taint inherent in absolute power is not its inhumanity but its antihumanity.

3

To make of human affairs a coherent, precise, predictable whole, one must ignore or suppress man as he really is and treat human nature as a mere aspect of nature. The theoreticians do it by limiting the shaping forces of man's destiny to nonhuman factors: providence, the cosmic spirit, geography, climate, economic or physiochemical factors. The practical men of power try to eliminate the human variable by inculcating iron discipline or blind faith, by dissolving the unpredictable individual in a compact group, by subjecting the individual's judgment and will to a ceaseless barrage of propaganda, and by sheer coercion. It is by eliminating man from their equation that the makers of history can predict the future and the writers of history can give a pattern to the past. There is an element of misanthropy in all determinists. To all of them, man as he really is is a nuisance, and they strive to prove by various means that there is no such thing as human nature.

Even in the freest society, power is charged with the impulse to turn men into precise, predictable automatons. When watching men of power in action it must be always kept in mind that, whether they know it or not, their main purpose is the elimination or neutralization of the independent individual—the independent voter, consumer, worker, owner, thinker—and that every device they employ aims at turning man into a manipulatable "animated instrument," which is Aristotle's definition of a slave.

On the other hand, every device employed to bolster individual freedom must have as its chief purpose the impairment of the absoluteness of power. The indications are that such an impairment is brought about not by strengthening the individual and pitting him against the possessors of power, but by distributing and diversifying power and pitting one category or unit of power against another. Where power is one, the defeated individual, however strong and resourceful, can have no refuge and no recourse.

There is no doubt that of all political systems the free society is the most "unnatural." It embodies, in the words of Bergson, "a mighty effort in a direction contrary to that of nature." Totalitarianism, even when it goes hand in hand with a modernization of technique, constitutes a throwback to the primitive and a return to nature. It is significant that "back to nature" movements since the day of Rousseau, though generous and noble in origin, have tended to terminate in absolutism and the worship of brute force.

Considering the complexity and unpredictability of man, it is doubtful whether effective social management can be based on expert knowledge of human nature. Societies are likely to function tolerably well either under a total dictatorship, which need not take human nature into account, or when least interfered with by government. Both absolute government and nominal government are ways of avoiding the necessity of having to deal with human nature.

4

Power, whether exercised over matter or over man, is partial to simplification. It wants simple problems, simple solutions, simple definitions. It sees in complication a product of weakness— the tortuous path compromise must follow.

Now, whereas in the realm of matter the great simplifiers are the great scientists and technologists, in human affairs the great simplifiers are the great coercers—the Hitlers and Stalins. To some extent, Hitler and Stalin were scientists of man the way the physicist and the chemist are scientists of matter. Their policies and crimes were motivated as much by the scientist's predilection for simplification, predictability, and experimentation as by doctrinaire tenets or sheer malevolence. Even their murderous intolerance of dissenters had a "scientific" aspect: a dissenter is to the absoluteness of power what an exception is to the validity of a formulated scientific rule—both must be dealt with and somehow eliminated.

It is no coincidence that the men of absolute power in Soviet Russia have been so intrigued by the social implications of the Pavlovian experiments on dogs, and that concentration camps in Germany and Communist countries became factories of dehumanization, in which men were reduced to the state of animals and were experimented on the way scientists experiment on rats and dogs. Absolute power produces not a society but a menagerie—even if it be what D'Argenson called a "menagerie of happy men."

The full savor of power comes not from the mastery of nature but from the mastery of men. It is questionable whether he who can move mountains and tell rivers whither to flow has as exquisite a sense of power as he who can command the multitude and turn human beings into animated robots. Hence we find that a spectacular increase of man's power over nature is likely to be followed by passionate attempts to master men—to use the power gained by victory over nature in the enslavement of men.

Such a diversion is first discernible in the transition from the Late Neolithic to the totalitarianism of the ancient river-valley civilizations in the Near East. The Late Neolithic Age saw something like an industrial revolution; the era of civilization that followed was mainly preoccupied with the taming of man by coercion and magic.

The scientific and industrial revolution of modern times represents the next giant step in the mastery over nature; and here, too, an enormous increase in man's power over nature is followed by an apocalyptic drive to subjugate man and reduce human nature to the status of nature. Even where enslavement is employed in a mighty effort to tame nature, one has the feeling that the effort is but a tactic to legitimize total subjugation. Thus, despite its spectacular achievements in science and technology, the twentieth century will probably be seen in retrospect as a century mainly preoccupied with the mastery and manipulation of men. Nationalism, socialism, communism, fascism, and militarism, cartelization and unionization, propaganda and advertising are all aspects of a general relentless drive to manipulate men and neutralize the unpredictability of human nature. Here, too, the atmosphere is heavy-laden with coercion and magic.

5

On the whole, the unnaturalness of human nature is more strikingly displayed in the weak of the human species than in the strong. The strong are as a rule more simple, direct, and comprehensible—in a word, more natural. The indications are that in the process of tearing loose from nature it was the weak who took the first steps. Chased out of the forest by the strong, they first essayed to walk erect, and first uttered words, and first grabbed a stick to use as weapon and tool. The weak's singular capacity for evolving substitutes for that which they lack suggests that they played a chief role in the evolvement of technology.

Man is most peculiarly human when he cannot have his way. His momentous achievements are rarely the result of a clean forward thrust but rather of a soul intensity generated in front of an apparently insurmountable obstacle which bars his way to a cherished goal. It is here that potent words and explosive substitutes have their birth, and the endless quest, and the stretching of the soul which encompasses heaven and earth. The impulse to escape an untenable situation often prompts human beings not to shrink back but to plunge ahead.

It is the unique glory of the human species that its rejected do not fall by the wayside but become the building stones of the new, and that those who cannot fit into the present should become the shapers of the future. Those like Nietzsche and D. H. Lawrence, who see in the influence of the weak a taint that might lead to decadence and degeneration, are missing the point. It is precisely the peculiar role played by its weak that has given the human species its uniqueness. One should see the dominant role of the weak in shaping man's fate not as a perversion of natural instincts and vital impulses but as the starting point of the deviation which led man to break away from, and rise above, nature—not as degeneration but as the generation of a new order of creation.

The weak are not a noble breed. Their sublime deeds of faith, daring, and self-sacrifice usually spring from questionable motives. The weak hate not wickedness but weakness, and one instance of their hatred of weakness is hatred of self. All the passionate pursuits of the weak are in some degree a striving to escape, blur, or disguise an unwanted self. It is a striving shot through with malice, envy, self-deception, and a host of petty impulses, yet it often culminates in superb achievements. Thus we find that people who fail in everyday affairs often become responsive to grandiose schemes and will display unequaled steadfastness, formidable energies, and a special fitness in the performance of tasks which would stump superior people. It seems paradoxical that defeat in dealing with the possible should embolden people to attempt the impossible, but a familiarity with the mentality of the weak reveals that what seems a path of daring is actually an easy way out. It is to escape the responsibility for failure that the weak so eagerly throw themselves into grandiose undertakings.

The inept and unfit also display a high degree of venturesomeness in welcoming and promoting innovations in all fields. It is not usually the successful who advocate drastic social reforms, plunge into new undertakings in business and industry, go out to tame the wilderness, or evolve new modes of expression in literature, art, or music. People who make good usually stay where they are and go on doing more and better what they know how to do well. The plunge into the new is often an escape from an untenable situation and a maneuver to mask one's ineptness. To adopt the role of the pioneer and the avant-garde is to place oneself in a situation where ineptness and awkwardness are acceptable and even unavoidable; for experience and know-how count for little in tackling the new, and we expect the wholly new to be ill-shapen and ugly.

Now to point to the discrepancy between questionable motives and imposing achievements is not to decry humanity but to extol it. For the outstanding characteristic of man's creativeness is the ability to transmute petty and trivial impulses into momentous consequences. The alchemist's notion about the transmutation of metals is absurd with reference to nature, but it corresponds to the actualities of human nature. There is in man's soul a flowing equilibrium between good and evil, the noble and the base, the sublime and the ridiculous, the beautiful and the ugly, the weighty and the trivial. To look for a close correspondence between the quality of an achievement and the nature of the motive which gave it birth is to miss a most striking aspect of man's uniqueness. The greatness of man is in what we can do with petty grievances and joys, and with common physiological pressures and hungers. "When I have a little vexation," wrote Keats, "it grows in five minutes into a theme for Sophocles." To the creative individual, all experience is seminal—all events are equidistant from new ideas and insights—and his inordinate humanness shows itself perhaps mainly in the ability to make the trivial and common reach an enormous way.

6

The significant fact is that the attributes which are at the root of man's uniqueness are also the main factors in the release of his creative energies. As we have seen, it was man's unfinishedness—his being an incomplete animal—which started him on his unique course. This unfinishedness consists not only in the lack of specialized organs and organic adaptations but also in the imperfection of man's instincts and in an inability to grow up and mature. Now, each of these defects plays a vital role in the release of the creative flow. If the lack of specialized organs started the groping toward tools and weapons, then the lack of instinctual automatism introduced into man's behavior the seminal pause of hesitation. In animals, action follows on perception mechanically with almost chemical swiftness and certainty, but in man there is an interval of faltering and groping; and this interval is the seedbed of the images, ideas, dreams, aspirations, irritations, longings, and forebodings which are the warp and woof of the creative process. Finally, it is the retention of youthful characteristics in adult life that endows man with the perpetual playfulness so fruitful of insights and illuminations.

It is to be expected that the pattern of unfinishedness should be most pronounced in the autonomous individual. Nothing on earth or in heaven is so poignantly and chronically incomplete as the individual on his own. In the individual totally integrated with others in a compact group, human uniqueness is considerably blurred. Fusion with others completes, stabilizes, and de-fuses. A compact collective body displays a submissiveness, predictability, and automatism reminiscent of nonhuman nature. Thus the emergence of the unattached individual must have been a crucial step in the attainment of human uniqueness. Yet the indications are that this step was not the end result of a slow process of social growth and maturing but the by-product of catastrophe and disaster. The first individual was a lone survivor, a straggler, an outcast, a fugitive. Individual selfhood was first experienced not as something ardently wished for but as a calamity which befell the individual: he was separated from the group. All creative phases in history were preceded by a shattering or weakening of communal structures, and it was the individual debris who first set the creative act in motion. Fugitives seem to have been at the birth of everything new. They were the first free men, the first founders of cities and civilizations, the first adventurers and discoverers; they were the seed of Israel, of Greece, of Rome, of America.

The severing of the individual from a compact group is an operation from which the individual never fully recovers. The individual on his own remains a chronically incomplete and unbalanced entity. His creative efforts and passionate pursuits are at bottom a blind striving for wholeness and balance. The individual striving to realize himself and prove his worth has created all that is great in literature, art, music, science, and technology. The individual, also, when he can neither realize himself nor justify his existence by his own efforts, is a breeding cell of frustration and the seed of the convulsions which shake a society to its foundations. These convulsions, being in essence a flight from the burdens of an individual existence, often terminate in totalitarian bodies dominated by absolute power.

It is a strangely moving spectacle this: the individual wearying of the burden of human uniqueness, shifting the load on his shoulders, and finally dropping it. For as he turns about, he finds himself one of a vast army with flags flying and drums beating, marching back to unbounded submissiveness and certitude—back to being a crumb of the rock of ages and an anonymous particle of a monolithic whole.

Yet it is part of the fantastic quality of man's nature that this passionate retreat should have often turned out to be but a stepping back preliminary to a leap ahead. In the modern Occident there has been a continuous tug of war between individualist and anti-individualist tendencies. The chauvinist and Socialist collectivism of the twentieth century is to the individualism of the nineteenth what Jacobinism was to the age of the Enlightenment and what the Reformation was to the Renaissance. And every time, until now, the resourceful Occidental individual somehow managed to reassert himself and come out on top. He managed to convert the enthusiasm released by the anti-individualist movements into a stimulus of his own creative capacities and an aid in his striving for self-realization and self-advancement. Thus we see again and again during the past four hundred years how the aftermath of every anti-individualist movement was marked by an outburst of individual creativeness in literature and art, and an upswing in individual venturesomeness and enterprise.

7

Nothing so baffles the scientific approach to human nature as the vital role words play in human affairs. How can one deal with a physiochemical complex in which reactions are started and checked, accelerated and slowed down, by the sound or image of a word—usually a meaningless word?

It is of interest that the practice of magic where nature is concerned—the attempt to manipulate nature by words—rested on the assumption that nature is not unlike human nature, that methods of proven effectiveness in the manipulation of human affairs may be equally potent when applied to nonhuman nature. It can be seen that such an assumption is the mirror image of, and not infinitely more absurd than, the assumption implied in the scientific approach that human nature is merely an aspect of nature.

We know that words cannot move mountains, but they can move the multitude; and men are more ready to fight and die for a word than for anything else. Words shape thought, stir feeling, and beget action; they kill and revive, corrupt and cure. The "men of words"—priests, prophets, intellectuals—have played a more decisive role in history than military leaders, statesmen, and businessmen.

Words and magic are particularly crucial in time of crisis when old forms of life are in dissolution and man must grapple with the unknown. Normal motives and incentives lose then their efficacy. Man does not plunge into the unknown in search of the prosaic and matter-of-fact. His soul has to be stretched by a reaching out for the fabulous and unprecedented. He needs the nurse of magic and breathtaking fairy tales to lure him on and sustain him in his faltering first steps. Even modern science and technology were not in the beginning a sober pursuit of facts and knowledge. Here, too, the magicians—alchemists, astrologers, visionaries—were the pioneers. The early chemists looked not for prosaic acids and salts but for the philosopher's stone and the elixir of life. The early astronomers and discoverers, too, were animated by myths and fairy tales. Columbus went looking not only for gold and fabulous empires but also for the Garden of Eden. When he saw the Orinoco he was sure it was Gihon, one of the four rivers of Eden. He wrote back to Spain about all the tokens and virtues and mathematical calculations which forced him to the conclusion that "Paradise is to be found in these parts."

It is indeed questionable whether we can make sense of critical periods in history without an awareness of the role words and magic play in them. This is particularly true of the century we live in—a century dominated on the one hand by the scientific spirit and a superb practical sense and on the other by the black magic of chauvinism, racialism, fascism, and communism. The rapid transformation of millions of peasants into urban industrial workers, which often meant a leap from the Neolithic Age into the twentieth century, could not be realized without soul-stirring myths and illusions about an impending national, racial, or social millennium.

There is a widespread feeling that mankind has come to a fateful turning point. The feeling stems partly from the threat of a nuclear holocaust and partly from the fear that in a drawn-out contest with the Communist powers we shall unavoidably be shaped in the image of the totalitarianism we loathe, and slay our hope even as we battle for it. More ominous perhaps are the signs that the weak of the species are about to be elbowed out of their role as pathfinders and shapers of the future. The new revolution in science and technology which has so enormously increased man's power over nature has also enormously reduced the significance of the average individual. With the advent of automation and the utilization of atomic energy, it might soon be possible for a relatively small group of people to satisfy all of a country's needs and fight its wars too without the aid of the masses. Man's destiny is now being shaped in fantastically complex and expensive laboratories staffed by supermen, and the new frontier has no place for the rejected and unfit. Instead of being the leaven of history and the mainspring of the ascending movement of man, the weak are likely to be cast aside as a waste product. One is justified in fearing that the elimination of the weak as shaping factors may mean the end of history—the reversion of history to zoology.

2   CAVE PAINTINGS

IT IS A STORY WORTH RETELLING. In 1879 the Spanish amateur archaeologist Marquis de Sautuola and his little daughter Maria discovered the breathtaking paintings of bison and other animals on the ceiling of the cave at Altamira. The Marquis was forty-eight years old, sparely built, reticent, not strikingly original, but with a consuming hunger for distinction. It was actually little Maria who discovered the paintings. The Marquis did what other prehistorians were doing at the time: he dug and puttered just inside the entrance of the cave, looking for stone tools, bone needles, and pieces of carved mammoth ivory. But the twelve-year-old Maria, who held the torch to give light to the Marquis, strayed some distance from the entrance, and waving the torch playfully over her head she suddenly saw a herd of bison galloping on the ceiling and cried out, "¡Toros, toros!"

The Marquis recognized immediately the significance of the discovery for prehistory and for himself. Here was a heaven-sent chance to land him in one jump in the front ranks of prehistorians. He was going to write a monograph on the paintings, magnificently illustrated, and the name of Sautuola would forever mark an epochal change in our conception of Paleolithic man.

Everything went swimmingly for a while. The Marquis wrote to his friend Professor Vilanova of the University of Madrid. The

---

This essay appeared under the title "Man's Most Useful Occupation" in *First Things, Last Things*.

Professor came, saw the paintings, and was swept off his feet. The Madrid newspapers had front-page stories and photographs of the momentous discovery. King Alfonso XII visited the cave and stayed at the Marquis's castle in Santillana-del-Mar. The Marquis had sometime earlier befriended a destitute French painter, afflicted with dumbness, who had been stranded in the neighborhood, and he now put him to making the sketches for his treatise.

Then disaster struck out of the blue. At the congress of prehistory in Lisbon in 1880 the assembled experts and scholars denied the authenticity of the Altamira paintings. Professor Émile Cartailhac of the University of Toulouse thought it was all a hoax perpetrated by the Marquis to obtain cheap renown and make fools of the experts. Anti-Altamira articles began to appear in the press. Professor Vilanova eventually went over to the experts. The Marquis tried again at the next congress, held in Algiers in 1882. No one would listen to him. The Marquis retired to his estates and died in 1888 at the relatively early age of fifty-seven.

The denouement is interesting. Fifteen years after the death of the Marquis, Professor Émile Cartailhac of the University of Toulouse published a beautifully illustrated monograph on the paintings under the title *La Caverne d'Altamira*.

2

The story is told here not to demonstrate the fallibility of experts. Actually the experts could not help themselves. These paintings supposedly done by Paleolithic savages who lived fifteen to thirty thousand years ago had nothing primitive, crude, or awkward about them. They were masterpieces, and closer to the feeling and understanding of modern man than any other ancient art. Moreover, the oil colors, deep reds and the blackest black, were vivid and fresh and felt damp to the touch. It was natural to suspect that the paintings were the work of a living painter—probably of the French painter in the Marquis's employ.

Equally crucial was the picture the experts had of the Paleolithic savage. He was at least as primitive as the most primitive tribes in various parts of the world today—at least as primitive as the Australian aborigines. Paleolithic man had only the most rudimentary tools. He could not make a pot, weave cloth, or work metals. He had no domesticated animals, not even a dog. What

connection could there be between such an utterly primitive creature and works of art which are among the greatest achievements
of mankind?

We know that eventually the experts changed their minds
about the paintings. Was this due to a drastic revision of their
thought on the nature and life of early man? Not that you can
notice it. Pick up an armful of books on prehistoric man and you
still find the Paleolithic hunter depicted as wholly absorbed in a
perpetual cruel struggle for sheer survival, always only one step
ahead of starvation, always facing the problem of how to eat without being eaten, never knowing when he fell asleep whether he
would be there in the morning. Why then the paintings? They
were, we are told, an aid in the eternal quest for food; they reflect
the deep anxiety of the hunter community about the animals on
whose meat they depended for very life; they were part of the
magical rites connected with the capture and killing of game. The
savage, we are told, had noticed that by imitating, by disguising
himself as an animal, he could lure and kill his prey, which led
him to believe that likeness was the key to mysterious powers by
which to control other creatures. The more lifelike the likeness,
the greater the magic. Hence the marvelous realism of the paintings.

3

Now, one can admit the magical connotations of the cave
paintings and yet reject the suggestion that Paleolithic art had its
origin in magic. Giotto and Michelangelo painted for the church
and many of their paintings had a religious purpose, but no one
would maintain that religion was at the root of the impulse, drive,
preoccupation, and aspiration which animated these artists. We
know that the shaman, medicine man, and priest make use of the
artist; they subsidize him and enable him to execute momentous
works. But magic and religion do not bring forth the artist. The
artist is there first. The Paleolithic artists engraved, carved, and
modeled in clay long before they executed the animal frescoes in
the caves. The artistic impulse is likely to emerge where there are
leisure, a fascination with objects, and a delight in tinkering and
playing with things.

The first thing I do when I get a book on prehistoric man is go to the index to see whether it has the word *play*. It is usually not there. You find Plato but not play. The experts take it for granted that man's ability to master his environment was the product of a grim, relentless struggle for existence. Man prevailed because he was more purposeful, determined, and cunning than other creatures. Yet whenever we try to trace the origin of a skill or a practice which played a crucial role in the ascent of man, we usually reach the realm of play.

The first domesticated animal—the dog puppy—was not the most useful but the most playful animal. The hunting dog is a rather late development. The bow, we are told, was a musical instrument before it became a weapon. Man first used clay to mold figurines rather than make pots.

Seen thus, it is evident that play has been man's most useful occupation. It is imperative to keep in mind that man painted, engraved, carved, and modeled long before he made a pot, wove cloth, worked metals, or domesticated an animal. Man as an artist is infinitely more ancient than man as a worker. Play came before work, art before production for use.

When grubbing for necessities, man is still in the animal kingdom. He becomes uniquely human and is at his creative best when he expends his energies, and even risks his life, for that which is not essential for sheer survival. Hence it is reasonable to assume that the humanization of man took place in an environment where nature was bountiful, and man had the leisure and the inclination to tinker and play. The ascent of man was enacted in an Eden-like playground rather than on a desolate battleground.

4

Let us return to the Paleolithic hunters who painted the cave masterpieces. Was their life an endless cruel struggle for sheer survival? Actually they lived in a hunter's paradise, a crossroad of the seasonal migrations of huge herds of bison, reindeer, wild horses, musk-ox, and deer. The animals filed past in their thousands along well-defined routes. Food was almost no problem. The hunters lived mostly in skin tents and were clad in sable, arctic fox, and other fancy furs. Judged by their fine bone needles, the Paleolithic hunters were expert tailors. They sported

swagger sticks of mammoth ivory beautifully carved and engraved. They wore necklaces of shell and perforated animal teeth,
and engraved pendants made of ivory, bone, horn, or baked clay.
They were sportsmen, their life rich with leisure yet not without
tensions and passionate preoccupations. They had leisure to develop and exercise subtle skills not only in carving, engraving, and
painting but also in elaborating the sophisticated art of fishing
with bone fishhooks and sinew lines. They probably had secret
societies which met in cave hideouts adorned with engravings and
paintings of animals. The shaman injected himself into these
sporting activities and gradually endowed them with a pronounced magical connotation.

I said that the artistic impulse is likely to arise where there is a
fascination with objects. In the case of the Paleolithic hunter, the
objects were animals. Almost all the engravings, carvings, and
paintings of Paleolithic man were of animals. What was his attitude toward animals? He adored and worshiped them. They were
his betters. Man among the animals is an amateur among superbly
skilled and equipped specialists, each with a built-in tool kit. Man
has neither claws nor fangs nor horns to fight with, neither scales
nor hide to shield him, no special adaptations for burrowing,
swimming, climbing, or running. He craved the strength, speed,
and skill of the superior animals around him. When he boasted,
he likened himself unto an elephant, a bull, a deer. He watched
the adored animals with the total absorption of a lover and could
paint them in vivid detail even on the ceiling of a dark cave.

Man's being an unfinished, defective animal has been the root
of his uniqueness and creativeness. He is the only animal not satisfied with being what he is. His ideal was a combination of the
perfections he saw in the animals around him. His art, dances,
songs, rituals, and inventions were born of his groping to compensate himself for what he lacked as an animal. His spirituality had
its inception not in a craving to overcome his animality but in a
striving to become a superior animal. In the cave of Trois Frères,
the sorcerer painted high on a ledge above the ground seems to
rule over the world of animals depicted on the walls below, and
this sorcerer, whose face is human, is a composite of animals: he
has the antlers of a stag, the ears of a wolf, the eyes of an owl, the
paws of a bear, the tail of a horse, and the genitalia of a wildcat.

5

The most crucial consequence of man's incurable unfinishedness is of course that he cannot truly grow up. Man is the only perpetually young thing in the world, and the playground is the ideal milieu for the unfolding of his capacities and talents. It is the child in man that is the source of his uniqueness and creativeness.

I have always felt that five is a golden age. We are all geniuses at the age of five. The trouble with the juvenile is not that he is not yet a man but that he is no longer a child. If maturing is to have meaning, it must be a recapturing of the capacity for total absorption and the avidity to master skills characteristic of a five-year-old. But it needs leisure to be a child. When we grow up, the world steals our hours and the most it gives us in return is a sense of usefulness. Should automation rob us of our sense of usefulness, the world will no longer be able to steal our hours. Banned from the marketplace, we shall return to the playground and resume the task of learning and growing. Thus to me the coming of automation is the coming of a grand consummation, the completion of a magic circle. Man first became human in an Eden playground, and now we have a chance to attain our ultimate destiny, our fullest humanness, by returning to the playground.

3   THE PLAYFUL MOOD

I HAVE ALWAYS FELT that the world has lost much by not preserving the small talk of its great men. The little that has come down to us is marked by a penetration and a directness not usually conspicuous in formal discourse or writing, and one is immediately aware of its universality and timelessness. It seems strange that men should so effortlessly attain immortality in their playful moments. Certainly, some have missed immortality as writers by not writing as they talked. Clemenceau is a case in point. His books make dull and difficult reading, yet he could not open his mouth without saying something memorable. The few scraps we have of his small talk throw a more vivid light on the human situation than do shelves of books on psychology, sociology, and history. Toward the end of his life Clemenceau is reported to have exclaimed, "What a shame that I don't have three or four more years to live—I would have rewritten my books for my cook." It is also worth noting that the New Testament and the *Lun Yü* are largely records of impromptu remarks and sayings, and that Montaigne wrote as he spoke. ("I speak to my paper as I speak to the first person I meet.")

We are told that a great life is "thought of youth wrought out in ripening years"; and it is perhaps equally true that "great" thinking consists in the working out of insights and ideas which come to us in playful moments. Archimedes' bathtub and Newton's apple suggest that momentous trains of thought may have their inception in idle musing. The original insight is most likely to come when elements stored in different compartments of the mind drift into the open, jostle one another, and now and then coalesce to form new combinations. It is doubtful whether a mind that is pinned down and cannot drift elsewhere is capable of formulating new questions. It is true that the working out of ideas and insights requires persistent hard thinking, and the inspiration necessary for such a task is probably a by-product of single-minded application. But the sudden illumination and the flash of discovery are not likely to materialize under pressure.

Men never philosophize or tinker more freely than when they know that their speculation or tinkering leads to no weighty results. We are more ready to try the untried when what we do is inconsequential. Hence the remarkable fact that many inventions had their birth as toys. In the Occident the first machines were mechanical toys, and such crucial instruments as the telescope and microscope were first conceived as playthings. Almost all civilizations display a singular ingenuity in toy making. The Aztecs did not have the wheel, but some of their animal toys had rollers for feet. It would not be fanciful to assume that in the ancient Near East, too, the wheel and the sail made their first appearance as playthings, or that the first domesticated animals were children's pets. Planting and irrigating, too, were probably first attempted in the course of play. (A girl of five once advised me to plant hair on my bald head.) Even if it could be shown that a striking desiccation of climate preceded the first appearance of herdsmen and cultivators, it would not prove that the concept of domestication was born of a crisis. The energies released by a crisis usually flow toward sheer action and application. Domestication could have been practiced as an amusement long before it found practical application. The crisis induced people to make use of things which amused them.

2

When we do find that a critical challenge has apparently evoked a marked creative response, there is always the possibility that the response came not from people cornered by a challenge but from people who in an exuberance of energy went out in search of a challenge. It is highly doubtful whether people are capable of genuine creative responses when necessity takes them by the throat. The desperate struggle for existence is a static rather than a dynamic influence. The urgent search for the vitally necessary is likely to stop once we have found something that is more or less adequate, but the search for the superfluous has no end. Hence the fact that man's most unflagging and spectacular efforts were made not in search of necessities but of superfluities. It is worth remembering that the discovery of America was a by-product of the search for ginger, cloves, pepper, and cinnamon. The utilitarian device, even when it is an essential ingredient of our daily life, is most likely to have its ancestry in the nonutilitarian. The sepulcher, temple, and palace preceded the utilitarian house; ornament preceded clothing; work, particularly teamwork, derives from play. Some authorities believe that the subtle craft of fishing originated in a period when game was abundant—that it was the product not so much of grim necessity as of curiosity, speculation, and playfulness. We know that poetry preceded prose, and it may be that singing came before talking.

On the whole it seems to be true that the creative periods in history were buoyant and even frivolous. One thinks of the light-heartedness of Periclean Athens, the Renaissance, the Elizabethan Age, and the age of the Enlightenment. Nehru tells us that in India "during every period when her civilization bloomed, we find an intense joy in life and nature and a pleasure in the art of living." One suspects that much of the praise of seriousness comes from people who have a vital need for a façade of weight and dignity. La Rochefoucauld said of solemnity that it is "a mystery of the body invented to conceal the defects of the mind." The fits of deadly seriousness we know as mass movements, which come bearing a message of serious purpose and weighty ideals, are usually set in motion by pedants possessed of a murderous hatred for festive creativeness. Such movements bring in their wake meager-mindedness, fear, austerity, and sterile conformity. Hardly one of the world's great works in literature, art, music, and pure science was conceived and realized in the stern atmosphere of a mass movement. It is only when these movements have spent themselves, and their pattern of austere boredom begins to crack and the despised present dares assert its claims to trivial joys, that the creative impulse begins to stir amidst the grayness and desolation.

Man shares his playfulness with other warm-blooded animals, with mammals and birds. Insects and reptiles do not play. Clearly, the division of the forms of life into those that can play and those that cannot is a significant one. Equally significant is the duration of the propensity to play. Mammals and birds play only when young, while man retains the propensity throughout life. My feeling is that the tendency to carry youthful characteristics into adult life, which renders man perpetually immature and unfinished, is particularly pronounced in the creative individual. Youth has been called a perishable talent, but perhaps talent and originality are always aspects of youth, and the creative individual is an imperishable juvenile. When the Greeks said, "Whom the gods love die young," they probably meant, as Lord Sankey suggested, that those favored by the gods stay young till the day they die: young and playful.

4   THE BIRTH OF CITIES

I<small>T HAS BEEN GENERALLY ASSUMED</small> that the birth of the city came at the culmination of a technological revolution which took place in Mesopotamia between 4000 and 3000 B.C. V. Gordon Childe maintained that not only the domestication of plants and animals but also the invention of the wheel, sail, plow, irrigation, brick-making, metallurgy, the calendar, and even the invention of writing preceded the coming of the city; that all these momentous inventions and discoveries were made in the sticks, in some rudimentary settlements or villages.

To anyone even vaguely acquainted with the nature of the creative situation, such an assumption will seem absurd. Whoever heard of anything new coming out of a village! All through the millennia the village has been a bastion of deadly conservatism. Even at this moment, in many parts of the world, villages are still stuck in the Neolithic Age. A crucial characteristic of backward, stagnant countries is that the village and not the city is the basic unit of society. People who live close to nature have little occasion to experience continuous progress toward something new and better. They are immersed in the endless recurrence of similar events. The village is equally inhospitable to strange people and strange ways.

From the point of view of the creative milieu, it is difficult to see how the subtly creative act of plant domestication was con-

From *First Things, Last Things.*

ceived in the sticks and, as most prehistorians believe, by food-collecting women driven by the necessity to stave off starvation. The creative milieu is characterized not only by a considerable degree of leisure and the absence of pressing necessity, which stifles the impulse to tinker and play, but also by the interaction of people with different ways and bents. Where in any village can you find a human situation distantly approaching such a milieu?

It has long been taken for granted that the farming village preceded the city, that the earliest village must be far more ancient than the earliest city, and that some villages grew into cities. When some years ago Kathleen Kenyon at Jericho and James Mellaart at Çatal Hüyük unearthed walled cities which antedated by several millennia any excavated ancient village, they upset many archaeological applecarts. Indeed, Miss Kenyon suggested that the breakthrough from food collecting to food production took place in walled cities like Jericho.[1] At Çatal Hüyük the presence of wall paintings of hunting scenes and of large hunting weapons suggested to Mr. Mellaart that here was a link between the fabulous hunter–cave painters of the upper Paleolithic Age and the new order of food production.[2]

2

Domestication of seed plants was first achieved in the Near East after the end of the last Ice Age. There is no evidence that the melting of the ice cap in Europe and other northern latitudes about 10,000 B.C., which brought about poignant changes in the life of the Paleolithic hunters, caused crucial climatic changes in the lands of the fertile crescent. In other words, domestication of plants did not come as a response to climatic change. Climatic conditions in the Near East were probably as favorable for the growth of seed plants before 10,000 B.C. as they were after. Nor was domestication prompted by a shrinkage of the food supply. The abundance of wild barley, wheat, and other edible grasses made the Near East an ideal place for intensive grain collecting. Some time ago, the American archaeologist Jack R. Harlan tested

[1] Kathleen M. Kenyon, *Digging Up Jericho* (New York: Frederick A. Praeger, 1957).

[2] James Mellaart, *Çatal Hüyük* (New York: McGraw-Hill, 1967).

the harvesting of wild grain on a mountainside in southern Turkey. He used a reconstructed sickle with a flint blade. He estimated that "a family group beginning harvesting near the base of the mountain and working slowly upslope as the season progressed, could easily collect over a three-week span, without ever working too hard, more grain than the family could possibly consume in a year."[3] There is no reason to assume that conditions were substantially different in prehistoric days. Moreover, hunting with bow and arrow was a long-established practice among Near Eastern food collectors and, judging by the enormous quantities of gazelle bones, a highly rewarding one. In short, domestication of plants was first attempted by people living in an economy of plenty.

What then was the event after 10,000 B.C. which prompted expert grain collectors living in a region rich in wild grains to plant the seed they had in their leather pouches and storage bins? Something momentous must have happened in the Near East a millennium or so after the melting of the ice cap in Europe. One ought to look for traces of some upheaval that shattered and churned the long-established communes of grain collectors and threw their human debris together in places of refuge where, pressed against each other and with time on their hands, they talked, reflected, tinkered, and experimented. It was probably in such a stockade or sanctuary that grain production was first conceived and attempted.

What could have been the cause of such an upheaval?

3

In Europe, the end of the last Ice Age had dramatic effects. The herds of migratory bison, reindeer, wild horse, and mammoth, already decimated by a continuously perfected hunting technique, disappeared completely. The land, free of ice, was soon covered with forest hospitable only to smaller solitary animals, such as deer and boar, which had to be hunted with bow and arrow. The hunters had to become food collectors living on these smaller animals and on fish, shellfish, and berries. The shift from the communal hunt of large game to food collecting drained

[3] *Archaeology*, vol. 20, no. 3 (June 1967), p. 197.

life of fierce joys, sharp exertions, instinctual satisfactions, and the exhilaration of communion. It is not at all unreasonable to assume that the proudest and most venturesome among the hunters began to drift eastward and southward in search of a new hunters' paradise.[4] Such a migration of hunters would be neither anomalous nor unprecedented, since we know of migrations even during the Ice Age when man first reached Australia and North America. Sometime in the ninth millennium the drifting bands of hunters reached the Near East, where they came up against the territorial rights of long-established, thriving communes of grain collectors. The resulting clash and protracted struggle must have been the event which set the stage for the invention of domestication.

The full emergence of agriculture may have been a slow evolution. But the idea of domestication came probably as a sudden illumination. Both the grain collectors and the hunter bands sought refuge in walled places near wells or rivers. These stockades were embyronic cities, where a mixed group of people, the debris of various communes, had the leisure, between forays to collect food and harass the enemy, to talk, tinker, and eventually hit upon the idea of producing food by planting grain in plots of ground.

It is of absorbing interest that the art of earliest Jericho and of Çatal Hüyük should call to mind the Late Paleolithic hunter–cave painters. It shows a naturalism and a refinement not found in other food-collecting areas. In Europe, Asia, and North Africa, the art of the food-collecting period is typified by schematic figures of animals and human beings and abstract geometric patterns, with not a trace of the superb realism which animated the Paleolithic cave paintings. In addition to the art there were also large hunting weapons and burial customs to indicate some continuity between the Paleolithic hunters and the postglacial Near East.

4

Earliest Jericho was a sanctuary adjacent to a copious well. It was occupied by hunters who made it a more or less permanent camping place. Some of the clay floors had stone sockets for the

---

[4] The Persian word *Pairidaize* means a hunting preserve.

placing of totem poles. There is evidence of the tentative beginning of agriculture dating from 8840 B.C. The presence of Anatolian obsidian indicates a link with northern regions.

The settlement grew rapidly in size during the eighth millennium and was heavily fortified with three super-imposed drystone walls, a huge watchtower with an internal staircase, and a deep rock-cut ditch outside the wall.

Toward the end of the eighth millennium Jericho was taken over by a different cultural group, possibly by the one against whom the massive fortifications had been erected. There is evidence that the city was deserted for a time previous to the takeover. The newcomers raised crops and domesticated the goat. Though they had no pottery, they knew how to make clay figurines of the Mother Goddess, and how to plaster skulls and mold them into faces of singular beauty. They fashioned beautiful stone vessels.

There is no telling whether the first settlers were natives or invading hunters. The fact that some were longheaded and some broadheaded may indicate a mixed population. Nor do we know whether the people who took over Jericho after the end of the eighth millennium, and who were more artistically gifted, were of the invading Paleolithic hunters. It is perhaps legitimate to assume that the first attempt to plant grain was made by grain collectors familiar with the life cycle of wild grain plants, and that the hunters appropriated the practice from them. One ought also to assume that the hunters from the north would not readily take to the life of an agriculturalist. Many of them would sooner or later turn northward again and resume the search for a hunter's paradise. They would carry with them the new mode of food production and a taste for living in a fortified city. It was probably such remnants of the Paleolithic hunters who built the city of Çatal Hüyük on the Konya plain in Anatolia.

Çatal Hüyük was a town of substantial size in the seventh millennium B.C., three or four thousand years before the famous cities of Mesopotamia. The dwellers of the town farmed and hunted. Since the Konya plain had no wild grain plants, the agriculture of Çatal Hüyük was imported from somewhere else, probably from Palestine, as Mellaart conjectures.

As late as 6000 B.C. the Konya plain teemed with wild life.

There were aurochs, wild pigs, several species of deer, two species of wild ass, wild sheep, and some gazelles. The people of Catal Hüyük made good use of the hunter's paradise. They also cultivated no less than fourteen food plants and raised sheep and goats. Since the houses were built one against the other, the city presented to the outside world a blank wall which gave it the appearance of a fortress.

As already mentioned, the upper Paleolithic heritage is clearly recognizable in Çatal Hüyük. There are the large hunting weapons, the realistic hunting scenes painted on walls, the modeling of animals wounded in hunting rites, the practice of red-ocher burials, and, finally, certain types of stone tools.

5

It is safe to assume that there were other early cities, foci of the earliest civilization. They lasted for millennia but for some unknown reason were abandoned late in the sixth millennium B.C. It was then (about 5000 B.C.) that drab farming villages began to dot the Near East. The prototype of the village was probably a suburb housing the dropouts who could not make it in the early city. When the city disappeared, the suburb continued as a village. The agricultural villages were, then, the end product of the decay of the first cities.

It is in areas where the remnants of cities are more ancient than the remnants of farming villages that domestication originated. Where cities are a late development, as in Egypt, Europe, and elsewhere, domestication was introduced from without.

The idea of two cycles of city building separated by several millennia is not as strange as it sounds. There are instances in history of precursors foreshadowing a momentous event long in advance. Thus the voyages of the Vikings, beginning in the eighth century, were forerunners of the voyages of discovery in the fifteenth and sixteenth centuries. Though there is no unquestionable evidence that Columbus benefited from the experience of the Vikings, there is no doubt that the Sumerians, who initiated the second cycle of city building in the fourth millennium, made full use of the agriculture and the crafts elaborated in the earliest cities and conserved in the villages of Mesopotamia. In the Sumerian language the words for farmer, herdsman, fisherman, plow, smith, carpenter, weaver, potter, mason, and perhaps even merchant are non-Sumerian.

The Sumerians were hunters who came into lower Mesopotamia, from the mountainous region to the northeast, sometime in the fourth millennium. We are so used to the idea that the village was a preliminary to the city that we assume the villager to have a greater affinity to city life than the hunter. Actually, the life of a band of hunters has many things in common with life in the city: adventurous vicissitudes, fabulous windfalls, meetings with strangers, ceaseless movement and ceaseless vying, and the exhilaration of communion. The drab Neolithic village was without the breath of freedom, and the human spirit lost there its swing and extravagance. Neolithic agriculture brought the curse of work to man and animal. Only in the city did the human spirit regain for a time the flight it knew in the Eden playground of the Paleolithic hunters. Moreover, no one doubts that the trader who is most at home in the city has in him more of the hunter than of the villager. Finally, the hunter's talent for organization places him way above the villager as a potential city builder. Hence, often in history, hunters have played a decisive role in the birth of cities. Aztec civilization was a fusion between that of the native Toltecs, skilled in crafts, and that of the invading Aztec hunter-warriors, skilled in organization. The word Toltec in Nahuatl means "master craftsman." Something similar might have taken place in Egypt, Greece, India, and China.

The cities built by the Sumerians, though based on agriculture, had a varied population. In addition to farmers and herdsmen there were fishermen, merchants, craftsmen, scribes, doctors, soldiers, and priests. The Sumerian city has been the prototype of the cities that have dotted the planet for five thousand years. We of the present, writhing in the grip of an apparently insoluble urban crisis, may be witnessing the end of the second cycle of city building begun by the Sumerians.

5   CITIES AND NATURE

I SPENT A GOOD PART OF MY LIFE close to nature as migratory worker, lumberjack, and placer miner. Mother Nature was breathing down my neck, so to speak, and I had the feeling that she did not want me around. I was bitten by every sort of insect and scratched by burrs, foxtails, and thorns. My clothes were torn by buckbrush and tangled manzanita. Hard clods pushed against my ribs when I lay down to rest, and grime ate its way into every pore of my body. Everything around me was telling me all the time to roll up and be gone. I was an unwanted intruder. I could never be at home in nature the way trees, flowers, and birds are at home in human habitations, even in the city. I did not feel at ease until my feet touched the paved road.

The road led to the city, and I knew with every fiber of my being that the man-made world of the city was man's only home on this planet, his refuge from an inhospitable nonhuman cosmos.

Vaguely at first then more distinctly I realized that man is an eternal stranger on this planet. He became a stranger when he cut himself off from the rest of creation and became human. From this incurable strangeness stems our incurable insecurity, our unfulfillable craving for roots, our passion to cover the planet with man-made compounds, our need for the city—a citadel against the encroachment of nature.

I did not have to be a scholar to recognize that man's greatest achievements were conceived and realized not in the bracing at-

A slightly altered version of the essay of the same title in *First Things, Last Things*.

mosphere of plains, deserts, forests, and mountaintops but in the crowded, noisy, and smelly cities of ancient Mesopotamia and Egypt, and of Jerusalem, Athens, Florence, Amsterdam, Vienna, Paris, London, and New York.

So true is it that the city is man's optimal creative milieu that even communion with the self is more attainable in the press and noise of the city than in the silence of the great outdoors. There is no genuine solitude outside the city.

2

There is in this country, particularly among the educated, a romantic, worshipful attitude toward nature. Nature is thought to be pure, innocent, serene, health-giving, the fountainhead of elevated thoughts and feelings. We are told how nature aids and guides us; how, like a stern mother, she nudges and pushes man to fulfill her wise designs. Coupled with this admiration of nature there is often a distaste for man and man's work. Man is a violator, a defiler and deformer.

My hunch is that the attitude of the educated American toward nature is shaped and colored by European literature. Europe is one of the tamest parts of the world. Nowhere else are man and nature so much in each other's confidence. Imagine a subcontinent without a desert or a rampaging river, without hurricanes and tornadoes, and where you are never too far from a road or even an inn. So unusual was the Lisbon earthquake in 1755 that it upset the moral, religious, and intellectual conceptions of a generation. Goethe said that "the demon of fright was abroad in the land."

Compare this with our savage continent. Open your newspaper any morning and you find reports of floods, tornadoes, hurricanes, hailstorms, sandstorms, pests, and droughts. Sometimes when reading about nature's terrible visitations and its massacre of the innocents you wonder whether North America is fit for human beings. Fly over this country and you see what we have done. We have cast a net of concrete roads over a snarling continent and proceeded to tame each square. Every now and then there is a heaving and rumbling, and the continent shakes us off its back.

Nevertheless, on the Berkeley campus generations of young

people, brainwashed by Wordsworth, Shelley, Tennyson, and other poets of a manicured little island, have gone up to the woods to make love and come back swollen with poison oak. They have as yet not realized that on this continent woods and meadows are not what the poets say they are.

It is worth noting that Thoreau, who loved nature "because she is not man but a retreat from man," lived in a tamed corner of America, where the meadows were fertile, the hills gentle, and the woods hospitable.

The miracle is that we have taken a continent almost unfit for human beings and made it a cornucopia of plenty. We are accused of ravaging and raping a continent. Actually, our mastery of nature is such that if we were so minded we could, in fifty years or so, regrow all the forests, replenish the soil, cleanse the rivers and the air of pollution, have buffalo herds again thundering on the plains, and make the continent as virgin as when we got here.

If this nation declines and decays it will be not because we have raped and ravaged a continent, but because we do not know how to build and maintain viable cities. America's destiny will be decided in the cities.

3

It is particularly grotesque to hear Latin-American or African intellectuals mouth clichés about nature they picked up during their student days in Paris or London. Several years ago I had a visitor from Peru. He said he was a professor of sociology and also a novelist and poet. He was traveling as a guest of the State Department. I let him talk. It was unfortunate, he said, that this country was so far ahead technologically. The effort to catch up with us distorts and cripples other countries. He had all the right phrases about the evils of our materialism, how it stifles and crushes the countries below the Rio Grande. I asked him how he liked San Francisco. He liked it fine, but he was disgusted with the Golden Gate Park. How dared we play tricks upon nature! The artifical lakes, creeks, mountains, and waterfalls were a blasphemy. We lacked all reverence and made nature jump at our bidding.

I said, "You come from a country where nature has repossessed all that the Incas built with infinite toil through the centuries. All the wonderful terraces, canals, roads, bridges, and cities have become a wilderness. Nature is snatching the bread from your mouth. Your one and only problem is how to cope with nature, and your wildest dream should be a Peru turned into a Golden Gate Park."

Not surprisingly, he stood up, a picture of outraged dignity. The Peruvian student from Berkeley who did the translating had a twinkle in his eyes, and we exchanged winks. Sometime later I came upon a speech delivered by Fernando Belaunde Terry, then President of Peru, when he opened a network of rural roads. The last sentence of the speech read, "In Peru nature is the enemy."

As to Africa: we tend to forget that in Africa the battle that has to be won is not against colonialism but against nature—primeval, relentless, and aggressive. The central task in Africa is the taming of the forests, rivers, and deserts, the banishing of diseases and pests, and the dispelling of the fear of nature embodied in brutalizing superstitions and rituals.

1

There are many who warn us that a cocky attitude toward nature spells trouble. Yet it is questionable whether a society awed by nature can be truly free. For freedom is basically freedom from nature, from the iron necessities and the implacable determinism which dominate nature. Moreover, a society awed by nature tends to equate power with nature and would no more revolt against despotic power than it would against a natural calamity.

Equally vital is the fact that a society awed by nature is not likely to develop an effective technology for mastering nature. Man had to separate himself from nature, had to hole up in the city, a citadel against the encroachment of nature, before he could evolve a technology that liberated him from the animal imprisonment of nature with its wants, its menace, and its bondage. Only in the city could man become truly Promethean, in perpetual revolt against the iron laws which imprison all other forms of life.

Yet in Asia, where cities first made their appearance, the liberating role of the city was shortlived. The outburst of discoveries and inventions in the earliest days of city building betokened a free, venturesome, questioning spirit. The people who were behind that onrush of achievements were more like us than any in the intervening historic generations. But this self-reliant, venturesome spirit did not last. It was stifled by the domination of kings, priests, and scribes, and for millennia the cities of Asia stagnated in superstition and resignation. The civilizations of Asia functioned as if the answers were there before the questions.

In the Occident, self-governing cities have been for centuries nurseries of the human spirit, havens of welcome for strangers, stages of pageantry and high drama, the seedbed of freedom, art, literature, science, and technology. But they have also been the abode of the devil, of the forces of corruption and dehumanization. In the Occident the city has been the greatest opportunity and the worst influence: a place of creation and decay, of freedom and subjection, of riches and poverty, of splendor and misery, of communion and lonesomeness—an optimal milieu for talent, character, vice, and corruption.

For nature is both around and within us. Though the city has been the headquarters of the great movement of the human spirit to emancipate itself from the tyranny of matter, it has also been the place where man has been losing his battle with the nature that is sealed within him. The city has not freed man from the tyranny of his lusts, his savage impulses, his ferocious malice, and the dark destructive forces that lie in wait in the cellars of his psyche. If God is that which makes man human, and the devil that which dehumanizes him, then it is in the city and not in heaven that God and the devil are in perpetual combat.

5

Just now the devil is gaining the upper hand. In the past, cities decayed because they lost the battle with nature around them and could no longer support themselves. Our cities are decaying at a moment when our victory over nature seems almost total, and affluence is widely diffused. It is inside our cities that nature is striking back at us, pushing us back into the jungle and turning us into primitive savages. For many Americans the city has become an environment as threatening as a neighboring tract of jungle is for an Asian or African villager. The words of Baltasar

Gracián have never sounded more true than they do now: "The real wild beasts exist where most men live."

We are up against a predicament of the human condition: the impossibility of coordinating the two fronts of man's battle with nature. Worse still, victory on one front is unavoidably followed by defeat on the other front. The moment we have gained mastery over things, we are faced with the unsavory task of mastering men. Up to now in free societies, the mastery of men has been the automatic by-product of the effort to master things; social discipline has been a function of scarcity. Thus anarchy and terror in the cities make it questionable whether affluent societies can remain free.

The choice before us at present seems to be between two types of nonfree societies: (a) our present society with its constitutional guarantees of individual freedom and its helplessness against willful individuals who mug, rob, rape, murder, bomb, riot, and disrupt our institutions; or (b) a dictatorship which deprives individuals of many freedoms but maintains order and security in the cities. It is clear that a society in the grip of fear is not free no matter how numerous the freedoms its constitution guarantees. There are already many people in this country who would surrender certain of their civil rights for a feeling of personal security.

Still, a dictatorship is not an acceptable solution of the apparent incompatibility between affluence and order. My hunch is that, to keep stable and healthy, a free affluent society must become a creative society. The destructive forces released by affluence must serve to fuel the creative process. There are indications that creativeness has its source in the tension between that which is most human and most unhuman in us. Paul Valéry defines social peace as "the state of things in which the natural hostility of man toward man is manifested by creation instead of destruction. . . . It is the period of creative competition and the struggle of inventions."

The sublimity of man manifests itself not in the purity and nobility of his impulses and motives but in the alchemy of his soul, which transmutes meanness and savagery into things of beauty and into thoughts and visions which reach unto heaven. The primordial slime is always within us, and we become uniquely human as we process it. We cope best with the devil not by fighting but by using him.

I ONCE HEARD a brilliant young professor of political science wonder what it would be like if one were to apply the law of the diffusion of gases to the diffusion of opinion. The idea seemed to him farfetched, yet he was eager to play with it.

It occurred to me, as I listened, that to a Galileo or a Kepler the idea would not have seemed at all fantastic. For both Galileo and Kepler really and truly believed in a God who had planned and designed the whole of creation—a God who was a master mathematician and technician. Mathematics was God's style, and whether it was the movement of the stars, the flight of a bird, the diffusion of gases, or the propagation of opinions, they all bore God's mathematical hallmark.

It sounds odd in modern ears that it was a particular concept of God that prompted and guided the men who were at the birth of modern science. They felt in touch with God in every discovery they made. Their search for the mathematical laws of nature was to some extent a religious quest. Nature was God's text, and the mathematical notations were his alphabet.

The book of nature, said Galileo, is written in letters other than those of our alphabet—"these letters being triangles, quadrangles, circles, spheres, cones, pyramids, and other mathematical figures." So convinced was Kepler that in groping for the laws that govern the motions of the heavenly bodies he was trying to

From *The Ordeal of Change.*

decipher God's text, he later boasted in exaltation that God the author had to wait six thousand years for his first reader. Leonardo da Vinci paused in his dissection of corpses to pen a prayer: "Would that it might please the Creator that I were able to reveal the nature of man and his customs even as I describe his figure." Leonardo's interest in anatomy may have arisen from his work as an artist, but he was eventually driven mainly by the curiosity of the scientist and the mechanic. Living creatures were wondrous machines devised by a master mechanic, and Leonardo was taking them apart to discover how they were built and how they worked. By observing them and tinkering with them, man could himself become a maker of machines. One could perhaps eventually build a seeing mechanism, a hearing mechanism, a flying machine, and so on. The making of machines would be a second creation: man's way of breathing will and thought into matter.

2

The concept of God as a master mathematician and craftsman accounts perhaps for the striking difference between the revival of learning and the revival of science in the sixteenth and seventeenth centuries. Whereas the revival of learning was wholly dominated by the ideas and examples of antiquity, the revival of science, though profiting from Greek writing, manifested a marked independence from the beginning. The vivid awareness of God's undeciphered text spread out before them kept the new scientists from expending their energies in the exegesis and imitation of ancient texts. In this case, a genuine belief in God was a factor in the emergence of intellectual independence.

It is of course conceivable that modern science and technology might have developed as they did without a particular conception of God. Yet one cannot resist the temptation to speculate on the significance of the connection. It is as if the Occident had first to conceive a God who was a scientist and a technician before it could create a civilization dominated by science and technology.

It is perhaps not entirely so, though it has often been said, that man makes his God in his own image. Rather does he create him in the image of his cravings and dreams—in the image of what man wants to be. God making could be part of the process by which a society realizes its aspirations: it first embodies them in the conception of a particular god and then proceeds to imitate that god. The confidence requisite for attempting the unprecedented is most effectively generated by the fiction that in realizing the new we are imitating rather than originating. Our preoccupation with heaven can be part of an effort to find precedents for the unprecedented.

For all we know, one of the reasons that other civilizations, with all their ingenuity and skill, did not develop a machine age is that they lacked a god whom they could readily turn into an all-powerful engineer. For has not the mighty Jehovah performed from the beginning of time the feats that our machine age is even now aspiring to achieve? He shut up the sea with doors and said, "Hitherto shalt thou come but no further; and here shall thy proud waves be stayed." He made pools of water in the wilderness and turned the desert into a garden. He numbered the stars and called them by name. He commanded the clouds and told rivers whither to flow. He measured the waters in the hollow of his hand, and meted out the heavens with the span, and comprehended the dust in a measure, and weighed the mountains in scales.

3

The momentous transition that occurred in Europe after the late Middle Ages was in some degree also a transition from the imitation of Christ to the imitation of God. The new scientists felt close to the God who had created the world and set it going. They stood in awe of him, yet felt as if they were of his school. They were thinking God's thoughts and, whether they knew it or not, aspired to be like him.

The imitation of God was undoubtedly a factor in the release of the dynamism which marked the modern Occident from its birth and set it off from other civilizations. Not only the new scientists but the artists, explorers, inventors, merchants, and men of affairs felt that, in the words of Alberti, "men can do all things if they will." When Columbus exclaimed, *"Il mondo è poco!"* he was expressing triumph rather than despair. The momentous discoveries and achievements implied a downgrading of God. For there is vying in imitation, and the impulse is to overtake and overcome the model we imitate. With its increased mastery over things, the Occident began to feel that it was catching up with God, that it was taming God's creation and making it subservient to a man-made world. The Occident was harking back to the generation of the flood that set out to storm the heavens and felt that "nothing will be restrained from them which they have imagined to do."

7   THE PRIMACY OF MAN

THERE IS PROBABLY in all professions some discrepancy between words and performance. Usually the words are the more impressive and noble. But in the case of certain architects the opposite seems to be true: their performance is more original and pregnant with meaning than their words. I know several excellent architects who usually speak feelingly and reverentially about nature: how we must harmonize and blend with nature and never violate it. To hear them talk you would think that if they built a house on the side of a hill they would so blend it with nature that you could not see the house until you bumped against it. Actually, they do no such thing. As genuine creators they know that harmony with nature must be achieved on human terms; that when they bring man and nature together, man is the host and nature his guest. The primacy of man must be patent. When a gifted architect finishes his task, a gate built between two ancient trees will look as if the gate were there first and the trees planted afterward. If he builds a house over a creek, the beholder ought not to have the least doubt that the house was there first and the creek brought in later. You do not violate or demean nature by making her your guest. From the beginning of time, trees, grass, flowers, birds, and animals have felt wholly at home in human habitations, even the city, whereas nature has always been a stern and grudging host.

Whenever I talk with architects, I tell them about the British

A slightly longer version of this essay appeared in *In Our Time*.

general Charles Granville Bruce, who when he first gazed at the prodigious massif of that great Himalayan peak Nanga Parbat, clad in eternal snow, felt that he wasn't there and that it did not matter whether he existed. That a human being, the greatest prodigy of the universe, who has all continents, all oceans, and all mountains within him, should feel that he doesn't exist when he gazes at a pile of mindless, soulless rock and snow seems to me outrageous. Architects, if they are any good, ought to be able to build a bungalow on the Himalayas so that Nanga Parbat and all the other peaks would seem but a background for it. Pascal expressed it beautifully: "All the bodies, the firmament, the stars, the earth are not equal in value to the lowest human being. From all bodies together not the slightest thought and not a single impulse of charity can be obtained."

I also find my own experience reflected in the saying of another Frenchman, Henry de Montherlant: "However wonderful the stars may be, I still prefer the light made by man." Compare this with the words of the great humanitarian Bertrand Russell: "The sea, the stars, the wind in waste places mean more to me than even the human beings I love best." I can guess, more or less, what Russell felt when he listened to the wind in waste places. He was lifted out of the paltriness and transitoriness of an individual existence by communion with nature's eternal recurrence, and by feeling one with sea, stars, and the whispering wind. But it may fare ill with mankind if ever power falls into the hands of the Bertrand Russells.

II

INNOVATION AND
THE INTELLECTUALS

MAN'S LONGINGS are the raw material of his creativeness, his dreams, his excesses, his self-sacrifice, his urge to build and to destroy. A man's soul is pierced as it were with holes, and as his longings flow through each they are transmuted into something specific. The flow through one outlet affects the flow through all the others. Creativeness is a leak; so are dissipation, self-sacrifice, acquisitiveness; the fever of building and the frenzy of destruction; the love of women, of God, and of humanity.

Σ

The soul intensity induced by an inner inadequacy constitutes a release of energy, and it depends on a person's endowments and on attending circumstances whether the released energy works itself out in discontent, in desire, in sheer action, or in creativeness.

The chemistry of dissatisfaction is as the chemistry of some marvelously potent tar. In it are the building stones of explosives, stimulants, poisons, opiates, perfumes, and stenches.

Σ

There is perhaps no better way of measuring the natural endowment of a soul than by its ability to transmute dissatisfaction into a creative impulse. The genuine artist is as much a dissatisfied person as the revolutionary, yet how diametrically opposed are the products each distills from his dissatisfaction.

Σ

The discrepancy between trivial causes and momentous consequences is a crucial trait of human uniqueness, and it is particularly pronounced in the creative individual. It is the mark of the creator that he makes something out of nothing.

It has been said that all places are equidistant from heaven, and all eras equidistant from eternity. It is also true that all experiences are equidistant from the regularity they illustrate. But only to a creative mind can a common occurrence be the key to a revelation.

Σ

The genuine creator creates something that has a life of its own, something that can exist and function without him. This is true not only of the writer, artist, and scientist but of creators in other fields. The creative teacher is he who, in the words of Comenius, "teaches less and his students learn more." A creative organizer creates an organization that can function well without him. When a genuine leader has done his work, his followers will say, "We have done it ourselves," and feel that they can do great things without great leaders. With the noncreative it is the other way around: in whatever they do, they arrange things so that they themselves become indispensable.

Σ

It is a juvenile notion that a society needs a lofty purpose and a shining vision to achieve much. Both in the marketplace and on the battlefield, men who set their hearts on toys have often displayed unequaled initiative and drive. And one must be ignorant of the creative process to look for a close correspondence between motive and achievement in the world of thought and imagination.

The romantic view which sees grandiose conceptions at the root of great deeds stems from an unrealized passion for impressive action, just as the romantic view of love thrives on sexual frustration.

Σ

The sense of uniqueness inherent in the creative process has often inclined the writer and the artist to see themselves as the center of the universe and as the bearers of a destiny shaped by cosmic forces. Hence their fascination with coincidences, omens, and signs. It is a conceit which requires a high capacity for self-dramatization—a capacity indigenous to the juvenile mentality. It is amazing how much phoniness is needed to produce a grain of originality.

Σ

Familiarity blurs and flattens. Both the artist and the thinker are preoccupied with the birth of the ordinary and the discovery of the unknown. They both conserve life by recapturing the childhood of things.

Σ

They who lack talent expect things to happen without effort. They ascribe failure to a lack of inspiration or ability, or to misfortune, rather than to insufficient application. At the core of every true talent there is an awareness of the difficulties inherent in any achievement, and the confidence that by persistence and patience something worthwhile will be realized. Thus talent is a species of vigor.

Σ

To have an exceptional talent and the capacity to realize it is like having a powerful appetite and the capacity to enjoy it. In both cases there is an impatience with anything that hampers free movement, and the feeling that the world is one's oyster.

Σ

It is the stretched soul that makes music, and souls are stretched by the pull of opposites—opposite bents, tastes, yearnings, loyalties. Where there is no polarity—where energies flow smoothly in one direction—there will be much doing but no music.

Σ

We acquire a sense of worth either by realizing our talents, or by keeping busy, or by identifying ourselves with something apart from us—be it a cause, a leader, a group, possessions, or the like. Of the three, the path of self-realization is the most difficult. It is taken only when other avenues to a sense of worth are more or less blocked. Men of talent have to be encouraged and goaded to engage in creative work. Their groans and laments echo through the ages.

Action is a highroad to self-confidence and esteem. Where it is open, all energies flow toward it. It comes readily to most people, and its rewards are tangible. The cultivation of the spirit is elusive and difficult, and the tendency toward it is rarely spontaneous. Where the opportunities for action are many, cultural creativeness is likely to be neglected. The cultural flowering of New England came to an almost abrupt end with the opening of the West. The relative cultural sterility of the Romans might perhaps be explained by their empire rather than by an innate lack of genius. The best talents were attracted by the rewards of administrative posts just as the best talents in America have been attracted by the rewards of a business career.

The conditions optimal for cultural creativeness seem to be a marked degree of individual autonomy; a modicum of economic well-being; absence of mass fervor whether religious, patriotic, revolutionary, business or war; a paucity of opportunities for action; a milieu which recognizes and rewards merit; and a degree of communal discipline.

The last point needs elucidation.

When people are free to do as they please, they usually imitate each other. Originality is deliberate and forced, and partakes of the nature of a protest. A society which gives unlimited freedom to the individual, more often than not attains a disconcerting sameness. On the other hand, where communal discipline is strict but not ruthless—"an annoyance which irritates, but not a heavy yoke which crushes"—originality is likely to thrive. It is true that when imitation runs its course in a wholly free society it results in a uniformity which is not unlike a mild tyranny. Thus the fully standardized free society has perhaps enough compulsion to challenge originality.

Σ

The vigor of a society shows itself partly in the ability to borrow copiously without ill effects and without impairing its identity. The Occident borrowed profusely from other civilizations and thrived on it. It is startling to realize that between A.D. 1400 and 1800 the Eastern influence on the West was greater than the Western influence on the East. Had it not been for the Eastern influence, Columbus might not have set out to discover America. Moreover, the East gave us the instruments—gunpowder, the compass, the astrolabe—with which to subdue it.

Early in history, Egypt, Crete, India, and others, borrowed freely from Sumer yet developed unique, vigorous civilizations.

Contrary to what one would expect, it is the more ancient civilizations that can assimilate borrowings from others without ill effects. The more distinct and unassailable the identity of a society, the more easily and safely it can imitate foreign models. Japan's copious borrowings from China did not make it less uniquely Japanese. The same is true of Japan's borrowings from the Occident. China, too, did not become less Chinese by adopting Communism.

The Phoenicians invented the alphabet and the Greeks borrowed it from them. Yet how great the discrepancy between what the Phoenicians did with that which they originated and what the Greeks did with that which they borrowed. Perhaps our originality manifests itself most strikingly in what we do with that which we did not originate. To discover something wholly new can be a matter of chance, of idle tinkering, or even of the chronic dissatisfaction of the untalented.

Σ

When the genuinely creative imitate, they end up making the model a poor imitation of themselves.

Σ

Total innovation is the refuge of the untalented and the innately clumsy. It offers them a situation where their ineptness is acceptable and natural. For we are all apprentices when we tackle the wholly new, and we expect the new to show the apprentice's hand—to be clumsy and ill-shapen.

Yet, however untalented and clumsy, the innovators have a vital role to play. For it is the fate of every great achievement to be pounced upon by pedants and imitators who drain it of life and turn it into an orthodoxy which stifles all stirrings of originality. The avant-garde counteracts this deadening influence, and fulfills the vital role of keeping the gates open for the real talents who will eventually sweep away the inanities of the experimenters and build the new with a sure hand.

Σ

The link between ideas and action is rarely direct. There is almost always an intermediary step in which the idea is overcome. De Tocqueville points out that it is at times when passions start to govern human affairs that ideas are most obviously translated into political action. The translation of ideas into action is usually in the hands of people least likely to follow rational motives. Hence it is that action is often the nemesis of ideas, and sometimes of the men who formulated them.

Σ

There are people who need the sanction—or rather the incantation—of an idea in order to be able to act. They want to command, manage, and conquer; but they must feel that in satisfying these passions and hungers they do not cater to the despised self but are engaged in the solemn ritual of making the word become flesh. Usually, such people are without the capacity to originate ideas. Their special talent lies rather in the deintellectualization of ideas—the turning of ideas into slogans and battle cries which beget action.

Σ

It is by their translation into mere words that ideas stir people and move them to action. The deintellectualization of ideas is the work of self-styled intellectuals who are impotent with pen and ink and hunger to write history with sword and blood.

Σ

Action is released by emotion, and emotion is stirred by words. What, then, is the role of thought in the release of action? For all we know, its role is as an instrument in the production of potent words.

Σ

Words have ruined more souls than any devil's agency. It is strange that the word, which is a chief ingredient of human uniqueness, should also be a chief instrument of dehumanization. The realm of magic is the realm of the invisible and the domain of the word.

Σ

Add a few drops of malice to a half truth and you have an absolute truth.

Σ

We often use strong language not to express a powerful emotion but to evoke it in us. It is not only other people's words that can rouse feeling in us. We can talk ourselves into a rage or an enthusiasm.

Σ

We lie loudest when we lie to ourselves.

Σ

Lack of self-awareness renders us transparent. A soul that knows itself is opaque; like Adam after he ate from the tree of knowledge, it uses words as fig leaves to cover its nakedness and shame.

Σ

One might equate growing up with a mistrust of words. A mature person trusts his eyes more than his ears. Irrationality often manifests itself in upholding the word against the evidence of the eyes.

Children, savages, and true believers remember far less what they have seen than what they have heard.

Σ

The uncompromising attitude is more indicative of an inner uncertainty than of deep conviction. The implacable stand is directed more against the doubt within than the assailant without.

Σ

To attach people to words is to detach them most effectively from life and possessions, and thus ready them for reckless acts of self-sacrifice. Men will fight and die for a word more readily than for anything else.

They are dangerous times when words are everything.

Σ

Those who proclaim the brotherhood of men fight every war as if it were a civil war.

Σ

Elitist intellectuals hug the conviction that talent and genius are rare exceptions. They are inhospitable to any suggestion that the mass of people are lumpy with unrealized potentialities. Yet there is evidence that the masses are a mine rich in all conceivable talents. We have as yet no expertise of talent mining but must wait for chance to wash nuggets out of hidden veins.

Σ

Elitists never tire of repeating that only the chosen few matter; the majority are pigs. Yet it does happen that a he pig marries a she pig and a Leonardo is born.

Σ

To perform well, elites need tending and nurturing. They need attention, and would rather be persecuted than ignored. With the masses it is the other way around—like weeds, they thrive best when left alone.

Σ

The ignorant are a reservoir of daring. It almost seems that those who have yet to discover the known are particularly equipped for dealing with the unknown. The unlearned have often rushed in where the learned feared to tread, and it is the credulous who are tempted to attempt the impossible. They know not whither they are going, and give chance a chance. Often in the past, the wise were unaware of the great mutations which were unfolding before their eyes. How many of the learned knew in the early decades of the nineteenth century that they had an industrial revolution on their hands? The discovery of America hardly touched the learned but inflamed the minds of common folk.

Σ

It would be difficult to exaggerate the degree to which anonymous examples triggered creative outbursts or were the seed of new styles in the fields of action, thought, and imagination. A minor versifier, a minor composer, a mediocre writer, painter, or teacher, an untalented tinkerer may be the seed of momentous developments in art, literature, technology, science, or politics. Many who have shaped history are buried in unmarked and unvisited graves.

It is a mark of a creative milieu that lesser people can become instruments for things greater than themselves.

1 THE ROLE OF

THE UNDESIRABLES

IN THE WINTER OF 1934, I spent several weeks in a federal transient camp in California. These camps were originally established
by Governor Rolph in the early days of the Depression to care for
the single homeless unemployed of the state. In 1934 the federal
government took charge of the camps for a time, and it was then
that I first heard of them.

How I happened to get into one of the camps is soon told. Like
thousands of migrant agricultural workers in California, I then
followed the crops from one part of the state to the other. Early in
1934 I arrived in the town of El Centro, in the Imperial Valley. I
had been given a free ride on a truck from San Diego, and it was
midnight when the truck driver dropped me on the outskirts of El
Centro. I spread my bedroll by the side of the road and went to
sleep. I had hardly dozed off when the rattle of a motorcycle
drilled itself into my head and a policeman was bending over me
saying, "Roll up, mister." It looked as though I was in for something; it happened now and then that the police got overzealous
and rounded up the freight trains. But this time the cop had no
such thought. He said, "Better go over to the federal shelter and
get yourself a bed and maybe some breakfast." He directed me to
the place.

I found a large hall, obviously a former garage, dimly lit and
packed with cots. A concert of heavy breathing shook the thick
air. In a small office near the door, I was registered by a middle-
aged clerk. He informed me that this was the "receiving shelter"

where I would get one night's lodging and breakfast. The meal was served in the camp nearby. Those who wished to stay on, he said, had to enroll in the camp. He then gave me three blankets and excused himself for not having a vacant cot. I spread the blankets on the cement floor and went to sleep.

I awoke with dawn amid a chorus of coughing, throat clearing, the sound of running water, and the intermittent flushing of toilets in the back of the hall. There were about fifty of us, of all colors and ages, all more or less ragged and soiled. The clerk handed out tickets for breakfast, and we filed out to the camp located several blocks away, near the railroad tracks.

From the outside, the camp looked like a cross between a factory and a prison. A high fence of wire enclosed it, and inside were three large sheds and a huge boiler topped by a pillar of black smoke. Men in blue shirts and dungarees were strolling across the sandy yard. A ship's bell in front of one of the buildings announced breakfast. The regular camp members—there was a long line of them—ate first. Then we filed in through the gate, handing our tickets to the guard.

It was a good, plentiful meal. After breakfast our crowd dispersed. I heard some say that the camps in the northern part of the state were better, that they were going to catch a northbound freight. I decided to try this camp in El Centro.

My motives in enrolling were not crystal clear. I wanted to clean up. There were shower baths in the camp and washtubs and plenty of soap. Of course I could have bathed and washed my clothes in one of the irrigation ditches, but here in the camp I had a chance to rest, get the wrinkles out of my belly, and clean up at leisure. In short, it was the easiest way out.

A brief interview at the camp office and a physical examination were all the formalities for enrollment. There were some two hundred men in the camp. They were the kind I had worked and traveled with for years. I even saw familiar faces—men I had worked with in orchards and fields. Yet my predominant feeling was one of strangeness. It was my first experience of life in intimate contact with a crowd. For it is one thing to work and travel with a gang, and quite another thing to eat, sleep, and spend the greater part of the day cheek by jowl with two hundred men.

I found myself speculating on a variety of subjects: the reason for their chronic bellyaching and beefing—it was more a ritual than the expression of a grievance; the amazing orderliness of the men; the comic seriousness with which they took their games of cards, checkers, and dominoes; the weird manner of reasoning one overheard now and then. Why, I kept wondering, were these men within the enclosure of a federal transient camp? Were they people temporarily hard up? Would jobs solve all their difficulties? Were we indeed like the people outside?

Up to then I was not aware of being one of a specific species of humanity. I had considered myself simply a human being—not particularly good or bad, and on the whole harmless. The people I worked and traveled with I knew as Americans and Mexicans, Whites and Negroes, Northerners and Southerners, and so on. It did occur to me that we were a group possessed of peculiar traits and that there was something—innate or acquired—in our make-up which made us adopt a particular mode of existence.

It was a slight thing that started me on a new track.

I got to talking to a mild-looking elderly fellow. I liked his soft speech and pleasant manner. We swapped trivial experiences. Then he suggested a game of checkers. As we started to arrange the pieces on the board I was startled by the sight of his crippled right hand. I had not noticed it before. Half of it was chopped off lengthwise, so that the horny stump with its three fingers looked like a hen's leg. I was mortified that I had not noticed the hand until he dangled it, so to speak, before my eyes. It was, perhaps, to bolster my shaken confidence in my powers of observation that I now began paying close attention to the hands of the people around me. The result was astounding. It seemed that every other man had been mangled in some way. There was a man with one arm. Some men limped. One young good-looking fellow had a wooden leg. It was as though the majority of the men had escaped the snapping teeth of a machine and left part of themselves behind.

It was, I knew, an exaggerated impression. But I began counting the cripples as the men lined up in the yard at mealtime. I found thirty (out of two hundred) crippled either in arms or legs. I immediately sensed where the counting would land me. The simile preceded the statistical deduction: we in the camp were a human junk pile.

I began evaluating my fellow tramps as human material, and for the first time in my life I became face-conscious. There were some good faces, particularly among the young. Several of the middle-aged and the old looked healthy and well-preserved. But the damaged and decayed faces were in the majority. I saw faces that were wrinkled, or bloated, or raw as the surface of a peeled plum. Some of the noses were purple and swollen, some broken, some pitted with enlarged pores. There were many toothless mouths (I counted seventy-eight). I noticed eyes that were blurred, faded, opaque, or bloodshot. I was struck by the fact that the old men, even the very old, showed their age mainly in the face. Their bodies were still slender and erect. One little man over sixty years of age looked a mere boy when seen from behind. The shriveled face joined to a boyish body made a startling sight.

My diffidence had now vanished. I was getting to know everybody in the camp. They were a friendly and talkative lot. Before many weeks I knew some essential fact about practically everyone.

And I was continually counting. Of the two hundred men in the camp there were approximately as follows:

Cripples	30
Confirmed drunkards	60
Old men (fifty-five and over)	50
Youths under twenty	10
Men with chronic diseases: heart, asthma, TB	12
Mildly insane men	4
Constitutionally lazy men	6
Fugitives from justice	4
Apparently normal	70

(The numbers tally up to more than two hundred, since some of the men were counted twice or even thrice—as cripples and old, or as old and confirmed drunks, etc.)

In other words, less than half the camp inmates (seventy normal, plus ten youths) were unemployed workers whose difficulties would be at an end once jobs were available. The rest (60 percent) had handicaps in addition to unemployment.

I also counted fifty war veterans and eighty skilled workers representing sixteen trades. All the men (including those with chronic diseases) were able to work. The one-armed man was a wizard with a shovel.

I did not attempt any definite measurement of character and intelligence. But it seemed to me that the intelligence of the men in the camp was certainly not below the average. And as for character, I found much forbearance and genuine good humor. I never came across one instance of real viciousness. Yet, on the whole, one would hardly say that these men were possessed of strong characters. Resistance, whether to one's appetites or to the ways of the world, is a chief factor in the shaping of character; and the average tramp is, more or less, a slave of his few appetites. He generally takes the easiest way out.

The connection between our makeup and our mode of existence as migrant workers presented itself now with some clarity. The majority of us were incapable of holding a steady job. We lacked self-discipline and the ability to endure monotonous, leaden hours. We were probably misfits from the very beginning. Our contact with a steady job was not unlike a collision. Some of us were maimed, some got frightened and ran away, and some took to drink. We inevitably drifted in the direction of least resistance—the open road. The life of a migrant worker is varied and demands only a minimum of self-discipline. We were now in one of the drainage ditches of ordered society. We could not keep a footing in the ranks of respectability and were washed into the slough of our present existence.

Yet, I mused, there must be in this world a task with an appeal so strong that were we to have a taste of it we would hold on and be rid for good of our present restlessness.

2

My stay in the camp lasted about four weeks. Then I found a haying job not far from town, and finally, in April, when the hot winds began blowing, I shouldered my bedroll and took the highway to San Bernardino.

It was the next morning, after I got a lift to Indio by truck, that a new idea began to take hold of me. The highway out of Indio led through waving date groves, fragrant grapefruit orchards, and lush alfalfa fields; then, abruptly, it passed into a desert of white sand. The sharp line between garden and desert was striking. The turning of white sand into garden seemed to me an act of magic. This, I thought, was a job one would jump at—even the men in the transient camps. They had the skill and the ability of the average American. But their energies, I felt, could be quickened only by a task that was spectacular, that had in it something of the miraculous. The pioneer task of making the desert flower would certainly fill the bill.

Tramps as pioneers? It seemed absurd. Every man and child in California knows that the pioneers were giants, men of boundless courage and indomitable spirit. However, as I strode on across the white sand I kept mulling over the idea.

Who were the pioneers? Who were the men who left their homes and went into the wilderness? A man rarely leaves a soft spot and goes deliberately in search of hardship and privation. People become attached to the places they live in; they sink roots. A change of habitat is a painful act of uprooting. A man who has made good and has a standing in his community stays put. The successful businessmen, farmers, and workers usually stayed where they were. Who then left for the wilderness and the unknown? Obviously those who had not made good: men who went broke or never amounted to much; men who though possessed of abilities were too impulsive to stand the daily grind; men who were slaves of their appetites—drunkards, gamblers, and women chasers; outcasts—fugitives from justice and ex-jailbirds. There were no doubt some who went in search of health—men suffering with TB, asthma, heart trouble. Finally, there was a sprinkling of young and middle-aged in search of adventure.

All these people craved change, some probably actuated by the naïve belief that a change in place brings with it a change in luck. Many wanted to go to a place where they were not known and there make a new beginning. Certainly they did not go out deliberately in search of hard work and suffering. If in the end they shouldered enormous tasks, endured unspeakable hardships, and accomplished the impossible, it was because they had to. They became men of action on the run. They acquired strength and skill in the inescapable struggle for existence. It was a question of do or die. And once they tasted the joy of achievement, they craved more.

Clearly the same types of people which now swelled the ranks of migratory workers and tramps had in former times made up the bulk of the pioneers. As a group the pioneers were probably as unlike the present-day "native sons"—their descendants—as one could well imagine. Indeed, were there to be today a new influx of typical pioneers, twin brothers of the forty-niners only in modern garb, the citizens of California would consider it a menace to health, wealth, and morals.

With few exceptions, this seems to be the case in the settlement of all new countries. Convicts were the vanguard in the settling of Australia. Exiles and convicts settled Siberia. In this country, a large portion of our earlier and later settlers were failures, fugitives, and felons. The exceptions seem to be those who were motivated by religious fervor, such as the Pilgrims and the Mormons.

Although quite logical, the train of thought seemed to me then a wonderful joke. In my exhilaration I was eating up the road in long strides, and I reached the oasis of Elim in what seemed almost no time. A passing empty truck picked me up just then, and we thundered through Banning and Beaumont, all the way to Riverside. From there I walked the seven miles to San Bernardino.

Somehow, this discovery of a family likeness between tramps and pioneers took a firm hold on my mind. For years afterward it kept intertwining itself with a mass of observations which on the face of them had no relation to either tramps or pioneers. And it moved me to speculate on subjects in which, up to then, I had had no real interest, and of which I knew very little.

I talked with several old-timers—one of them over eighty and a native son—in Sacramento, Placerville, Auburn, and Fresno. It was not easy, at first, to obtain the information I was after. I could not make my questions specific enough. "What kind of people were the early settlers and miners?" I asked. They were a hardworking, tough lot, I was told. They drank, fought, gambled, and wenched. They wallowed in luxury or lived on next to nothing with equal ease. They were the salt of the earth.

Still it was not clear what manner of people they were.

If I asked what they looked like, I was told of whiskers, broadbrimmed hats, high boots, shirts of many colors, suntanned faces, horny hands. Finally I asked, "What group of people in present-day California most closely resembles the pioneers?" The answer, usually after some hesitation, was invariably the same: "The Okies and the fruit tramps."

I tried also to evaluate the tramps as potential pioneers by watching them in action. I saw them fell timber, clear firebreaks, build rock walls, put up barracks, build dams and roads, handle steam shovels, bulldozer, tractors, and concrete mixers. I saw them put in a hard day's work after a night of steady drinking. They sweated and growled, but they did the work. I saw tramps elevated to positions of authority as foremen and superintendents, and in those cases I noticed a remarkable physical transformation: a seamed face gradually smoothed out, and the skin showed a healthy hue; an indifferent mouth became firm and expressive; dull eyes cleared and brightened; voices actually changed; there was even an apparent increase in stature. In almost no time these promoted tramps looked as if they had been on top all their lives. Yet sooner or later I would meet up with them again in a railroad yard, on some skid row, or in the fields—tramps again. It was usually the same story: they got drunk or lost their temper and were fired, or they got fed up with the steady job and quit. Usually, when a tramp becomes a foreman he is careful in his treatment of the tramps under him; he knows the day of reckoning is never far off.

In short, it was not difficult to visualize the tramps as pioneers. I reflected that if they were to find themselves in a single-handed life-and-death struggle with nature, they would undoubtedly display persistence. For the pressure of responsibility and the heat of battle steel a character. The inadaptable would perish, and those who survived would be the equal of the successful pioneers.

I also considered the few instances of pioneering engineered from above—that is to say, by settlers possessed of lavish means, who were classed with the best where they came from. In these instances, it seemed to me, the resulting social structure was inevitably precarious. For pioneering de luxe usually results in a plantation society, made up of large landowners and peon labor, either native or imported. Very often there is a racial cleavage between the two. The colonizing activities of the Teutonic barons in the Baltic, the Hungarian nobles in Transylvania, the English in Ireland, the planters in our South, the Spanish in Latin America, the

British and Dutch in their plantation colonies are cases in point. Whatever their merits, such societies are characterized by poor adaptability. They are likely eventually to be broken up either by a peon revolution or by an influx of typical pioneers—who are usually of the same race or nation as the landowners.

3

There is in us a tendency to judge a race, a nation, or an organization by its least worthy members. The tendency is manifestly perverse and unfair; yet it has some justification. For the quality and destiny of a nation are determined to a considerable extent by the nature and potentialities of its inferior elements. The inert mass of a nation is in its middle section. The industrious, decent, well-to-do, and satisfied middle classes—whether in cities or on the land—are worked upon and shaped by minorities at both extremes: the best and the worst.

The superior individual, whether in politics, business, industry, science, literature, or religion, undoubtedly plays a major role in the shaping of a nation. But so do the individuals at the other extreme: the poor, the outcasts, the misfits, and those who are in the grip of some overpowering passion. The importance of these inferior elements as formative factors lies in the readiness with which they are swayed in any direction. This peculiarity is due to their inclination to take risks ("not giving a damn") and their propensity for united action. They crave to merge their drab, wasted lives into something grand and complete. Thus they are the first and most fervent adherents of new religions, political upheavals, patriotic hysteria, gangs, and mass rushes to new lands.

And the quality of a nation—its innermost worth—is made manifest by its dregs as they rise to the top: by how brave they are, how humane, how orderly, how skilled, how generous, how independent or servile; by the bounds they will not transgress in their dealings with a man's soul, with truth, and with honor.

The average American of today bristles with indignation when he is told that this country was built, largely, by hordes of undesirables from Europe. Yet, far from being derogatory, this statement, if true, should be a cause for rejoicing, should fortify our pride in the stock from which we have sprung.

This vast continent with its towns, farms, factories, dams,

aqueducts, docks, railroads, highways, powerhouses, schools, and parks is the handiwork of common folk from the Old World, where for centuries men of their kind had been beasts of burden, the property of their masters—kings, nobles, and priests—and with no will and no aspirations of their own. When on rare occasions one of the lowly had reached the top in Europe he had kept the pattern intact and, if anything, tightened the screws. The stuffy little corporal from Corsica harnessed the lusty forces released by the French Revolution to a gilded state coach and could think of nothing grander than mixing his blood with that of the Hapsburg masters and establishing a new dynasty. In our day a bricklayer in Italy, a house painter in Germany, and a shoemaker's son in Russia have made themselves masters of their nations; and what they did was to re-establish and reinforce the old pattern.

Only here, in America, were the common folk of the Old World given a chance to show what they could do on their own, without a master to push and order them about. History contrived an earth-shaking joke when it lifted by the nape of the neck lowly peasants, shopkeepers, laborers, paupers, jailbirds, and drunks from the midst of Europe, dumped them on a vast virgin continent, and said, "Go to it; it is yours!"

And the lowly were not awed by the magnitude of the task. A hunger for action, pent up for centuries, found an outlet. They went to it with ax, pick, shovel, plow, and rifle; on foot, on horse, in wagons, and on flatboats. They went to it praying, howling, singing, brawling, drinking, and fighting. Make way for the people! This is how I read the statement that this country was built by hordes of undesirables from the Old World.

Small wonder that we in this country have a deeply ingrained faith in human regeneration. We believe that, given a chance, even the degraded and the apparently worthless are capable of constructive work and great deeds. It is a faith founded on experience, not on some idealistic theory. And no matter what some anthropologists, sociologists, and geneticists may tell us, we shall go on believing that man, unlike other forms of life, is not a captive of his past—of his heredity and habits—but is possessed of infinite plasticity, and his potentialities for good and for evil are never wholly exhausted.

2   THE PRACTICAL SENSE

Nowadays we take the practical attitude for granted. We seem to think that there is in most people an inborn inclination to make use of every device and circumstance to facilitate their work and further their ends. Yet it needs but a moment's reflection to realize that, so far from being natural, the practical sense has been throughout history a rare phenomenon. Its prevalence in our time is a peculiarity of the Occident, and here, too, it has asserted itself only during the last two hundred years.

There was a period of superb practicalness in the Near East during the Late Neolithic Age (4000–3000 B.C.). It saw the harnessing of oxen and asses; the invention of the plow, wheeled cart, sailboat, calendar, and script; the discovery of metallurgy, artificial irrigation, brickmaking, fermentation, and other fundamental techniques and devices. One has the impression that the coming of civilization about 3000 B.C. tapered off a brilliant practical era.

From their first appearance, civilizations almost everywhere were preoccupied with the spectacular, the fantastic, the sublime, the absurd, and the playful—with hardly a trickle of ingenuity seeping into the practical and useful. The prehistoric discoveries and inventions remained the basis of everyday life in most countries down to our time. Technologically, the Neolithic Age lasted even in Western Europe down to the end of the eighteenth century.

From *The Ordeal of Change.*

In Europe as late as the seventeenth century the view still prevailed that there was something preposterous and unseemly in using sublime knowledge for practical ends. We are told that when the inventor Salomon de Caus tried to interest Richelieu in the possibility of a jet engine, he was locked up as a madman in an asylum. People who came forward with practical plans for increasing output by the use of more powerful and efficient machines were considered queer. It was only in the late seventeenth and early eighteenth centuries that some sort of liaison began to be established between "sublime" knowledge and practical application. Fontenelle eulogized the military engineer Vauban for bringing down mathematics from the skies and attaching it "to various kinds of mundane utility." By the eve of the revolution, the French government was welcoming proposals for increasing output even when they were advanced by obvious cranks.

The rise of the practical sense in Europe was not only slow but uneven. Spurts of preoccupation with practical arts were followed by periods of stagnation or by a diversion of energies to other fields. During the High Middle Ages, in the wake of the Crusades, there was not only a marked expansion of commerce but also a striking increase in the use of waterwheels and windmills in manufacture; an increased proficiency in the mining, extraction, and working of metals; and an expansion of arable land by clearing of forests and draining of marshes. The Black Death (1349), which killed off a third of the population, and the Hundred Years' War, which drained the resources of England and France, brought to an end a period which had some of the earmarks of an industrial revolution. The revival came in the fifteenth century and had its center in Italy and Germany. It saw not only the introduction of printing and paper, and an unprecedented advance in the art of navigation, but a venturesomeness in all crafts and industries. This was a passionately creative age, and its practical activities consisted in more than mere adaptation of devices and practices from the Muslim world and the Far East. One has the feeling that its passionate pursuits—the voyages of discovery; the pursuit of beauty, excellence, power, and pleasure; the bent for religious and social reforms; the pursuit of the practical—were all aspects of one and the same drive. The fading faith in a beyond released a fervent groping and searching for a heaven on earth. The explorers were looking for the lost paradise; beauty, excellence, power, and pleasure are the ingredients of an earthly paradise; the reformers were out to recast earthly life into a perfect shape; and the practical inventors tried to make the world over by work.

The wars in Italy between Spain and France, and the savage religious wars in Germany, put a halt to this flourishing period. It was not until the end of the eighteenth century that the practical sense finally came into its own, and the modern Occidental took up where the late Neolithic craftsman left off.

2

There is some evidence that the rise of the practical sense is linked with a diffusion of individual freedom. It is the "breath of democracy," as Bergson calls it, which urges the spirit of invention onward and gives it the necessary scope. The impulse to make use of every resource and device to facilitate and expand the world's work is lodged in the individual who is more or less on his own and has to prove his worth by his own work. Where compact collective unity blurs the awareness of individual separateness, the present is seen as a mere link between past and future and the details of everyday life as too trivial to bother with. This was as true of the Middle Ages as it is of contemporary collectivist societies. On the other hand, to the individual on his own the present looms large, with everyday affairs the main content of life and every undertaking a test and a trial. He is eager to utilize everything within reach to advance his ends.

Wherever we find a quickening of the human spirit, we are perhaps justified in tracing it back to a situation in which the individual has been released, if but for a short time, from the dominance of the group—its observations, formulas, and ideas. The significant point is that where such a situation occurs, its earliest phase is as a rule marked by an alertness to practical affairs. In most cases, the practical phase is of relatively short duration; it is terminated either by stagnation or by a diversion of energies to other fields.

There are indications that the outburst of practical ingenuity in the Near East during the Late Neolithic period was a function of individual activity. In both Mesopotamia and Egypt the era was marked by a conflict of unknown origin that shattered village communities, clans, and tribes and filled the land with their debris. The cities which first took shape during this period, and which set the stage for the emergence of civilization, were probably to begin with places of refuge for the remnants of broken communal bodies. Such a conglomerate population was for a time without fixed traditions and customs, and during this fluid phase the individual had elbow room to follow his bents and exercise his initiative. Civilization, as it evolved round temple and royal household, was an effort to impose collective compactness on a heterogeneous multitude and herd it back into the communal corral.

We come upon a somewhat similar situation toward the end of the second millennium B.C. This was a time of tumult and trouble on the eastern coast of the Mediterranean. Invasions and migrations churned and heaved whole populations in Greece, Asia Minor, Syria, and even in the delta region of Egypt. Out of this turbulence eventually crystallized the city-states of Greece, the Ionian settlements in Asia Minor, the Philistine towns on the coast of Palestine, Greek and Etruscan settlements in Italy, and the Phoenician colonies in North Africa and Spain. The practical phase of this period saw the introduction and spread of the phonetic alphabet, the diffusion of the technique of iron smelting, and the invention of coined money.

A peculiar variant of the situation is to be found in the emergence of a Muslim civilization in the wake of the Arab conquest. Here we have a release of the individual by conversion—a conversion that was more convenient than heartfelt. Millions of people found themselves, almost overnight, stripped of age-old traditions and practices without as yet being encased by a new orthodoxy. For the talented individual in particular, the conversion to Islam was the opening of the door to opportunity. Almost all the outstanding personalities of the Muslim renaissance were non-Arabs. They were Persians, Turks, Jews, Greeks, Berbers, and Spaniards. The bearers of the new culture, known as "the people of the pen," were so notoriously impious that orthodox Muslims refused to break bread with them.[1]

---

[1] S. D. Goitein, *Jews and Arabs* (New York: Schocken Books, 1955), p. 104.

In its early phase, lasting two to three centuries, Muslim civilization displayed a remarkable ingenuity in putting to practical use theories and processes borrowed from near and far. Paper factories, sugar refineries, manufactories of textiles, leather, glazed tile, steel, and chemicals dotted the Muslim world from Spain to Central Asia. For the first time there was a systematic employment of the waterwheel and windmill. Artesian wells were bored in North Africa and other semiarid regions, and there was a development of vast irrigation projects. The magnetic compass, the astrolabe, and Indian arithmetic were put to practical use. All crafts flourished. Stagnation set in, with a hardening of orthodoxy, and finally disintegration in the wake of the Mongol incursion in the East and the Christian reconquest in Spain.

The impulse toward practical application given by the Crusades was also the product of the individual's release from constraints and ties. The sight of the sun-drenched world of the Near East with its fabulous cities, its exotic fashions in dress and food, and its flamboyant everyday life must have stirred the feeling in many of the crusaders that the present was not the vale of tears and place of exile the Church had made it out to be. The observation of a thriving Muslim civilization in action could not but give birth to the realization that Europe, too, had possibilities. Still, the mere contact with the Muslim world probably was not decisive. Byzantium and Spain had such a contact for centuries, yet it did not release in them an impulse toward experimentation and innovation. What counted more was the fact of movement—the pulling out of thousands of individuals from the familiar routing of a parochial world.

It would be difficult to exaggerate the role played by immigrants, exiles, and refugees in the awakening of the Western world. It is plausible, for instance, that if the Reformation was a crucial factor in the rise of the modern Occident, it was due less to the effect of its doctrines than to the fact that the religious persecutions it set in motion filled Western Europe with refugees and voluntary emigrants. The rise of the Netherlands to economic eminence in the sixteenth century was in no small degree due to the influx of exiles from Spain, Portugal, and France. Similarly, the foundations of England's industrial prowess were laid by exiles and emigrants—both Protestant and Catholic—from Spain, Portugal, France, and the Netherlands. America is a classic example of energy released by the influx of emigrants from the Old World and the ceaseless movement of population inside the continent.

3

The question is: why did not classical Greece, with its considerable individual differentiation and its appreciation of the present, canalize its intelligence and ingenuity into practical pursuits? Despite its breathtaking uniqueness, Greek civilization shared a contempt for practicalness with other civilizations. It believed that a preoccupation with practical affairs "renders the body, soul, and intellect of free persons unfit for the exercise of virtue."

The first answer to suggest itself is that what counts most in the rise of the practical sense is the extent of individualism. Where individualism is exclusive, as it was in Greece, the individual can prove his worth by leadership or by cultivating his talents rather than by work. The 30,000 autonomous individuals who set the tone in Athens did not have to spend their energies on the mechanics of everyday life because most of the work was done by some 200,000 slaves. On the other hand, in the modern Occident, where individualism is diffused in the mass, there is inevitably an intimate contact between the individual and the world's work, and he will use everything on earth and in heaven to advance his undertakings.

Still, this does not tell the whole story. The neglect of the practical in Greece was also due to the fact that it was a society in which the influence of the intellectual was paramount. There is considerable evidence of the intellectual's age-long hostility to the utilitarian point of view. The antagonism made itself felt at a very early stage in history—almost with the invention of writing. Writing was first developed in the Near East for a practical purpose: to facilitate accounting in storerooms and treasuries. The earliest examples we have of writing are inventories and tallies. Writing was one of the crafts attached to the temple and royal household, but from the very beginning the men who practiced the craft of writing were in a category by themselves. The scribe, unlike the potter, weaver, or carpenter, did not produce anything tangible and of unquestioned usefulness. Furthermore, the scribe was from the beginning an adjunct of management rather than a member of the labor force. Inevitably, this special position induced in the scribe attitudes and biases which could not but have a profound effect on the outlook of any society in which he played a paramount role. His lack of an unequivocal sense of usefulness set his face against practicalness and usefulness as tests of worth. His penchant for exclusiveness, too, reinforced his antipractical bias. Since the realm of the practical is probably the only one in which the common run of humanity has as much chance of attaining excellence as the educated, it was natural for the scribe to limit the proof of individual worth to fields inaccessible to the masses.

On the whole it seems to be true that where the equivalents of the intellectual constitute a dominant class, there is little likelihood of ingenuity's finding wide application in practical affairs. The inventiveness which now and then breaks through in such social orders is diverted into the fanciful, magical, and playful. Hero's steam engine was used to work tricks in temples and divert people at banquets. According to Plutarch, Archimedes considered the work of an engineer ignoble and vulgar and looked on his ingenious mechanical inventions as playthings. In Mandarin-dominated China the potent inventions of the magnetic compass, gunpowder, and printing hardly affected daily life. The compass was used to find a desirable orientation for graves, gunpowder was used to frighten off evil spirits, and printing was employed mainly to multiply amulets, playing cards, and paper money. The exceptional arithmetical achievements of the Brahmin intellectuals did not have the slightest effect on the management of practical affairs, nor did it occur to Buddhist intellectuals to use their ingenuity to lighten the burden of daily tasks. They invented the waterwheel not to mill grain but to grind out prayers. In the Occident, too, the elite of clerks during the Middle Ages, and the early humanists of the Renaissance, decried revolutionary innovations in the way of doing things. The humanists were hostile to the invention of printing and ignored the great geographical discoveries.

It is of interest that the intellectual's disdain of the practical seems to persist even when he is apparently up to his neck in purely practical affairs. In the Communist countries the dominant intelligentsia is preoccupied with the highly practical task of industrializing a vast expanse of the globe's surface. Yet despite their fervor for factories, mines, and powerhouses, they are permeated with a disdain for the practical aspects of these works. Their predilection is for the monumental, grandiose, spectacular, and miraculous. They have no interest in the merely useful, and it is not at all strange that they should have left the details of housing, food, clothing, and other components of everyday life in a relatively primitive state.

The exceptional prominence given to the practical in America stems partly from the fact that we have had here, for the first time in history, a civilization that operated its economy and government, and satisfied most of its cultural needs, without the aid of the typical intellectual. One wonders whether the fact of the country's current dependence for its defense and progress on pure science and the performance of scientific theoreticians might presage a lessening of the cult of the practical, whether here as in other things our world is coming full circle. In the seventeenth century, Vauban was eulogized for bringing mathematics down from the stars and applying it to mundane affairs. Perhaps now, with the orbiting of man-made stars, our intelligence and ingenuity are being diverted from practical affairs and directed back to the skies.

3 SCRIBE, WRITER, AND REBEL

It is often stated that the invention of writing about 3000 B.C. marked an epoch in man's career because it revolutionized the transmission of knowledge and ideas. Actually, as I have said, writing was invented not to write books but to keep books, and it was not until the first millenium B.C. that people began to write down their observations and thoughts. Nevertheless, the invention of writing had an immediate and fateful effect by giving rise to the class of the educated. Though the scribe started out as a craftsman, he found himself from the beginning associated not with the working force but with the supervisory personnel. In the tomb painting of Egypt, the scribe with his scroll and pen stands alongside the overseer with his whip—both facing the common folk who did the world's work. The career of a scribe became, therefore, an avenue by which common people could gain entrance into the privileged segment of society, and it inevitably drew unto itself talent and ambition which might have flowed into more practical crafts and occupations. Thus the invention of writing initiated a change in the direction of the flow of social energies, and such a change is a crucial event often characteristic of turning points in history.

2

Ever since the invention of writing, the educated minority has been a factor in social stability. Where the educated make

From *The Ordeal of Change*.

common cause with those in power, there is little likelihood of social unrest and upheaval, since only the educated can supply the catalyst of words that turns grievances into disaffection and revolt. On the other hand, a ruling class of vigor and merit may be swept away if it does not know how to win and hold the allegiance of the educated. With few exceptions, wherever we find a long-lived social organization there is either an absence of an educated class or a close alliance between the educated and the prevailing dispensation. This was true of Sumer with its scribes, Egypt with its literati, India with its Brahmins, China with its mandarins, Judaism with its rabbis and scholars, the Roman Empire with its Roman and Greek intellectuals, Byzantium with its kritoi and sekretoi, and the Catholic Church with its clerks. The Chinese sage Mo Ti said of the ruling classes of Chi and Chu that "they lost their empire and their lives because they would not employ their scholars." Stalin the Terrible echoed this truth when he said, "No ruling class can endure without its intelligentsia."

If society is to win and hold the allegiance of the educated, they must be given a chance to live purposeful and prestigious lives; and almost all long-lived social bodies solved the problem by absorbing the educated into bureaucratic hierarchies. Since he is not an actual producer, the scribe needs a clearly marked status to certify his worth, some connection with the world's work to prove his usefulness, and some arrangement of automatic promotion to give him a sense of growth. All these needs are ideally fulfilled by the status and function of a civil servant. Ensconced in his bureaucratic niche, the scribe looked at his world and saw that it was good. He had no grievances and dreamed no dreams.

3

At what point did the scribe make his appearance as a writer?

For centuries after the invention of writing the scribe exercised his craft solely in matters connected with his employment as a civil servant. He kept records, took dictation, copied documents and religious texts. Literature was the domain of bards and storytellers who no more thought of writing down their stock-in-trade than any other craftsmen would the secrets of their craft.

When we note the approximate dates at which literature made

its first appearance in several of the ancient civilizations we detect a certain regularity. In Egypt, the earliest examples of literary writing are from the later part of the third millennium B.C., the period of confusion which marked the breakdown of the Old Kingdom—the first catastrophic crisis since the birth of civilization. In Sumer, the oldest literary records are from the early part of the second millennium B.C., after the fall of the Third Dynasty of Ur—"the most glorious age of Sumer." Sir Leonard Woolley remarks on the strangeness of the fact "that the great days of the Third Dynasty of Ur have left virtually no trace of any lterary record." It is only when the great age was brought to an abrupt end by the invading Amorites and Elamites that we find a period of genuine literary activity. It was then (around 2000 B.C.) that "Sumerian scribes took it in hand to record the glories of the great days that had passed away."[1] In Greece, written literature begins after the fall of the highly bureaucratized social organization of the Mycenean age, and in Palestine after the breakdown of the centralized Solomonic kingdom. Finally, in China, literature begins in the sixth century B.C. during the chaotic period of "the contending states" which followed the dissolution of the Chou Empire.

The recurring connection between social debacle and the birth of literature might suggest that it needed the apocalyptic spectacle of a world coming to an end to release the creative flow in the scribe. Still, granting that he was deeply moved by the sight of an eternal order dissolving in violence and anarchy, it is quesionable whether it was the spectacle as such, however soul-stirring, that started the scribe writing. The dissolution of the social order had a personal significane for the scribe, more so than for any other segment of the population. The aristocracy and the priesthood weathered the social breakdown without experiencing a radical change in their standing. Indeed, in Egypt and China the breakdown of the empire resulted in the creation of numerous feudal states in which the power and prestige of the aristocracy and the priesthood were unimpaired or even enhanced. The masses, submerged in age-long subjection, continued as they were irrespective of a change of masters. Not so the scribe: he who had been so

[1] C. Leonard Woolley, The Sumerians (Oxford: The Clarendon Press, 1929), p. 178.

snugly in his bureaucratic berth, secure in his worth and usefulness, found himself suddenly abandoned and unemployed. We
hear an echo of the scribe's "private ail" in one of the earliest
examples of Egyptian literature, written by the treasury official
Ipuwer: "They pay taxes no more by reason of the unrest. . . . The
magistrates are hungry and suffer need. . . . The storehouse is bare
and he that kept it is stretched out on the ground. The splendid
judgment hall, its writings are taken away, the secret place is laid
bare . . . public offices are opened and their lists are taken away.
. . . Behold the officers of the land are driven out through the
land."[2]

Stripped of his official identity, the scribe not only reached out
for a new role as sage, prophet, and teacher, but had a desperate
need to shine again in the use of his skill with pen, stylus, or
brush. Thus Neferrohn, "a scribe with cunning fingers . . .
stretched out his hand to the box of writing materials and took
him a scroll and pen-and-ink case, and then he put in writing."
He wrote: "Up my heart that thou mayest bewail this land
whence thou are sprung. . . . Rest not! Behold, it lieth before your
face. . . . The whole land hath perished, there is naught left, and
the black of the nail surviveth not what should be there."[3] He
goes on lamenting and admonishing in the manner of his contemporary Ipuwer.

In Palestine and Greece the social debacle coincided with a
diffusion of literacy due to the introduction of the simplified alphabet. The increase in the number of literate persons at a time
when there were only meager opportunities for their adequate
employment added to the unrest. Amos, a shepherd, and Hesiod,
a farmer, mastered the art of writing and were gripped by the
impluse to instruct and admonish their fellow men.

In China, many of the hereditary scribe families sank into the
masses during the period of social disintegration, and carried the
art of writing with them. Confucius came from such a family.[4] It
is often the descendants of families that have come down in the

---

[2] Adolph Erman, *The Literature of the Ancient Egyptians* (London: Methuen &
Co., 1927), pp. 97–99.

[3] Ibid., p. 112.

[4] Liv Wu-chi, *Confucius, His Life and Time* (New York: Philosophical Library,
1955), p. 27.

world who act as a creative ferment. The memory of past splendor is like fire in their veins and it is likely to leak out in romancing, philosophizing, and prophesying.

So long as the scribe was kept busy as a civil servant, there was little likelihood that he would start writing. The creative impulse is often born of a thwarted desire for commanding action. It was the hankering for a busy, purposeful life which forced the energies of the disinherited scribe into creative channels.

4

It should be obvious that the circumstances which started the scribe writing could have equally turned him into a sheer rebel. The revolutionary, whatever be his cause or ideology, is often a man thwarted in his consuming passion for purposeful and imposing action. "Next to love," wrote Bakunin, "action is the highest form of happiness." He may spend most of his life talking and arguing, but once he gets his chance he reveals himself as a superb man of action.

In Palestine and China, the writer and the revolutionary appeared simultaneously and were often embodied in the same person. The prophets, as Renan suggested, were the first radical journalists, while in China the roving bands of unemployed clerks that were a feature of the period of "the contending states" cultivated both literature and subversion. It has been alleged that Confucius was "inciting the feudal lords against each other in the course of his wandering from one state to another, with the intention of somewhere coming into power himself."[5] The scribe ancestry of the revolutionary manifests itself in the fact that when he comes into power he creates a social pattern ideally suited to the aspirations and talents of the scribe—a regimented social order planned, managed, and supervised by a horde of clerks.

Still, despite their common ancestry, there is a fundamental difference between the writer's and the rebel's attitude toward the word. To the genuine writer the word is an end in itself and the center of his existence. He may dream of spectacular action and be lured to play an active role, but in the long run he does not

[5] Wolfram Eberhard, A *History of China* (Berkeley: University of California, 1950), p. 38.

feel at home in the whirl of a busy life. However imposing and successful his action, he feels in his innermost being that he is selling his birthright for a mess of pottage. It is only when the creative flow within him materializes in serried ranks of words that he feels at home in the world.

Not so the rebel: to him words remain a means to an end; and the end is action. His eyes remain fixed on the denied goal, and his energies keep pressing against the obstacle. He cannot derive a sense of fulfillment from the sheer manipulation of words and inevitably drifts toward the zone where words turn into action. Ideas have significance for him only as a prelude to action. Theorizing, philosophizing, and writing are a means for hurdling or exploding the obstacles on the road to action.

There is thus a certain antagonism between the writer and the revolutionary. In general it is probably true that by how much the writer is a revolutionary, by so much less is he a writer. At bottom it is perhaps a question of inner endowment: the genuine writer can write his rebellion while the revolutionary can only live it. In the rare instances where outstanding capacities for revolutionary activity and for creativeness are present in the same person, the two capacities do not manifest themselves simultaneously. In Milton, Trotsky, Koestler, Silone, and others, writing came to the fore in periods of enforced or voluntary inaction. Trotsky knew that "Periods of high tension and social passions leave little room for contemplation and reflection." He also recognized that to a true rebel writing is an anemic substitute for action. In his *Diary in Exile*, Trotsky says of Lassale that he would have gladly left unwritten what he knew if only he could have accomplished at least part of what he felt able to do, and he adds, "Any revolutionary would feel the same way."

5

Nothing is so unsettling to a social order as the presence of a mass of scribes without suitable employment and an acknowledged status. The spread of literacy in an illiterate society is, therefore, a critical process, and it has probably been an element in many turning points in history. Perhaps, in retrospect, the present convulsions in the underdeveloped countries will be seen mainly as the by-product of a sudden increase in the number of literate persons. One hears a lot about the revolt of the masses, but, aside from the rise of the United States, it would be difficult to point to a single historical development in which the masses were a prime mover and chief protagonist. Neither in the underdeveloped nor in the advanced countries are the masses restless, militant, and vainglorious. The explosive component in the contemporary scene is not the noise of the masses but the self-righteous claims of a multitude of graduates from schools and universities. This army of scribes clamors for a society in which planning, regulation, and supervision are paramount—and the prerogative of the educated. They hanker for the scribe's golden age, for a return to something like the scribe-dominated societies of ancient Egypt, China, and the Europe of the Middle Ages. There is little doubt that the trend in both new and renovated countries toward social regimentation stems partly from the need to create adequate employment for a large number of scribes. And since the tempo of the production of the literate is continually increasing, the prospect is of ever-swelling bureaucracies. Obviously, a high ratio between the supervisory and the productive force spells economic inefficiency. Yet where social stability is an overriding need, the economic waste involved in providing suitable positions for the educated might be an element of social efficiency.

It has been often stated that a social order is likely to be stable so long as it gives scope to talent. Actually, it is the ability to give scope to the untalented that is most vital in maintaining social stability. For not only are the untalented more numerous but, since they cannot transmute their grievances into a creative effort, their disaffection will be more pronounced and explosive. Thus the most troublesome problem which confronts social engineers is how to provide for the untalented and, what is equally important, how to provide against them. For there is a tendency in the untalented to divert their energies from their own development into the management, manipulation, and probably frustration of others. They want to police, instruct, guide, and meddle. In an adequate social order, the untalented should be able to acquire a sense of usefulness and of growth without interfering with the development of talent around them. This requires, first, an abundance of opportunities for purposeful action and self-advancement; and, secondly, a wide diffusion of technical and social skills so that people will be able to work and manage their affairs with a minimum of tutelage. The scribe mentality is best neutralized by canalizing energies into purposeful and useful pursuits and by raising the cultural level of the whole population so as to blur the dividing line between the educated and the uneducated. If such an arrangement lacks provisions for the encouragement of the talented, it yet has the merit of not interfering with them. We do not know enough to suit a social pattern to the realization of all the creative potentialities inherent in a population. But we do know that a scribe-dominated society is not optimal for the full unfolding of the creative mind.

4   THE TRADER

I<small>T</small> <small>SEEMS STRANGE</small> that we know so little of the history of the trader, for he preceded the cultivator and the herder, and he is probably more ancient than the hunter and the warrior. He and the artist are probably of equal antiquity; certainly he, like the artist, is uniquely human. There are animal hunters and warriors, and some ant species engage in activities reminiscent of cultivating and herding, but nowhere in the animal world is there anything remotely equivalent to the trader and the artist.

The trader was probably the first individual. He became an individual not by choice but by circumstances. He was either a straggler left behind or a fugitive or a sole survivor. Earliest trade was foreign trade— the trader was a foreigner—and it was trade in luxuries; trade in necessities was a late development. I can see the first trader, and outsider, approaching a strange human group, bearing a gift of something new and desirable, and then going on from group to group exchanging gifts.

2

Considering the trader's antiquity and the vital role he played in the evolution of civilization, it is difficult to understand the scorn and disdain he evoked in other human types, particularly in the warrior and the scribe. To the warrior who made history

Part of this essay is from the essay titled "The Trader" in *In Our Time;* the remainder was first published as the second half of the essay titled "The Practical Sense" in *The Ordeal of Change.*

and the scribe who recorded it, the trader was the embodiment of greed, dishonesty, cowardice, dishonor, mendacity, and corruption in general. Yet it was the trader who first gave weapons to the warrior and there is evidence that it was the trader who first conceived the idea of script. As we have seen, writing was invented to keep track of the income and outgo of wares. It originated not in houses of learning but in warehouses. Tags and marks of ownership preceded clay tablets and papyrus rolls.

Once writing came into the keeping of the scribe he set his face against any simplification and practical perfection of the art. For two millennia after its invention, writing remained a cumbersome, complex affair the mastery of which required a lifetime of application. Indeed, where the influence of the scribe remained unchallenged, as it was in Egypt, Mesopotamia, and China, there is evidence of a retrograde evolution: a tendency to overburden writing with all manner of artificial inflections. In short, the scribe was not interested in the elaboration of a practical script but in keeping writing a prerogative of the privileged few. He had a vested interest in complexity and difficulty. The simplification of writing by the introduction of the phonetic alphabet was the work of outsiders—the Phoenician traders.

It is often stated that it was the economic background of Mesopotamia and Egypt—payment of tribute to the temple, and the management of a vast irrigation system—which gave rise to the invention of writing. Actually, the economic background by itself does not seem enough. The empire of the Incas had no writing although its economic situation was not unlike that of Mesopotamia and Egypt. Where a preliterate society succeeds in perfecting an all-embracing bureaucratic system there is little likelihood that it will hit upon the idea of script. The preliterate equivalent of the scribe neither looks for nor welcomes practical devices such as writing and coinage, which would enormously simplify his task. He, too, has a vested interest in complexity and difficulty. What seems decisive for the appearance of writing is the presence of the free trader. We are told that "beyond local barter there was no trade in Inca times, since the movement and distribution of food and other commodities was controlled by the state."[1] By the same token we are justified in assuming the widespread presence of the

[1] G. H. S. Bushnell, *Peru* (New York: Praeger, 1957), p. 128.

free trader in Mesopotamia and the Delta region of Egypt during the Late Neolithic.

In scribe-dominated Egypt the free trader was as rare as in the Inca Empire. "We do not meet the word 'merchant' until the second millennium B.C., when it designates the official of a temple privileged to trade abroad." [2] Similarly in Mesopotamia the trade routes were for centuries the concern of the central government, and at all times the state had a tight control on trade. The Mesopotamian merchant, no matter how much he prospered, did not see himself as an independent agent and would not assert himself against the central power. In China, the free trader could assert himself only during the breakdown of the bureaucratic apparatus toward the end of the Chou dynasty.

We know less about the origins of the trader than we do about the origins of the scribe. But as we watch the present goings on inside the Communist world, the realization is forced upon us that trading is a form of self-assertion congenial to common people—a sort of subversive activity; undoctrinaire, unheroic, and uncoordinated, yet ceaselessly undermining and frustrating totalitarian domination. The trader probably did not initiate the downfall of the ancient totalitarian systems, but he was quick to lodge himself in any cracks which appeared in the monolithic walls, and did all he could to widen them. Thus despite his trivial motivation and questionable practices the trader has been a chief agent in the emergence of individual freedom and the canalization of ingenuity and energies into practical application.

It is true that where the trader feels himself supreme he may become as ruthless as any other ruling class. The institution of slavery which rotted the fiber of the ancient world was promoted and perpetuated by the trader as much as by king, priest, and scribe. It is also true that in the past commerce settled into a traditional stagnant routine over long periods of time. But on the whole, trade has been a catalyst of movement and change, and of government by persuasion rather than by coercion. The trader has neither the words nor the venom to transmute his grievances into an abso-

---

[2] Henri Frankfort, *The Birth of Civilization in the Near East* (New York: Doubleday Anchor Books, 1956), p. 118. See also J. E. Manchip White, *Ancient Egypt* (New York: Thomas Y. Crowell Co., 1955), p. 124: "Coined money did not appear in Egypt until the Persians introduced the silver shekel of Darius."

lute truth and impose it upon the world. In a trader-dominated society, the scribe is usually kept out of the management of affairs, but is given a more or less free hand in the cultural field. By frustrating the scribe's craving for commanding action, the trader draws upon himself the scribe's wrath and scorn, but unintentionally he also releases the scribe's creative powers. It was not a mere accident that the prophets, the Ionian philosophers, Confucius, and Buddha made their appearance in a period in which traders were conspicuous and often dominant. The same was of course true of the birth of the Renaissance, and of the growth of science, literature, and art in modern times.

In a scribe-dominated society, the trader is regulated and regimented off the face of the earth. When the scribe comes into power he derives a rare satisfaction from tearing tangible things out of the hands of practical people and harnessing these people to the task of achieving the impossible, and often killing them in the process.

The toleration of the scribe in a trader-dominated society means of course the toleration of an articulate opposition capable of giving voice to grievances, and breeding disaffection and revolt. Thus, until recently, the antagonism between trader and scribe has led to beneficent results—they cracked each other's monopoly. The trader cracked the scribe's monopoly of learning by introducing the simplified alphabet and printing, and by promoting popular education. On the other hand, the scribe has been in the forefront of every movement which set out to separate the trader from his wealth. In the process, both knowledge and riches leaked out to wider sections of the population.

5 THE INTELLECTUAL
AND THE MASSES

THE INTELLECTUAL as a champion of the masses is a relatively recent phenomenon. Education does not naturally waken in us a concern for the uneducated. The distinction conferred by education is more easily maintained by a sharp separation from those below than by a continued excellence of achievement. When Gandhi was asked by an American clergyman what worried him most, he replied, "The hardness of heart of the educated."

In almost every civilization we know of, the intellectuals have been either allied with those in power or members of a governing elite—and consequently indifferent to the fate of the masses. In ancient Egypt and imperial China the literati were magistrates, overseers, stewards, tax-gatherers, secretaries, and officials of every kind. They were in command and did not lift a finger to lighten the burden of the lower orders. In India the intellectuals were members of the uppermost caste of the Brahmins. Gautama Buddha, who preached love of service for others and the mixing of castes, was by birth not an intellectual but a warrior; and the attempt to translate Buddha's teaching into reality was made by another warrior—Emperor Asoka. The Brahmin intellectuals, far from rallying to the cause, led the opposition to Buddhism and finally drove it out of India. In classical Greece the intellectuals were at the top of the social ladder: philosophers and poets were also legislators, generals, and statesmen. This intellectual elite had

---

From *The Ordeal of Change.*

an ingrained contempt for the common people who did the world's work, regarding them as no better than slaves and unfit for citizenship. In the Roman Empire, the intellectuals, whether Greek or Roman, made common cause with the powers that be and kept their distance from the masses. In medieval Europe, too, the intellectual was a member of a privileged order—the Catholic Church—and did not manifest undue solicitude for the under-privileged.

In only one society prior to the emergence of the modern Occident do we find a group of "men of words" raising their voices in defense of the weak and oppressed. For many centuries, the small nation of the ancient Hebrews on the eastern shore of the Mediterranean did not differ markedly in its institutions and spiritual life from its neighbors. But in the eighth century B.C., owing to an obscure combination of circumstances, it began to develop a most strange deviation. Side by side with the traditional men of words—priests, counselors, soothsayers, scribes—there emerged a series of extraordinary men who pitted themselves against the ruling elite and the prevailing social order. These men, the prophets, were in many ways the prototype of the modern militant intellectual. Renan speaks of them as "open-air journalists" who recited their articles in the street and marketplace and at the city gate: "The first article of irreconcilable journalism was written by Amos about 800 B.C." Many of the characteristic attitudes of the modern intellectual—his tendency to see any group he identifies himself with as a chosen people and any truth he embraces as the one and only truth; the envisioning of a millennial society on earth—are clearly discerned in the prophets. The ideals, also, and the holy causes that the intellectuals preach and propagate today, were fully formulated during the three centuries in which the prophets were active.

We know too little about these remote centuries to explain the rise of the prophets. The temptation is great to look for circumstances not unlike those which attended the rise of the militant men of words in the modern Occident. One wonders whether a diffusion of literacy in the ninth century B.C. was not one of the factors. We have seen that it was at about this time that the Phoenicians perfected the alphabet, and considering the close relations which prevailed then between Phoenicians and Hebrews it would not be unreasonable to assume that the latter were quick to adopt it. Particularly during the reign of Solomon (960–925 B.C.), the intimate link with Phoenicia and the need for an army of scribes to run a centralized administration must have resulted in a sharp rise in the number of literate Hebrews. Such an increase in literacy was fraught with consequences for Hebrew society. In Phoenicia the new alphabet was primarily an instrument of commerce, and the sudden increase in the number of literate persons presented no problem, for they were rapidly absorbed in far-flung trade organizations. But the chiefly agricultural Hebrew society would have been swamped by a horde of unemployed scribes when the bureaucratic apparatus crumbled at Solomon's death. The new unattached scribes found themselves suspended between the privileged clique, whose monopoly on reading and writing they had broken, and the illiterate masses, to whom they were allied by birth. Since they had neither position nor adequate employment, it was natural that they should align themselves against established privilege and become self-appointed spokesmen of their inarticulate brethren. Such at least might have been the circumstances at the rise of the earliest prophets—of Amos the shepherd of Tekoa and his disciples. They set the pattern, and the road trodden by them was later followed by men from all walks of life, even by Isaiah the aristocrat.

The rise of the militant intellectual in the Occident was brought about not by a simplification of the art of writing but by the introduction of paper and printing. Undoubtedly the Church's monopoly of education was considerably weakened in the late Middle Ages. But it was the introduction of paper and printing that finished the job. The new men of words, like those of the eighth century B.C., were on the whole unattached—allied with neither church nor government. They had no clear status and no self-evident role of social usefulness. In the social orders evolved by the modern Occident, power and influence were, and to a large extent still are, in the hands of industrialists, businessmen, bankers, landowners, and soldiers. The intellectual feels himself on the outside. Even when he is widely acclaimed and highly rewarded, he does not feel himself part of the ruling elite. He finds himself almost superfluous in a civilization which is largely his handiwork. Small wonder that he tends to resent those in power as intruders and usurpers.

Thus the antagonism between men of words and men of action which first emerged as a historical motif among the Hebrews in the eighth century B.C., and made of them a peculiar people, reappeared in the sixteenth century in the life of the modern Occident and set it, too, apart from other civilizations. The unattached intellectual's unceasing search for a recognized status and a useful role has brought him to the forefront of every movement of change since the Reformation, not only in the West but wherever Western influence has penetrated. He has consistently sought a link with the underprivileged, be they bourgeois, peasants, proletarians, persecuted minorities, or the natives of colonial countries. So far, his most potent alliance has been with the masses.

2

The coming together of the intellectual and the masses has proved itself a formidable combination, and there is no doubt that it was largely instrumental in bringing about the unprecedented advancement of the masses in modern times. Yet, despite its achievements, the combination is not based on a real affinity.

The intellectual goes to the masses in search of weightiness and a role of leadership. Unlike the man of action, the man of words needs the sanction of ideals and the incantation of words in order to act forcefully. He wants to lead, command, and conquer, but he must feel that in satisfying these hungers he does not cater to a petty self. He needs justification, and he seeks it in the realization of a grandiose design and in the solemn ritual of making the word become flesh. Thus he does battle for the downtrodden and disinherited and for liberty, equality, justice, and truth, though, as Thoreau pointed out, the grievance which animates him is not mainly "his sympathy with his fellows in distress, but, though he be the holiest son of God, is his private ail." Once his "private ail" is righted, the intellectual's ardor for the underprivileged cools considerably. His cast of mind is essentially aristocratic. Like Heraclitus he is convinced that "ten thousand [of the masses] do not turn the scale against a single man of worth" and that "the many are mean; only the few are noble." He sees himself as a leader and master.[1] Not only does he doubt that the masses could do anything worthwhile on their own, but he would resent it if they made the attempt. The masses must obey. They need the shaping force of discipline in both war and peace. It is indeed doubtful that the typical intellectual would feel wholly at home in a society where the masses got their share of the fleshpots. Not only would there be little chance for leadership where people were almost without a grievance, but we might suspect that the cockiness and the airs of an affluent populace would offend his aristocratic sensibilities.

There is considerable evidence that when the militant intellectual succeeds in establishing a social order in which his craving for a superior status and social usefulness is fully satisfied, his view of the masses darkens, and from being their champion he becomes their detractor. The struggle initiated by the prophets in the eighth century B.C. ended, some three hundred years later, in the complete victory of the men of words. After the return from the Babylonian captivity, the scribes and the scholars were supreme and the Hebrew nation became "a people of the book." Once dominant, these scribes, like the Pharisees who succeeded them, flaunted their loathing for the masses. They made of the word for common folk, "am-ha-aretz," a term of derision and scorn—even the gentle Hillel taught that "no am-ha-aretz can be pious." Yet these scribes had an unassailable hold on the masses they despised. The noble carpenter from Galilee could make no headway when he challenged the pretension of the solemn scholars, hair-splitting lawyers, and arrogant pedants and raised his voice in defense of the poor in spirit. He was ostracized and anathematized, and his teachings found a following chiefly among non-Jews. Yet the teachings of Jesus fared no better than the teachings of the prophets when they came wholly into the keeping of dominant intellectuals. They were made into a vehicle for the maintenance and aggrandizement of a vast hierarchy of clerks, while the poor in spirit, instead of inheriting the earth, were left to sink into serfdom and superstitious darkness.

---

[1] In 1935 a group of students at Rangoon University banded themselves together into a revolutionary group and immediately added the prefix "Thakin" (master) to their names.

In the sixteenth century, we see the same pattern again. When Martin Luther first defied the Pope and his councils, he spoke feelingly of "the poor, simple, common folk." Later, when allied with the German princelings, he lashed out against the rebellious masses with unmatched ferocity: "Let there be no half-measures! Cut their throats! Transfix them! Leave no stone unturned! To kill a rebel is to destroy a mad dog." He assured his aristocratic patrons that "a prince can enter heaven by the shedding of blood more certainly than others by means of prayer."

It is the twentieth century, however, which has given us the most striking example of the discrepancy between the attitude of the intellectual while the struggle is on, and his role once the battle is won. Marxism started out as a movement for the salvation of both the masses and the intellectuals from the degradation and servitude of a capitalist social order. The *Communist Manifesto* condemned the bourgeoisie not only for pauperizing, dehumanizing, and enslaving the toiling masses but also for robbing the intellectual of his elevated status. "The bourgeoisie has stripped of its halo every occupation hitherto honored and looked up to with reverent awe." Though the movement was initiated by intellectuals and powered by their talents and hungers, it yet held up the proletariat as the chosen people—the only carrier of the revolutionary idea and the chief beneficiary of the revolution to come. The intellectuals, particularly those who had "raised themselves to the level of comprehending theoretically the historical movement as a whole," were to act as guides—a composite Moses—during the long wanderings in the desert. Like Moses, the intellectuals would have no more to do once the promised land was in sight. "The role of the intelligentsia," said Lenin, "is to make special leaders from among the intelligentsia unnecessary."

The Marxist movement has made giant strides in the twentieth century. It has created powerful political parties in many countries, and it is in possession of absolute power in the vast stretch of land between the Elbe and the China Sea. In Russia, China, and adjacent smaller countries, the revolution envisaged by Marxism has been consummated. What, then, is the condition of the masses and the intellectuals in these countries?

In no other social order, past or present, has the intellectual so completely come into his own as in the Communist regimes. Never before has his superior status been so self-evident and his social usefulness so unquestioned. The bureaucracy which manages and controls every field of activity is staffed by people who consider themselves intellectuals. Writers, poets, artists, scientists, professors, journalists, and others engaged in intellectual pursuits are accorded the high social status of superior civil servants. They are the aristocrats, the rich, the prominent, the indispensable, the pampered and petted. It is the wildest dream of the man of words come true.

And what of the masses in this intellectual's paradise? They have found in the intellectual the most formidable taskmaster in history. No other regime has treated the masses so callously as raw material, to be experimented on and manipulated at will, and never before have so many lives been wasted so recklessly in war and in peace. On top of all this, the Communist intelligentsia has been using force in a wholly novel manner. The traditional master uses force to exact obedience and lets it go at that. Not so the intellectual. Because of his professed faith in the power of words and the irresistibility of the truths which supposedly shape his course, he cannot be satisfied with mere obedience. He tries to obtain by force a response that is usually obtained by the most perfect persuasion, and he uses terror as a fearful instrument to extract faith and fervor from crushed souls.

3

One cannot escape the impression that the intellectual's most fundamental incompatibility is with the masses. He has managed to thrive in social orders dominated by kings, nobles, priests, and merchants but not in societies suffused with the tastes and values of the masses. The trespassing by the masses into the domain of culture and onto the stage of history is seen even by the best among the intellectuals as a calamity. Heine viewed with horror the mass society taking shape on the North American continent—"that monstrous prison of freedom where the invisible chains would oppress me even more than the visible ones at home, and where the most repulsive of tyrants, the populace, holds vulgar sway." Nietzsche feared that the invasion of the masses would turn history into a shallow swamp. The masses, said Karl Jaspers, exert "an immense gravitational pull which seems again and again to paralyze every upward sweep. The tremendous forces of the masses, with their attributes of mediocrity, suffocate whatever is not in line with them." To Emerson, the masses were "rude, lame, unmade, pernicious in their demands and influence, and need not to be flattered but to be schooled. I wish not to concede anything to them, but to tame, drill, divide and break them up, and draw individuals out of them. . . . If government knew how, I should like to see it check, not multiply, the population." Flaubert saw no hope in the masses: they "never come of age, and will always be at the bottom of the social scale." He thought it of little importance "that many peasants should be able to read and no longer heed their priests; but it is infinitely important that men like Renan and Littré should be able to live and be listened to."

Renan himself, so wise and humane, could not hold back his loathing for the masses. He thought that popular education, far from making the masses wiser, "only destroys their natural amiability, their instincts, their innate sound reason, and renders them positively unendurable." After the debacle of 1870, Renan spent several months in seclusion writing his *Philosophical Dialogues*, in which he vented his spleen not on the political and cultural elite which was responsible for France's defeat but on democracy and the masses. The principle that society exists for the well-being of the mass of people did not seem to him consistent with the plan of nature. "It is much to be feared that the last expression of democracy may be a social state with a degenerate populace having no other aim than to indulge in the ignoble appetites of the vulgar." The purpose of an ideal social order is less to produce enlightened masses than uncommon people. "If the ignorance of the masses is a necessary condition for this end, so much the worse for the masses." He was convinced that a high culture was hardly to be imagined without the full subordination of the masses, and he envisaged a world ruled by an elite of wise men possessed of absolute power and capable of striking terror into the hearts of the vulgar. This dictatorship of the wise would have hell at its command: "not a chimerical hell of whose existence there is no proof, but a veritable hell." It would institute a preventive terror not unlike that instituted by Stalin sixty years later, "with a view to frighten people and prevent their defending themselves," and it would "hardly hesitate to maintain in some lost district in Asia a nucleus of Bashkirs and Kalmuks, obedient machines, unencumbered by moral scruples and prepared for every sort of cruelty."

It is remarkable how closely the attitude of the intellectual toward the masses resembles the attitude of a colonial functionary toward the natives. The intellectual groaning under the dead weight of the inert masses reminds us of sahibs groaning under the white man's burden. Small wonder that when we observe a regime of intellectuals in action we have the feeling that here colonialism begins at home.

4

There is a remarkable statement made in 1958 by the director of industry and commerce in the Indian state of Andhra Pradesh. "It is harder," he said, "to provide the members of a community with shelter, clothing, and food than to launch an artificial satellite." The words sound odd in our ears, but they underline a now familiar paradox: the revolutionary governments which have sprung up in recent decades in all parts of the world see themselves as the embodiment of the popular will, yet they do not know how to make the masses work. They know how to generate popular enthusiasm and how to induce in the masses a readiness to fight, but they seem helpless in anything which requires an automatic readiness on the part of the masses to work day in, day out. On the other hand, the same governments do not find it hard to create conditions favorable for the performance of scientists, professors, top technicians, and intellectuals in general. They know how to foster the exceptional skills requisite for the manufacture of complex machinery and instruments, even the harnessing of the atom and the launching of satellites.

There is little likelihood that the intellectuals who constitute the leading element in these new governments would be receptive to the idea that, in the case of the masses, there is a connection between individual freedom and the readiness to work; that individual freedom is a potent factor in energizing and activating the masses. To an intelligentsia preoccupied with planning, managing, and guiding, no idea will seem so patently absurd as that the masses, if left wholly to themselves, would labor and strive of their own accord.

The interesting thing is that the energizing effect of freedom seems confined to the masses. There is no unequivocal evidence that the intellectual is at his creative best when left wholly on his own. It is not at all certain that individual freedom is a vital factor in the release of creative energies in literature, art, music, and science. Many of the outstanding achievements in these fields were not realized in an atmosphere of absolute freedom. Certainly in this country, cultural creativeness has not been proportionate to our degree of individual freedom. There is a chronic insecurity at the core of the creative person, and he needs a milieu that will nourish his confidence and sense of uniqueness. Discerning appreciation and a modicum of deference and acclaim are probably more vital for his creative flow than freedom to fend for himself. Thus a despotism that recognizes and subsidizes excellence might be more favorable for the performance of the intellectual than a free society that does not take him seriously. Coleridge protested that "the darkest despotisms on the continent have done more for the growth and elevation of the fine arts than the English government. A great musical composer in Germany and Italy is a great man in society and a real dignity and rank are conceded him. So it is with the sculptor or painter or architect. . . . In this country there is no general reverence for the fine arts." It is of course conceivable that a wholly free society might become imbued with a reverence for the fine arts; but up to now the indications have been that where common folk have room enough there is not much room for the dignity and rank of the typical writer, artist, and intellectual.

The paradox is, then, that although the intellectual has been in the forefront of the struggle for individual freedom, he can never feel wholly at home in a free society. He finds there neither an unquestioned sense of usefulness nor favorable conditions for the realization of his talents. Hence the contradiction between what the intellectual professes while he battles the status quo, and what he practices once he comes to power. At present, in every part of the world, we see how revolutionary movements initiated by idealistic intellectuals and preserved in their keeping tend to crystallize into hierarchical social orders in which an aristocratic intelligentsia commands and the masses are expected to obey. Such social orders, as we have seen, are ideal for the performance of the intellectual but not for that of the masses. It is this circumstance rather than the corruption of power which has been turning idealistic intellectuals into strident, ruthless slave drivers.

The masses, then, are not likely to perform well in a social order shaped and run by intellectuals. Some measure of coercion, even of enslavement, is apparently needed to keep the masses working in such a regime. However, with the coming of automation it may eventually be possible for a ruling intelligentsia to operate a country's economy without the aid of the masses, and it is legitimate to speculate on what the intellectual may be tempted to do with the masses once they become superfluous. In *The Possessed*, Dostoevski, with his apocalyptic premonition of things to come, puts the following words in the mouth of an intellectual by the name of Lyamshin: "For my part, if I didn't know what to do with nine tenths of mankind, I'd take them and blow them up into the air instead of putting them in paradise. I'd only leave a handful of educated people, who would live happily ever afterwards on scientific principles." Now, it is highly unlikely that even the most ruthless intelligentsia would follow Lyamshin's recommendation, though one has the feeling that Mao Tse-tung's apparent unconcern about a nuclear holocaust was perhaps bolstered by the wish to rid his system of millions of superfluous Chinese. There is no reason, however, why the doctrine should not be propounded eventually that the masses are a poisonous waste product which must be kept under a tight lid and set apart as a caste of untouchables. That such a doctrine would not be alien to the mentality of the Communist intellectual is evident from pronouncements made by Communist spokesmen in East Germany after the rising of 1953. They maintained that the rebels, though they looked and behaved like workers, were not the working class known by Marx but a decadent mixture of unregenerate remnants of eliminated classes and types. The real workers, they said, were now in positions of responsibility and power. Bertolt Brecht suggested in an ironical vein that since the Communist government had lost confidence in the people, the simple thing to do was to dissolve the people and elect another.

Actually, the intellectual's dependence on the masses is not confined to the economic field. It goes much deeper. He has a vital need for the flow of veneration and worship that can come only from a vast, formless, inarticulate multitude. After all, God himself could have gotten along without men, yet he created them, to be adored, worshiped, and beseeched by them. What elation could the intellectual derive from dominating an aggregation of quarrelsome, backbiting fellow intellectuals? It is, moreover, the faith of the masses which nourishes and invigorates his own faith. Hermann Rauschning quotes a Nazi intellectual: "If I am disheartened and despairing, if I am dead beat through the eternal party quarrels, and I go to a meeting and speak to these simple, goodhearted, honest people, then I am refreshed again; then all my doubts leave me."

5

To sum up: the intellectual's concern for the masses is as a rule a symptom of his uncertain status and his lack of an unquestionable sense of social usefulness. It is the activities of the chronically thwarted intellectual which make it possible for the masses to get their share of the good things of life. When the intellectual comes into his own, he becomes a pillar of stability and finds all kinds of lofty reasons for siding with the strong against the weak.

It is, then, in the interest of the masses that the struggle between the intellectual and the prevailing dispensation should remain undecided. But can we justify a continuing state of affairs in which the most gifted part of the population is ever denied its heart's desire, while the masses go on from strength to strength?

Actually, an antagonism between the intellectual and the powers that be serves a more vital purpose than the advancement of the masses: it keeps the social order from stagnating. For the evidence seems clear that a society in which the educated are closely allied with the governing class is capable of a brilliant beginning but not of continued growth and development. Such a society often attains heights of excellence early in its career and then stops. Its history is in the main a record of stagnation and decline. This was true of the civilizations in Egypt, Mesopotamia, and China and of the younger civilizations in India, Persia, the Greco-Roman world, Byzantium, and the world of Islam. We also see that the first step in the awakening of a stagnant society is the estrangement of the educated minority from the prevailing dispensation, which is usually effected by the penetration of some foreign influence. This change in the relations between the educated and the governing class has been a factor in almost every renascence, including that of Europe from the stagnation of the Middle Ages.

The creativeness of the intellectual is often a function of a thwarted craving for purposeful action and a privileged rank. It has its origin in the soul intensity generated in front of an insurmountable obstacle on the path to action. The genuine writer, artist, and even scientist are dissatisfied persons—as dissatisfied as the revolutionary—but are endowed with a capacity for transmuting their dissatisfaction into a creative impulse. A busy, purposeful life of action not only diverts energies from creative channels but above all reduces the potent irritation which releases the secretion of creativity.

There is also the remarkable fact that where the intellectuals are in full charge they do not usually create a milieu conducive to genuine creativeness. The reason for this is to be found in the role of the noncreative pseudo-intellectual in such a system. The genuinely creative person lacks, as a rule, the temperament requisite for the seizure, the exercise, and, above all, the retention of power. Hence, when the intellectuals come into their own, it is usually the pseudo-intellectual who rules the roost, and he is likely to imprint his mediocrity and meagerness on every phase of cultural activity. Moreover, his creative impotence brews in him a murderous hatred of intellectual brilliance and he may be tempted, as Stalin was, to enforce a crude leveling of all intellectual activity.

Thus it can be seen that the chronic thwarting of the intellectual's craving for power serves a higher purpose than the well-being of common folk. The advancement of the masses is a mere by-product of the uniquely human fact that discontent is at the root of the creative process: the most gifted members of the human species are at their creative best when they cannot have their way, and must compensate for what they miss by realizing and cultivating their capacities and talents.

6 THE READINESS

TO WORK

I HAPPENED TO ASK MYSELF a routine question, one day, and stumbled on a surprising answer. The question was: what is the uppermost problem which confronts the leadership in a Communist regime? The answer: how to make people work—how to induce them to plow, sow, harvest, build, manufacture, work in the mines, and so forth. It is the most vital problem which confronts them day in, day out, and it shapes not only their domestic policies but their relations with the outside world.

I was struck by the strangeness of it: that a movement which set out to achieve a miraculous transformation of man and society should have succeeded in transforming into a miracle something which to us seems entirely natural and matter-of-fact. In the Occident the chief problem is not how to induce people to work but how to find enough jobs for people who want to work. We take the readiness to work almost as much for granted as the readiness to breathe. Yet this attitude toward work, so far from being natural and normal, is strange and unprecedented. It was its relatively recent emergence which, as much as anything else, gave modern Western civilization its unique character and marked it off from its predecessors.

In practically all civilizations we know of, and in the Occident too for many centuries, work was viewed as a curse, a mark of bondage, or, at best, a necessary evil. That free men should be

---

From *The Ordeal of Change*.

willing to work day after day, even after their vital needs are satisfied, and that work should be seen as a mark of uprightness and worth, is not only unparalleled in history but remains more or less incomprehensible to many people.

The Occident's novel attitude toward work is traced by some to the rules of Saint Benedict (*circa* A.D. 530) which prescribed manual labor (six hours a day in winter and seven hours in summer) for every monk in the Benedictine monasteries. Hereby the contemptuous attitude of the classical world toward work, as fit only for slaves, was turned into reverence. The new attitude penetrated the towns which usually grew around the monasteries, and from there was diffused farther afield. Still, the fact remains that in the Middle Ages people did not show any marked inclination to labor more than was necessary to maintain a fairly low standard of living. It was only in the sixteenth century that we see emerging a strange addiction to work.

According to Max Weber and others, it was Luther's idea of the sacredness of man's calling, and particularly Calvin's doctrine of predestination, which infused a new seriousness into man's daily doings. Calvin believed that salvation and eternal damnation are predestined from the foundation of the world. No one can know whether he is of the few predestined to everlasting life or of the many foreordained to everlasting death. But since it is natural to assume that the chosen will succeed in whatever they undertake while the damned will fail, one is spurred to strive with all one's might for worldly success as proof of one's salvation. Erich Fromm complements this theory by pointing out that the unbearable uncertainty induced by this doctrine would by itself drive people to "frantic activity and a striving to do something."

Still, it is highly doubtful whether the tremendous dynamism displayed by the Occident during the past four hundred years was fueled mainly by religious elements or derivatives. The decisive factor in the development of modern Western civilization was not the psychological effect of some religious idea or doctrine but the mass emergence of the autonomous individual. And it is plausible that the Reformation itself was a by-product of the process of individualization.

We are not concerned here with the manner in which the individual was released from the compact corporate pattern of the

Middle Ages. A fortuitous combination of circumstances, not the least of which was the spread of literacy by the introduction of paper and printing, brought about a cracking and crumbling of the feudal economy and a loosening of the grip of an all-embracing Catholic Church. Whether he willed it or not, the Western European individual, toward the end of the fifteenth century, found himself more or less on his own.

Now the separation of the individual from a collective body, even when it is ardently striven for, is a painful experience. The newly emerging individual is an unstable and explosive entity. This is true of the young who cut loose from the family and venture forth on their own; of persons who break away or are separated from a compact tribe, clan, community, party, or clique; of discharged soldiers separated from the corporate life of an army; even of freed slaves removed from the intimate corporate life of slave quarters. An autonomous existence is heavily burdened and beset with fears and can be endured only when bolstered by confidence and self-esteem. The individual's most vital need is to prove his worth, and this usually means an insatiable hunger for action. For it is only the few who can acquire a sense of worth by developing and employing their capacities and talents. The majority prove their worth by keeping busy. A busy life is the nearest thing to a purposeful life. But whether the individual takes the path of self-realization or the easier one of self-justification by action, he remains unbalanced and restless. For he has to prove his worth anew each day. It does not require the uncertainties of an outlandish doctrine of predestination to drive him to "frantic activity and a striving to do something."

The burst of effort and creativeness we know as the Renaissance was in full swing before Luther and Calvin entered the field. It was the individualization of a once corporate society which manifested itself as an awakening and a renascence. The Reformation itself was a by-product of this individualization—a reaction against it. For there are many who find the burdens, the anxiety, and the isolation of an individual existence unbearable. This is particularly true when the opportunities for self-advancement are relatively meager, and one's individual interests and prospects do not seem worth living for. Such persons sooner or later turn their backs on an individual existence and strive to acquire a sense of worth and of purpose by an identification with a cause, a leader, or a movement. The faith and pride they derive from such an identification serve them as substitutes for the unattainable self-confidence and self-respect. The movement of the Reformation was to begin with such an escape from the burden of an autonomous existence.

Luther and Calvin did not come to liberate the individual from the control of an authoritarian church. "The Reformation," says Max Weber, "meant not the elimination of the church's control over everyday life, but rather the substitution of a new form of control for the previous one. It meant the repudiation of a control which was very lax, at that time barely perceptible in practice, and hardly more than formal, in favor of a regulation of the whole conduct which, penetrating to all departments of private and public life, was infinitely burdensome and earnestly enforced."[1] The rule of Calvinism as enforced in Geneva and elsewhere was inimical to individual autonomy not only in religious matters but in all departments of life. Had Luther and Calvin had at their disposal the fearful instruments of coercion of a Hitler or a Stalin, they would have perhaps herded back the emerging individual into the communal corral and would have stifled the new Occident at its birth. As it was, the European individual mastered the Reformation and used it for his own ends. He used faith to lubricate his machine of action and legitimize his success. He rushed headlong down the thousand new paths to action and fortune opened by the discovery of new continents and trade routes and the development of new sciences and techniques. He reached out to the four corners of the earth, carrying his restlessness with him and infecting the whole world with it.

To an outside observer, an individualist society seems in the grip of some strange obsession. Its ceaseless agitation strikes him as a kind of madness. And, indeed, action is basically a reaction against loss of balance. To dispose a soul to action we must upset its equilibrium. And if, as Napoleon wrote to Carnot, "the art of government is not to let men go stale," then it is essentially an art of unbalancing. This is particularly true in an industrialized society which requires a population disposed to continued exertion

[1] Max Weber, *The Protestant Ethic and the Spirit of Capitalism* (London: G. Allen & Unwin, 1930), pp. 36–37.

and alertness. The crucial difference between the Communist regimes and the individualist Occident is thus perhaps in the methods of unbalancing by which their masses are kept active and striving.

The Communists started out as miracle workers. Not only were they to bring about a miraculous transformation of man and society but the material tasks, too, which they set themselves—the industrialization and modernization of vast territories—were to partake of the miraculous. These tasks were to be realized by the energies released by a creed, and they were to demonstrate the validity and superiority of this creed. To proceed soberly, after a careful mobilization of skill, equipment, and material, would have been to act in the manner of men of little faith. One had to plunge headlong into one grandiose project after another, heedless of the waste and suffering involved. Faith, dedication, and self-sacrifice were to accomplish the impossible.

Much has been said by all manner of people in praise of enthusiasm. The important point is that enthusiasm is ephemeral and hence unserviceable for the long haul. One can hardly conceive of a more unhealthy and wasteful state of affairs than where faith and dedication are requisite for the performance of unmiraculous everyday activities. The attempt to keep people enthusiastic once they have ceased to believe can produce the most destructive consequences. An enormous effort has to be expended to maintain the revivalist spirit and, inevitably, with the passage of time, the fuels used to generate enthusiasm become more crude and poisonous. The Communists started out with faith and extravagant hope, then passed to pride and hatred, and finally settled on fear. The use of terror to evoke enthusiasm was one of Stalin's most pernicious inventions. For he did succeed in extracting strength from crushed souls.

The Communists did not withhold their hand from other modes of unbalancing. The transportation of vast populations from one end of the land to another, the shifting of peasants to towns and of townspeople to farms, the periodic purges, the sudden changes in the party line—such were some of the crude jolts by which they tried to keep the masses from going stale.

There is no doubt that the Communists can point to industrial achievements. But even while Stalin was alive, it must have dawned on some of the leaders that the techniques of generating enthusiasm, despite their impressive potentialities, cannot achieve the smooth effortlessness which is the outstanding characteristic of a genuine machine age. If in order to keep the wheels turning you have to deafen ears with propaganda, crack the whip of terror, and keep pushing people around, you haven't got a machine civilization no matter how numerous and ingenious your machines.

2

In an individualist society, the mode of unbalancing is far more subtle and requires relatively little prompting from without. For the autonomous individual constitutes a chronically unbalanced entity. The confidence and sense of worth which alone can keep him on an even keel are extremely perishable and must be generated anew each day. An achievement today is but a challenge for tomorrow. And since it is mainly by work that the majority of individuals prove their worth and regain their balance, they must keep at it continuously. Hence the ceaseless hustling of an individualist society.

No one will claim that the majority of people in an individualist society, be they workers or managers, find fulfillment in their work. But they do find in it a justification of their existence. The ability to do a day's work and get paid for it gives one a sense of usefulness and worth. The paycheck and the profitable balance sheet are certificates of value. Where the job requires exceptional skill or tests a person's capacities, there is an additional sense of exhilaration. But even a job of the sheerest routine yields the individual something besides the wherewithal of a living.

The significance of a job in the life of the individual in such societies is made particularly clear by the state of mind of the unemployed. There is little doubt that the frustration engendered by unemployment is due more to a corrosive sense of worthlessness than to economic hardship. Unemployment pay, however adequate, cannot mitigate it. In individualist societies it is inaction rather than actual hardship which breeds discontent and disaffection. In America even the legitimate retirement after a lifetime of work constitutes a fearsome crisis. In the longshoremen's union in San Francisco, the award of a $200-a-month pension to men over sixty-five who had twenty-five years of service on the waterfront brought in its wake a sudden rise in the rate of death among the retired. It is now recognized that men must be conditioned for retirement so as to endow them with a specific kind of endurance. Herbert Hoover on his eighty-second birthday echoed a widespread feeling when he said that a man who retires from work "shrivels up into a nuisance to all mankind."

The remarkable thing is that the addiction to work in an individualist society is by no means synonymous with a love of work. The workingman actually has the illusion that he can kill work and be done with it. He "attacks" every job he undertakes and feels the ending of a task as a victory. Those who know that work is eternal tend to take it easy.

The individualist society which manifests a marked readiness to work is one in which individualism is widely diffused. It is the individual in the mass who turns to work as a means of proving his worth and usefulness. Things are different where individualism is exclusive, as it was in Greece. The exclusive individual will tend to prove his worth and usefulness by managing and leading others or by developing and exercising his capacities and talents. Work, though it be hard and unceasing, is actually an easy solution of the problems which confront the autonomous individual, and it is not surprising that the individual in the mass should take this easy way out.

It hardly needs emphasizing that the individualist society we are talking about is not one in which every individual is unique, with judgments, tastes, and attitudes distinctly his own. All that one can claim for the individual in such a society is that he is more or less on his own; that he chooses his course through life, proves himself by his own efforts, and has to shoulder the responsibility for what he makes of himself. It is obvious, therefore, that it is individual freedom which generates the readiness to work. On the face of it, this is rather startling. It means that when the masses of people are free to work or not to work, they usually act as if they are driven to work. Freedom releases the energies of the masses not by exhilarating but by unbalancing, irritating, and goading. You do not go to a free society to find carefree people. When we leave people on their own, we are delivering them into the hands of a ruthless taskmaster from whose bondage there is no escape. The individual who has to justify his existence by his own efforts is in eternal bondage to himself.

3

    The vital question is of course whether the masses, energized and activated by freedom, can create anything worthwhile on their own. Though the masses have been with us from the beginning of time, we know little about their creative potentialities. In all the fifty centuries of history, the masses had apparently only one chance to show what they could do on their own, without masters to push them around, and it needed the discovery of a new world to give them that chance. In his *Last Essays*, Georges Bernanos remarks that the French Empire was not an achievement of the masses but of a small band of heroes. It is equally true that the masses did not make the British, German, Russian, Chinese, or Japanese empires. But the masses made America. They were the vanguard: they infiltrated, shoved, stole, fought, incorporated, founded, and raised the flag—

> And all the disavouched, hard-bitten pack
> Shipped overseas to steal a continent
> With neither shirts nor honor to their back.[2]

It is this fact which gives America its utter newness. All other civilizations we know of were shaped by exclusive minorities of kings, nobles, priests, and the equivalents of the intellectual. It was they who formulated the ideals, aspirations, and values, and it was they who set the tone. America is the only instance of a civilization shaped and colored by the tastes and values of common folk. No elite of whatever nature can feel truly at home in America. This is true not only of the aristocrat proper but also of the intellectual, the military leader, the business tycoon, and even the labor leader.

    The deprecators of America usually point to its defects as being those of a business civilization. Actually they are the defects of the mass: worship of success, the cult of the practical, the identification of quality with quantity, the addiction to sheer action, the

[2]Stephen Vincent Benét, *John Brown's Body* (New York: Doubleday, Doran & Co., 1928).

fascination with the trivial. We also know the virtues: a superb dynamism, an unprecedented diffusion of skills, a genius for organization and teamwork, a flexibility which makes possible an easy adjustment to the most drastic change, an ability to get things done with a minimum of tutelage and supervision, an unbounded capacity for fraternization.

So much for the defects and the virtues. What of the creative potentialities? My feeling has always been that the people I work and live with are lumpy with talents. We do not know enough of the nature of the creative process to maintain that a sense of uniqueness is crucial to the creative flow. Certainly, a wariness of people with a claim to uniqueness is not synonymous with an aversion to excellence. The men I know perfect and polish their way of doing things, whether in work or in play, the way the French of the seventeenth century polished their maxims and aphorisms. The realization of the creative potentialities of the masses hinges on the possibility of a diffusion of expertise in literature, art, music, and science comparable with the existing wide diffusion of expertise in mechanics and sports.

We know of at least one instance in the past where the masses entered the field of cultural creativeness not as mere onlookers but as participators. We are told that Florence at the time of the Renaissance had more artists than citizens. Where did these artists come from? They were for the most part the sons of shopkeepers, artisans, peasants, and petty officials. Giotto and Andrea del Castagno were sheepherding boys, Ghirlandajo was the son of a goldsmith, Andrea del Sarto the son of a tailor, Donatello the son of a wool carder. Most of the artists served their apprenticeship with artisans and craftsmen. The art honored in Florence was a trade, and artists were treated as artisans. They dressed like artisans in long tunics with leather belts, and cloaks that came halfway down the leg. When Veronese was asked about his profession, he answered, "I am a laborer" (*"Sono lavoratore"*). One can hardly imagine a Florentine painter of that time making the remark, attributed to Marcel Duchamp, that "when painting becomes so low that laymen talk about it, it doesn't interest me." Even the greatest of the Florentine painters and sculptors had an intimate contact with the world's work. They lacked the disdain for the practical that is characteristic of the artists of ancient Greece and of our time. Verrocchio, Alberti, and Leonardo da Vinci had a passionate interest in practical devices, machines, and gadgets. They were no more fastidious and no less "materialistic" than artisans and merchants.

The sixteenth-century historian Benedetto Varchi expressed his surprise that the Florentines who had been accustomed from childhood to carry heavy bales of wool and baskets of silk, and who spent all day and a large part of the night glued to their looms, should harbor so great a spirit and such high and noble thoughts. Everyone in Florence seemed to know something about the procedures and techniques of the arts and could judge whatever work was in progress. There was also a sort of spotting system. Just as in this country there is little chance that if a boy in a back lot throws a ball with speed and deftness the performance will go unnoticed, so in Florence there were discerning eyes watching the young for marks of talent. When a sheepherding boy picked up a piece of charcoal from the pavement and started to draw on the wall, there was someone who saw it and asked the boy whether he would like to draw and paint; and in this way Andrea del Castagno became a painter.

There is thus no evidence that cultural creativeness is incompatible with relatively gross bents, drives, and incentives. Though it may be questioned whether the lesson of Florence is applicable to a country of millions, it does suggest that the businesslike atmosphere of the workshop is more favorable for the awakening and unfolding of the creative talents of the masses than the precious atmosphere of artistic cliques. Should the increase in leisure due to the spread of automation make the participation of the masses in cultural creativeness an element of social health and stability, such participation would seem more feasible if we think of turning the masses into creative craftsmen rather than into artists and literati.

7   DULL WORK

THERE SEEMS TO BE a general assumption that brilliant people cannot stand routine; that they need a varied, exciting life in order to do their best. It is also assumed that dull people are particularly suited for dull work.

Actually, there is no evidence that people who achieve much crave for, let alone live, eventful lives. The opposite is nearer the truth. One thinks of Amos the sheepherder, Socrates the stonemason, Omar the tentmaker. Jesus probably had his first revelations while doing humdrum carpentry work. Einstein worked out his theory of relativity while serving as a clerk in a Swiss patent office. Machiavelli wrote *The Prince* and the *Discourses* while immersed in the dull life of a small country town where the only excitement he knew was playing cards with muleteers at the inn. Immanuel Kant's daily life was an unalterable routine. The housewives of Königsberg set their clocks when they saw him pass on his way to the university. He took the same walk each morning, rain or shine. The greatest distance Kant ever traveled was sixty miles from Königsberg.

An eventful life exhausts rather than stimulates. Cellini's exciting life kept him from becoming the great artist he could have been. It is legitimate to doubt whether Machiavelli would have written his great books had he been allowed to continue in the diplomatic service of Florence and had he gone on interesting

---

From *In Our Time*.

missions. It is usually the mediocre poets and writers who go in search of stimulating events to release their creative flow.

It may be true that work on the assembly line dulls the faculties and empties the mind, the only cure being fewer hours of work at higher pay. But during fifty years as a workingman, I have found dull routine compatible with an active mind. I can still savor the joy I used to derive from the fact that while doing dull, repetitive work on the waterfront, I could talk with my partners and compose sentences in the back of my mind, all at the same time. Chances are that had my work been of absorbing interest I could not have done any thinking and composing on the company's time, or even on my own time after returning from work.

People who find dull jobs unendurable are often dull people who do not know what to do with themselves when at leisure. Children and mature people thrive on dull routine, while the adolescent, who has lost the child's capacity for concentration and is without the inner resources of the mature, needs excitement and novelty to stave off boredom.

8   AUTOMATION, LEISURE,

     AND THE MASSES

THE SPECTACULAR PROGRESS of mechanization on the San Francisco waterfront at first filled me with foreboding. It seemed to me that in almost no time the people I had lived and worked with all my life would become unneeded and unwanted. It did not seem too farfetched to assume that in a matter of decades our cities would stand packed with masses of superfluous humanity.

Now at one point in history, God and the priests seemed to become superfluous, yet the world went on as before. Then again the aristocrats became superfluous, and hardly anyone noticed their exit. In Russia, where they have capitalism without capitalists, businessmen are superfluous, yet things get done somehow. But when the masses become superfluous it means that humanity is superfluous, and this is something that staggers the mind.

2

The thing that worried me about the prospective numbers of unemployed was not that they would starve. I assumed that the superfluous population would be given the wherewithal for a good living, even enough to buy things and go fishing. What worried me was the prospect of a skilled and highly competent labor force living off the fat of the land without a sense of usefulness and worth. There is nothing more explosive than a skilled population condemned to inaction. Such a group is likely to become a hotbed of extremism and intolerance and be receptive to any

From *The Temper of Our Time.*

proselytizing ideology, however absurd and vicious, which promises vast action. In pre-Hitlerian Germany a population that knew itself admirably equipped was rusting away in idleness and gave its allegiance to a Nazi party which offered unlimited opportunities for action.

Yet it is part of the fantastic quality of human nature that the thwarted desire for action which may generate extremism and intolerance may also release a flow of creative energies. Thucydides was a passionate general. He did not want to be a writer; he wanted to command men in battle. But after losing a battle he was exiled and had to eat his heart out watching other generals fight the war. So he composed *The Peloponnesian War*, one of the finest histories ever written. Machiavelli was a born schemer. His ardent desire was to pull strings, negotiate, intrigue, caucus, go on missions, and so on. But he lost his job as a minor diplomat and had to go back to his native village, where he spent his days gossiping and playing cards at the village inn. In the evening he returned to his house, took off his muddy clothes, put on a toga, and sat down to write *The Prince* and *Discourses on Livy*.

One more example. During the reign of Louis XIV the French aristocracy produced a crop of remarkable writers: de Retz, Hamilton, Saint-Simon, La Rochefoucauld. If you ask why it happened in France and not in other countries, the answer is again—unemployment. While the aristocracies of England, Spain, Italy, and Germany were managing affairs, amassing fortunes, fighting wars, and even making and unmaking kings, the French aristocrats were taken off their estates, pulled out of the army, and brought to Versailles, where all they could do was watch each other and be bored to death.

3

It goes without saying that in addition to a thwarted desire for action there must be talent and a degree of expertise if a creative flow is to be released. People who have nothing to say or have no idea how to say it when they do have something to say will not start writing no matter how optimal the conditions. La Rochefoucauld obviously had talent and, what is equally important, a taste for a good sentence. The reign of Louis XIV has been called "a despotism tempered by epigram," and La Rochefoucauld also had the salons in which expression was practiced as a fine art. We can, therefore, expect unemployment to release a creative flow in the masses of America only if we assume that the masses are not less endowed with genius than other segments of the population, and that it is possible to bring about a diffusion of expertise in literature, art, science, and so on comparable to the existing wide diffusion of expertise in mechanics and sports.

The cliché that talent is rare is not founded on fact. All that we know is that there are short periods in history when genius springs up all over the landscape, followed by long periods of mediocrity and inertness. In the small city of Athens within the space of fifty years there sprang up a whole crop of geniuses—Aeschylus, Sophocles, Euripides, Phidias, Pericles, Socrates, Thucydides, Aristophanes. These people did not come from heaven. Something similar happened in Florence at the time of the Renaissance, in the Netherlands between 1400 and 1700 during the great period of Dutch-Flemish painting, and in Elizabethan England. What we know with certainty is not that talent and genius are rare exceptions but that all through history talent and genius have gone to waste on a vast scale. Stalin liquidated the most intelligent, cultivated, and gifted segment of the Russian population and made of Russia a nation of lesser peasants, yet no one will maintain that Russia is at present unendowed with talent. I would not worry, therefore, whether the American masses have talents worth realizing.

The problem is that where the development of talent is concerned we are still in the food-gathering stage. We do not know how to grow it. Up to now in this country when one of the masses starts to write or paint it is because he happens to bump into the right accident. In my case the right accident happened in the 1930s. I had the habit of reading from childhood, but very little schooling. I spent half my adult life as a migratory worker and the other half as a longshoreman. The Hitler decade started me thinking, but there is an enormous distance between thinking and the act of writing. I had to acquire a taste for a good sentence—taste it the way a child tastes candy—before I stumbled into writing. Here is how it happened. Late in 1936 I was on my way to do some placer mining near Nevada City, and I had a hunch that I would get snowbound. I needed something to read, something that would last me for a long time. So I stopped over in San Francisco to get a thick book. I did not really care what the book was about—history, theology, mathematics, farming, anything—so long as it was thick, had small print, and no pictures. There was at that time a large secondhand bookstore on Market Street called Lieberman's, and I went there to buy my book. I soon found one. It had about a thousand pages of small print and no pictures. The price was one dollar. The title page said these were *The Essays of Michel de Montaigne*. I knew what essays were, but I did not know Montaigne from Adam. I put the book in my knapsack and caught the ferry to Sausalito.

Sure enough, I got snowbound. I read the book three times until I knew it almost by heart. When I got back to the San Joaquin Valley I could not open my mouth without quoting Montaigne, and the fellows liked it. It got so that whenever there was an argument about anything—women, money, animals, food, death—they would ask, "What does Montaigne say?" Out came the book and I would find the right passage. I am quite sure that even now there must be a number of migratory workers up and down the San Joaquin Valley still quoting Montaigne. I ought to add that the Montaigne edition I had was the John Florio translation. The spelling was modern, but the style seventeenth century—the style of the King James Bible and of Bacon's *Essays*. The sentences have hooks in them which stick in the mind; they make platitudes sound as if they were new. Montaigne was not above anyone's head. Once, in a workers' barrack near Stockton, the man in the next bunk picked up my Montaigne and read it for an hour or so. When he returned it he said, "Anyone can write a book like this."

4

The attempt to realize the potentialities of the masses may seem visionary and extravagant, yet it is eminently practical when judged by the criterion of social efficiency. For the efficiency of a society should be gauged not only by how effectively it utilizes its natural resources but by what it does with its human resources. Indeed, the utilization of natural resources can be deemed efficient only when it serves as a means for the realization of the intellectual, artistic, and manipulative capacities inherent in a population. It is evident, therefore, that if we are to awaken and cultivate the talents dormant in a whole population, we must change our conceptions of what is efficient, useful, practical, wasteful, and so on. Up to now in this country we are warned not to waste our time, but we are brought up to waste our lives.

Does this mean that we have to eliminate or radically change our present free-enterprise system? Not at all. On the contrary, the state of affairs we are striving for might actually give more leeway to the people who operate and benefit from the present system. For we shall free them from responsibility for the unneeded and unwanted millions who will remove themselves to a place where they can experiment with a new way of life. In other words, we recommend here two social systems coexisting side by side, not in competition and strife but in amity and mutuality, and with absolute freedom of movement from one to the other.

Usually, when we try to think of a substitute for our present system, the choices offer themselves singly or in combination: society as a church, society as an army, society as a factory, society as a prison, society as a school. For our purpose the choice must be the last named—society as a school. I am not unmindful of the fact that so far, except in science and philosophy, schools have not been a forcing house of talent. The best of our literature, painting, sculpture, music, and so on has not come out of schools. It is also true that as we look around us we find that the most oppressive and ruthless ruling classes in our present world have a large number of former schoolteachers. This is true of the Communist countries and of the new nations in Asia and Africa. But we shall have to take the risk and provide against tyranny by schoolmasters.

I would start with a pilot state made up of a slice of northern California and a slice of southern Oregon and run by the University of California. I would call it the state of the unemployed, and anyone crossing into it would automatically become a student. The state would be divided into a large number of small school districts, each district charged with the realization and cultivation of its natural and human resources. Production of the necessities of life would be wholly automated, since the main purpose of life would be for people to learn and grow. I said that the school districts would be small, for I am convinced that the unfolding of human capacities requires a social unit in which people of different interests, skills, and tastes know each other, commune daily with each other, emulate, antagonize, and spur each other. The absolute freedom of movement from one system to the other and from one district to the other will result in a continued sorting out of people, so that eventually each system and each district will be operated by its most ardent adherents.

I am convinced that the coexistence of two social systems in one country would enhance our sense of freedom. For freedom is predicated on the presence of alternatives in the economic, cultural, and political fields. Even in the absence of tyranny, freedom becomes meaningless where there is abject poverty, political inertness, and cultural sameness. And certainly no alternative can be as productive of a sense of freedom as the alternative of two different social systems.

Finally, it would be particularly fitting if the new states of the unemployed were to be created in parts of the country that have been depleted and ravaged—where forests have been destroyed, mines worked out, the soil exhausted. The simultaneous reclamation of natural and human resources would add zest and a higher congruity to the new societies.

To sum up: the business of a society with an automated economy can no longer be business. The choice will be between a learning society and no society at all, between a society preoccupied with the realization and cultivation of its human resources and a society in the grip of chaos.

5

The great fear which possessed me at the progress of automation made me do things I never dreamed of doing. After years of hardly ever sticking my nose outside the waterfront, I found myself running around, shooting my mouth off, telling people of a turning point ahead as fateful as any since the origin of society, and warning them that woe betides a society that reaches such a turning point and does not turn.

As the months went by, myths and legends came floating into my mind and dovetailed into a pattern. They were telling a coherent story—a version of automation. Here it is.

When God created the world he immediately automated it, and there was nothing left for him to do. So in his boredom he began to tinker and experiment. Man was a runaway experiment. It was in a mood of divine recklessness that God created man. "In the image of God created he him," and it was a foregone conclusion that a creature thus made would try to emulate and surpass his creator. And, indeed, no sooner was man created than God was filled with misgivings and suspicions. He could not take his eyes off his last and strangest creation. I can see Jehovah leaning over a bank of clouds contemplating the strange creature as it puttered about under the trees in the garden of Eden, wondering what was going on in the creature's head—what thoughts, what dreams, what plans, and what plots. The early chapters of Genesis make it plain that God was worried and took no chances. The moment man ate from the tree of knowledge, God had his worst fears confirmed. He drove man out of Eden and cursed him for good measure.

But you do not stop a conspirator from conspiring by exiling him. I can see Adam get up from the dust after he had been bounced out, shake his fist at the closed gates of Eden and the watching angels, and mutter, "I will return." Though condemned to wrestle with a cursed earth for his bread and fight off thistles and thorns, man resolved in the depths of his soul to become indeed a creator—to create a man-made world that would straddle and tame God's creation. Thus all through the millennia of man's existence the vying with God has been a leading motif of his strivings and efforts. Much of the time the motif is drowned by the counterpoint of everyday life, but it is clear and unmistakable in times of great venturesomeness. In the fabulous Late Neolithic period, "when men began to multiply on the face of the earth" and in a burst of creativeness invented the wheel, sail, plow, brickmaking, metallurgy, and other momentous devices, they also set out to build "a tower, whose top may reach unto heaven." They said they were building the tower for the glory of it, to "make us a name," but God knew better. "Behold," he said to his retinue of angels, "this they begin to do: and now nothing will be restrained from them, which they have imagined to do." So he confounded their language and scattered them abroad upon the face of the whole earth. It was only six thousand years later that the modern Occident picked up where the builders of the tower of Babel left off.

It was the machine age that really launched the man-made creation. The machine was man's way of breathing will and thought into inanimate matter. Unfortunately, the second creation did not quite come off. Unlike God, man could not immediately automate his man-made world. He was not inventive enough. Until yesterday, the machine remained a half-machine: it lacked the gears and filaments of will and thought, and man had to use his fellowmen as a stopgap for inventiveness. He had to yoke men, women, and children with iron and steam. The machine age became an echo of the fearful tale of the Bull of Phalaris, which tells of an Athenian artist who made a brazen bull for the King of Phalaris. The bull was so lifelike that the artist was seized with a desire to make the bull come alive and bellow like a real bull. Of course he was not inventive enough to do it, but he hit on the idea of using human beings as a stopgap. He constructed the throat of the bull so that when a human being was placed inside the belly and a fire lit underneath, the shrieks and groans of the victim as they came through the specially constructed throat sounded like the bellowing of a live bull. Even so, during the past 150 years millions of human beings were scooped off the land and shoveled into the bellies of smoke-belching factories to make the Bull of Phalaris roar. There was no escape for the mass of people from the ravenous maws of factories and mines. If they crossed the ocean and came to America, the factories and mines were there waiting to receive them.

Then yesterday, almost unnoticed, the automated machine edged onto the stage. It was born in the laboratories of technical schools where mathematicians and engineers were trying to duplicate the human brain. And it was brought into the factory not to cure the disease of work, which has tortured humanity for untold generations, but to eliminate man from the productive process.

Power is always charged with the impulse to eliminate human nature, the human variable, from the equation of action. Dictators do it by terror or by the inculcation of blind faith, the military do it by iron discipline, and the industrial masters think they can do it by automation. But the world has not fallen into the hands of commissars, generals, or the National Association of Manufacturers. Even in totalitarian countries the demands of common folk are determining factors in economic, social, and political decisions. There is, therefore, a chance that the denouement of automation might be what we want it to be.

I shall not forget the day mechanization made its entrance on the San Francisco waterfront. Discharging newsprint used to be one of the hardest jobs. The rolls, some of them eight feet high and weighing almost a ton, were landed horizontally on a platform, rolled onto long-handled metal trucks, and then hauled away. You had to watch your step, strain every muscle to balance the load, and be continually on the run. Now the rolls come out upright, two at a time, and land themselves. The clamp bridle releases the rolls automatically when they land. Then a special lift runs up, puts its padded arms gently around the two rolls, lifts them up like a feather, backs into the dock, and stacks the rolls two high when necessary. All that first day I watched the rolls come out. All I had to do was steady the rolls with a pat and change the gear now and then. I said to myself, "The skirmish with God has now moved all the way back to the gates of Eden. Jehovah and his angels with their flaming swords are holed up in their Eden fortress, and we with our automated machines are hammering at the gates. And right there, in the sight of Jehovah and his angels, we shall declare null and void the ukase that with the sweat of his face man shall eat bread."

Certainly, this mood was not shared by many of my fellow longshoremen. They displayed an instinctive wariness, as if wanting to make sure the thing wouldn't bite them—this despite the fact that a contract with the employers protects us against a loss of earnings and against layoffs. In less-protected industries the reaction is probably more poignant.

The fact is that the mad rush of the last hundred years has left us out of breath. We have had no time to swallow our spittle. We know that the automated machine is here to liberate us and show us the way back to Eden; that it will do for us what no revolution, no doctrine, no prayer, and no promise could do. But we do not know that we have arrived. We stand there panting, caked with sweat and dust, afraid to realize that the seventh day of the second creation is here, and the ultimate sabbath is spread out before us.

III

THE ORDEAL

OF CHANGE

THE BIRTH of the new constitutes a crisis, and its mastery calls for a crude and simple cast of mind—the mind of a fighter—in which the virtues of tribal cohesion and fierceness and infantile credulity and malleability are paramount. Thus every new beginning recapitulates in some degree man's first beginning.

Σ

Intense desire can be a habit, a fashion, or a tradition. It is then apparently unconnected with self-dissatisfaction. Nevertheless, it still retains the structure of its original derivation, and many of the attitudes that are induced by stirring up discontent may also be induced by stimulating sheer desire. The proclivity for change, the receptivity to faith, and the readiness for self-sacrifice are strong both in those who are at war with things as they are and those who merely desire "more." The fact is that those with the habit of intense desire are only tenuously attached to their lives and possessions. They are, whether they know it or not, the antithesis of the conservative.

Σ

There is radicalism in all getting, and conservatism in all keeping. Lovemaking is radical, while marriage is conservative. So, too, get-rich-quick capitalism is radical, while a capitalism intent solely on keeping what it already has is conservative. Radicalism itself ceases to be radical when absorbed mainly in preserving its control over a society or an economy.

Σ

A push-button civilization has no feeling for change by growth—the change that proceeds quietly, and by degrees scarcely to be perceived.

Σ

The craving to change the world is perhaps a reflection of the craving to change ourselves. The untenability of a situation does not by itself always give rise to a desire for change. Our quarrel with the world is an echo of the endless quarrel proceeding within us. The revolutionary agitator must first start a war in every soul before he can find recruits for his war with the world.

Σ

The oppressed and injured do have an advantage over the fortunate and the free. They need not grope for a purpose in life nor eat their hearts out over wasted opportunities. Grievance and extravagant hope are meat and drink to their souls, and there is a hero's garment to fit any size, and an imperishable alibi to justify individual failure.

It is doubtful whether the oppressed ever fight for freedom. They fight for pride and for power—power to oppress others.

Σ

Though the reformer is seen as a champion of change, he actually looks down on anything that can be changed. Only that which is corrupt and inferior must be subjected to the treatment of change. The reformer prides himself on the possession of an eternal unchangeable truth. It is his hostility toward things as they are which goads him to change them; he is, as it were, inflicting on them an indignity. Hence his passion for change is not infrequently a destructive passion.

Σ

It could be that human nature is stubbornly resistant to drastic change. Hence the fact that they who set their hearts on realizing revolutionary changes are as a rule hostile to human nature; they become antihuman, so to speak. They will do all they can to turn men into soulless material.

Σ

De Tocqueville in his researches into the state of society in France before the revolution of 1789 found that "a people which had supported the most crushing laws without complaint, and apparently as if they were unfelt, throws them off with violence as soon as the burden begins to be diminished." In other words, a popular uprising is less likely when oppression is crushing than when it is relaxed. He tried to explain this apparent contradiction by pointing out the connection between discontent and hope: "The evils which are endured with patience as long as they are inevitable, seem intolerable as soon as a hope can be entertained of escaping from them." Despair and misery are static factors. The dynamism of an uprising flows from hope and pride. Not actual suffering but the hope of better things incites people to revolt.

The remarkable thing is that though the connection between discontent and hope is often observed, it somehow fails to impress itself on the mind. This is probably due to a confusion of the two types of hope: the immediate and the distant. It is the around-the-corner brand of hope that prompts people to action, while the distant hope acts as an opiate. For—to quote Paul's Epistle to the Romans—"if we hope for what we see not, then do we with patience wait for it."

Σ

To the child, the savage, and the Wall Street operator everything seems possible—hence their credulity. The same is true of people who live in times of great uncertainty. Both fear and hope promote credulity. And it is perhaps true that those who want to create a state of mind receptive to fantastic and manifestly absurd tenets should preach hope and also create a feeling of insecurity.

Σ

If what we do and feel today is not in harmony with what we want to be tomorrow, the meeting with our hope at the end of the trail is likely to be embarrassing or even hostile. Thus it often happens that a man slays his hope even as he battles for it.

Σ

The unpredictability inherent in human affairs is due largely to the fact that the by-products of a human process are more fateful than the product.

Σ

Often, that which strikes us as the defeat of a hope is actually its fulfillment.

Σ

When a society sets out to purge itself of iniquities and shortcomings, it should expect the worst and gird itself for a crisis that will test its stability and stamina. A just society must strive with all its might to right wrongs, even if righting wrongs is a highly perilous undertaking. But if it is to survive, a just society must be strong and resolute enough to deal swiftly and relentlessly with those who would mistake its goodwill for weakness.

Σ

There is no doubt that a chief function of social authority is to impose predictable behavior, and it is self-evident that too much authority impairs human uniqueness. But when authority becomes ineffectual, we are likely to be dehumanized by the unpredictability induced by anarchy.

Σ

The danger inherent in reform is that the cure may be worse than the disease. Reform is an operation on the social body; but unlike medical surgeons, reformers are not on guard against unpredictable side effects which may divert the course of reform toward unwanted results. Moreover, quite often the social doctors become part of the disease.

Σ

It seems that when we concentrate for a time on something that is new and difficult, we acquire a sense of foreignness which we carry over as we shift to familiar fields. Thus it happens that those who set their minds on tackling the wholly new often end up by seeing the familiar as if it were new and difficult, and expend their energies in directing and regulating affairs which usually function automatically.

Σ

However much we talk of the inexorable laws governing the life of individuals and of societies, we remain at bottom convinced that in human affairs everything is more or less fortuitous. We do not even believe in the inevitability of our own death. Hence the difficulty of deciphering the present, of detecting the seeds of things to come as they germinate before our eyes. We are not attuned to seeing the inevitable.

Σ

In times of drastic change one has to ask children and the ignorant for news of the future. The saying in the Talmud that, after the destruction of the temple, prophecy was taken from the wise and given to children and fools reflects the disarray and perplexity of a time of trouble. When things become unhinged, wisdom and experience are a handicap in discerning the shape of things to come.

Σ

The central task of education is to implant a will and facility for learning; it should produce not learned but learning people. The truly human society is a learning society, where grandparents, parents, and children are students together.

In a time of drastic change it is the learners who inherit the future. The learned usually find themselves equipped to live in a world that no longer exists.

1 DRASTIC CHANGE

It is my impression that no one really likes the new. We are afraid of it. It is not only as Dostoevski put it that "taking a new step, uttering a new word is what people fear most." Even in slight things the experience of the new is rarely without some stirring of foreboding.

Back in 1936 I spent a good part of the year picking peas. I started out early in January in the Imperial Valley and drifted northward, picking peas as they ripened, until I picked the last peas of the season in June, around Tracy. Then I shifted all the way to Lake County, where for the first time I was going to pick string beans. And I still remember how hesitant I was that first morning as I was about to address myself to the string bean vines. Would I be able to pick string beans? Even the change from peas to string beans had in it elements of fear.

In the case of drastic change, the uneasiness is of course deeper and more lasting. We can never be really prepared for that which is wholly new. We have to adjust ourselves, and every radical adjustment is a crisis in self-esteem: we undergo a test, we have to prove ourselves. It needs inordinate self-confidence to face drastic change without inner trembling.

The simple fact that we can never be fit and ready for that which is wholly new has some peculiar results. It means that a population undergoing drastic change is a population of misfits,

---

From *The Ordeal of Change*.

and misfits live and breathe in an atmosphere of passion. There is a close connection between lack of confidence and the passionate state of mind, and, as we shall see, passionate intensity may serve as a substitute for confidence. The connection can be observed in all walks of life. A workingman sure of his skill goes leisurely about his job and accomplishes much, though he works as if at play. On the other hand, the workingman new to his trade attacks his work as if he were saving the world, and so he must if he is to get anything done at all. The same is true of the soldier. A well-trained soldier will fight well even when not stirred by strong feeling. His morale is good because his thorough training gives him a sense of confidence. But the untrained soldier will give a good account of himself only when animated by faith and enthusiasm. Cromwell used to say that common folk needed "the fear of God before them" to match the soldierly cavaliers. Faith, enthusiasm, and passionate intensity in general are substitutes for the self-confidence born of experience and the possession of skill. Where there is the necessary skill to move mountains, there is no need for the faith that moves mountains.

As I said, a population subjected to drastic change is a population of misfits—unbalanced, explosive, and hungry for action. Action is the most obvious way by which to gain confidence and prove our worth, and it is also a reaction against loss of balance—a swinging and flailing of the arms to regain one's balance. Thus drastic change is one of the agencies which release man's energies, but certain conditions have to be present if the shock of change is to turn people into effective men of action: there must be an abundance of opportunities, and there must be a tradition of self-reliance. Given these conditions, a population subjected to drastic change will plunge into an orgy of action.

The millions of immigrants dumped on our shores after the Civil War underwent a tremendous change, and it was a highly irritating and painful experience. Not only were they transferred, almost overnight, to a wholly foreign world, but they were, for the most part, torn from the warm communal existence of a small town or village somewhere in Europe and exposed to the cold and dismal isolation of an individual existence. They were misfits in every sense of the word, and ideal material for a revolutionary explosion. But they had a vast continent at their disposal, and fabulous opportunities for self-advancement, and an environment which held self-reliance and individual enterprise in high esteem. And so these immigrants from stagnant small towns and villages in Europe plunged into action. They tamed and mastered a continent in an incredibly short time, and we are still in the backwash of that mad pursuit.

Things are different when people subjected to drastic change find only meager opportunities for action or when they cannot, or are not allowed to, attain self-confidence and self-esteem by individual pursuits. In this case, the hunger for confidence, for worth, and for balance directs itself toward the attainment of substitutes. The substitute for self-confidence is faith, the substitute for self-esteem is pride, and the substitute for individual balance is fusion with others into a compact group.

It needs no underlining that this reaching out for substitutes means trouble. In the chemistry of the soul, a substitute is almost always explosive if for no other reason than that we can never have enough of it. We can never have enough of that which we really do not want. What we want is justified self-confidence and self-esteem. If we cannot have the originals, we can never have enough of the substitutes. We can be satisfied with moderate confidence in ourselves and with a moderately good opinion of ourselves, but the faith we have in a cause has to be extravagant and uncompromising, and the pride we derive from an identification with a nation, race, leader, or party is extreme and overbearing. The fact that a substitute can never become an organic part of ourselves makes our holding on to it passionate and intolerant.

To sum up: when a population undergoing drastic change is without abundant opportunities for individual action and self-advancement, it develops a hunger for faith, pride, and unity. It becomes receptive to all manner of proselytizing and is eager to throw itself into collective undertakings which aim at "showing the world." In other words, drastic change, under certain conditions, creates a proclivity for fanatical attitudes, united action, and spectacular manifestations of flouting and defiance; it creates an atmosphere of revolution. We are usually told that revolutions are set in motion to realize radical changes. Actually, it is drastic change which sets the stage for revolution. The revolutionary mood and temper are generated by the irritations, difficulties, hungers, and frustrations inherent in the realization of drastic change.

Where things have not changed at all, there is the least likelihood of revolution.

2   IMITATION AND FANATICISM

At present, the modernization of a backward country is still largely a process of Westernization—the transplantation of practices, methods, and attitudes indigenous to Western Europe and America. This means that rapid modernization is above all a process of imitation, and it is legitimate to wonder whether there may not be something in the nature of imitation which renders rapid modernization so explosive and convulsive.

Contrary to what one would expect, it is easier for the advanced to imitate the backward than the other way around. The backward and the weak see in imitation an act of submission and a proof of their inadequacy. They must rid themselves of their sense of inferiority, must demonstrate their powers, before they will open their minds and hearts to all that the world can teach them. Most often in history it was the conquerors who learned willingly from the conquered. The backward, says De Tocqueville, "will go forth in arms to gain knowledge but will not receive it when it comes to them." Thus the grotesque truculence, posturing, conceit, brazenness, and defiance which usually assail our senses whenever a backward country sets out to modernize itself in a hurry stem partly from the desperate need of the weak for an illusion of strength and superiority if they are to imitate rapidly and easily.

Most immediate and decisive in communism's appeal to

From *The Ordeal of Change*.

emerging nations avid for modernization is the Communists' proven ability to ready a backward society for victory on the battlefield. Though it remains doubtful whether a Communist regime can instill in the masses an enduring readiness to work, there is no doubt that it knows how to mold a backward population into an effective army and instill it with a fanatical will to fight. The Western democracies, try as they may, cannot generate pride, enthusiasm, and a spirit of self-sacrifice in a population poignantly conscious of its backwardness and inferiority. Christianity and democracy did not take root in Asia and Africa because they did not come as instruments for the conversion of the weak into conquerors.[1] Nationalism and industrialization, two other gifts of the West, can serve such a purpose and have found a ready acceptance. It is significant that when the Jesuits first came to China to save souls they were asked by the Emperor to cast cannon and were made masters of ordnance.

Seen as a process of imitation, it becomes understandable why the Westernization of a backward country so often breeds a violent antagonism toward the West. People who become like us do not necessarily love us. The sense of inferiority inherent in the act of imitation breeds resentment. The impulse of the imitators is to overcome the model they imitate—to surpass it, leave it behind, or, better still, eliminate it completely. Now and then in history the last was done first: the imitators began by destroying the model and then proceeded to imitate it. We are apparently most at ease when we imitate a defeated or dead model.

It is of course to be expected that imitation will be relatively free of resentment when it is possible for the imitators to identify themselves wholeheartedly with their model. It is the great misfortune of our time that in the present surge of Westernization so many factors combine to keep the awakening countries from identifying themselves with the West they imitate. The fresh memory of colonialism, the color line, the difference in historical experience, the enormous gap in living standards, the fear of the educated minority in the backward countries that democracy and

[1] Islam came as such an agency, and its spread has been phenomenal in both Asia and Africa. Even at this moment it is still winning converts in the heart of Africa. One cannot help thinking that were the Muslim missionary to combine his religious preaching with technical know-how—link Islamization with industrialization—the spread of Islam might again become phenomenal.

free enterprise would rob them of their birthright to direct, plan, and supervise—all these combine to create an attitude of suspicion and antagonism toward the West.

Less obvious is the fact that imitation is least impeded when we are made to feel that our act of imitation is actually an act of becoming the opposite of that which we imitate. A religion or civilization is most readily transmitted to alien societies by its heretical offspring, which come into being as a protest and a challenge. Heresies have often served as vehicles for the transmission of ideas, attitudes, and ways of life. India influenced the Far East by a heresy it rejected (Buddhism), and Judaism impressed itself upon the world by a heresy it rejected (Christianity). Christianity itself, after it became the official religion of the Roman Empire, spread outside the core of the Greco-Roman world mainly by its heresies. The Nestorians were Semites, the Jacobites Egyptians, and the Donatists Berbers. And if communism seems likely to become a vehicle for the transmission of Western achievement to non-Western countries, it is partly due to the fact that communism is a Western, and particularly a capitalist, heresy which the West rejected.

Since I have called communism a capitalist heresy, it may not be out of place to consider here briefly the nature and genesis of heresies. A heresy can spring only from a system that is in full vigor. There is hardly an instance of a declining system giving birth to a heresy and being supplanted by it. At the birth of Christianity the militant spirit of Judaism was at a white heat, and Christianity was one of several Jewish heresies. Christianity itself was bursting with heresies during its youthful growth, and later during its militant ascendancy in the West. A time of great religious fervor is optimal not only for the rise of saints and martyrs but also for the pullulation of schisms and heresies. Where there is static orthodoxy or sheer indifference there is the least likelihood of fervent deviations and mutations. It is a measure of capitalism's vigor that it could produce so forceful a heresy. To call communism a Christian heresy, as Toynbee and others have done, is to shut one's eye to the present state of Christianity and misread the true nature of communism.

As I said, a heresy is a by-product of exuberance and ebullience. It is by exaggerating, overfulfilling, and reaching out for extremes that a heresy breaks away from the parent body. There is apparently no surer way of turning a thing into its opposite than by exaggerating it. Joseph Klausner said of Jesus that "by overfilling Judaism he caused his disciples to make of it non-Judaism"; and it is by "overfilling" capitalism that the Communists make of it non-capitalism. Ever since capitalism came into its own, we have caught glimpses of the capitalists' dream of omnipotence. It is a dream of total noninterference—of a "company state" rather than a company within a state. Some capitalists tried to realize this dream in distant colonies where they were unrestrained by the mores and traditions of their homeland. But only a Communist regime succeeds in making the wildest capitalist dream come true right in the home country. A monolithic company—the Communist party—takes possession of a whole nation. It not only owns every acre of land, every building and factory, but has absolute dominion over the bodies and souls of every man, woman, and child. The aim of this super-capitalist company is to turn the captive population into skilled mechanics and to shape their souls that they will toil from sunup to sundown, thankful to be alive and blessing their exploiters. It is only natural that such a "company state" should aspire to turn itself into a holding company of the whole planet.

Even when a Communist regime is wholly free of Stalinist viciousness it can still be seen as an attempt to overfulfill capitalism. In a capitalist system the productive process is hampered by the trivial motivation of the owner, the recalcitrance of the worker, and the capriciousness of the consumer. It needs a prodigious expenditure of energy and substance to counteract the vitiating effect of these factors. Communism, with one sweep, rids capitalism of the anarchic owner, worker, and consumer. It makes of production an uncompromising deity which brooks no interference from any quarter.

Finally, communism is repeating a pattern followed by other heresies when it strives to separate capitalism from the capitalists. The Christian heresy detached Judaism from the Jews, and the Protestant heresy separated Catholicism from the Catholic hierarchy. And remembering the battle cry of the Kronstadt uprising, it is permissible to predict that the slogan of an eventual Communist heresy will be "Communism without Communists."

2

An awareness that rapid modernization is essentially a process of imitation helps us not only to make sense of the turmoil in the backward countries but also to gauge the durability of all that is being achieved there. When we see how wholly different the social and political conditions are in the underdeveloped countries from what they were in Europe and America at the birth of the machine age, it is natural to wonder whether the transplantation of Western achievements to these countries is likely to be viable. However, when we keep in mind that what we are observing is an act of concerted imitation, the view changes completely. Conditions which are optimal for origination are not necessarily optimal for imitation. Origination requires a more or less loose social order in which the individual has leeway to tinker, follow his hunches, and run risks on his own. On the other hand, rapid imitation is facilitated by social compactness, regimentation, and concerted action. The individual who is a member of a compact group is more imitative than the individual who is on his own. The unified individual is without a distinct self, and, like the child, his mind is without guards against the intrusion of influences from without. The paradox is then that rapid modernization requires a primitivization of the social structure. The collectivist bias of the backward countries thus may be an aid rather than a hindrance in their race to catch up with the West.

3   A TIME OF JUVENILES

THERE WAS A WEEK some years ago during which the newspapers reported an epidemic of student riots spreading from Istanbul to Teheran, Bombay, Saigon, Seoul, Tokyo, and Mexico City. Most of the riots had an anti-American flavor. And I remember how, early one morning, while waiting for the bus that would take me to the waterfront, I saw the headline announcing still another riot and heard myself snorting with disgust, "History made by juvenile delinquents!"

The sound of my words had a peculiar effect on me. Inside the bus I did not look at the newspaper but sat staring in front of me. Who makes history? Is it the old? How much of a role do the young play in shaping events? Things were coming together in my mind. I remembered that years ago I had inserted in *The Passionate State of Mind* an aphorism which read, "History is made by men who have the restlessness, impressionability, credulity, capacity for make-believe, ruthlessness, and self-righteousness of children. It is made by men who set their hearts on toys. All leaders strive to turn their followers into children." This insight, which came to me from observing two willful godchildren in action, had been filed away in my mind and had not affected my thinking. Now it seemed to me that we can hardly know how things happened in history unless we keep in mind that much of the time it was juveniles who made them happen.

From *The Temper of Our Time*.

Until relatively recent times, man's span of life was short. Throughout most of history the truly old were a rarity. In an excavation of one of the world's oldest cemeteries, the skeletons showed that the average age of the population at death was twenty-five, and there is no reason to suppose that the place was unusually unhealthy. Thus it seems plausible that the momentous discoveries and inventions of the Neolithic Age—the domestication of animals and plants; the invention of the wheel, sail, and plow; the discovery of irrigation, fermentation, and metallurgy—were the work of an almost childlike population. Nor is it likely that the ancient myths and legends, with their fairy-tale pattern and erotic symbolism, were elaborated by burnt-out old men.

The history of less ancient periods, too, reveals the juvenile character of their chief actors. Many observers have remarked on the smallness of the armor which has come down to us from the Middle Ages. Actually, the men who wore this armor were not grown-ups. They were married at thirteen, were warriors and leaders in their teens, and senile at thirty-five or forty. The Black Prince was sixteen when he won fame in the battle of Crécy, and Joan of Arc seventeen when she took Orléans from the English. Without some familiarity with the juvenile mentality and the aberrations of juvenile delinquency, it would be difficult to make sense of the romanticism, trickery, and savagery which characterized the Middle Ages. The middle-aged were out of place in the Middle Ages; troubadours and chroniclers gave them no pity and no mercy. Nor did things change markedly in the sixteenth century. Montaigne tells us that he hardly ever met a man as old as fifty. Salvador de Madariaga says of Spain's great age (1550–1650) that in those days "boys of fifteen were men; men of forty were old men." He adds that when the dramatists of that age designated a man as old they meant a man of about forty—yellow-skinned, wrinkle-faced, and toothless. In the first half of the sixteenth century, Charles the Fifth became emperor at the age of twenty, Francis the First became king of France at twenty-one, and Henry the Eighth king of England at eighteen.

The question is whether the juvenile mentality is confined to adolescents. Do people automatically grow up as they grow older? Is not juvenility a state of mind rather than a matter of years? Are there not teenagers of every age? In 1503, Cardinal Giuliano della

Rovere was elected pope at the age of sixty. He took the name of Julius the Second in honor of Julius Caesar, whom he esteemed as the greatest man who ever lived and whose career he determined to emulate. So on the threshold of old age he put on a helmet and cuirass, mounted a horse, and set out to become a conqueror. Clearly, the juvenile mentality may persist or re-emerge in later life, even in old age.

In all times there are people who cannot grow up, and there are times when whole societies begin to think and act like juveniles. The twentieth century in particular has seen juvenilization on an almost global scale.

Arthur Koestler suggests that there is in the revolutionary "some defective quality" which keeps him from growing up. The indications are, however, that the trend toward juvenile behavior has been gathering force for over a century and has affected people who cannot be classed as revolutionaries. Such behavior was rampant on the frontier and in the gold-rush camps, and the American go-getter, though he has no quarrel with the status quo, is as much a perpetual juvenile as any revolutionary. Militant nationalism, too, though not primarily revolutionary in character, fosters juvenile manifestations in all sorts of people. Laurens Van der Post calls nationalism "the juvenile delinquency of the contemporary world." Clearly, the juvenile pattern is not confined to people with "some defective quality" which keeps them from growing up, but may arise or be induced in all types.

To understand the process of juvenilization, we must know something about the genesis of the juvenile mentality in the adolescent. We shall not get anywhere by looking for differences in the brain structure or the nervous system between adolescent and adult. I know of no demonstrable differences. The reasonable approach is to assume that the adolescent's behavior is induced largely by his mode of existence, by the situation in which he finds himself. This would imply that adults, too, when placed in a similar situation would behave more or less like juveniles.

Now, the chief peculiarity of the adolescent's existence is its in-betweenness: it is a phase of transition from childhood to adulthood, a phase of uprootedness and drastic change. If our assumption is correct, other types of drastic change should evoke a somewhat similar psychological pattern. There should be a family likeness between adolescents and people who migrate from one country to another, or are converted from one faith to another, or pass from one way of life to another—as when peasants are turned into industrial workers, serfs into free men, civilians into soldiers, and people in underdeveloped countries are subjected to rapid modernization. One should also expect active people— whether workingmen, farmers, businessmen, or generals—who retire abruptly to display proclivities and attitudes reminiscent of juveniles.

2

Let us have a close look at the experience of change. After the Second World War, backward countries in Asia and Africa began to modernize themselves in an atmosphere charged with passion and a deafening clamor. As a naïve American I asked myself why the sober, practical task of modernization—of building factories, roads, dams, schools, and so forth—should require the staging of a madhouse. In *The Ordeal of Change* I tried to find answers to this question. My central idea was that drastic change is a profoundly upsetting experience, that when we face the new and unprecedented our past experience and accomplishments are a hindrance rather than an aid. What Montaigne said of death is also true of the wholly new: "We are all apprentices when we come to it." We are all misfits when we have to fit ourselves to a new situation.

Now the fact is that the staging of a madhouse in the process of modernization is not peculiar to people in Asia and Africa. Long before the present awakening of backward countries, we had been living in an apocalyptic madhouse staged on a global scale by Germany, Russia, and Japan, which set out to modernize themselves at breakneck speed. Moreover, the mass movements, upheavals, and wars which are a by-product of change indicate that there is more to the experience of change than a state of unfitness, that the process involves the deeper layers of man's soul. After all, change such as the world has seen during the past hundred and fifty years is something wholly unprecedented and unique in mankind's experience. From the beginning of recorded history down to the end of the eighteenth century, the way of life of the average man living in the civilized centers of the earth had remained substantially unchanged. The technology developed during the Late Neolithic Age lasted almost unchanged down to the Industrial Revolution.

It would be legitimate, therefore, to assume that there is in man's nature a built-in resistance to change. It is not only that we are afraid of the new, but that deep within us there is the conviction that we cannot really change, that we cannot adapt ourselves to the new and remain our old selves, that only by getting out of our skin and assuming a new identity can we become part of the new. In other words, drastic change creates an estrangement from the self and generates a need for a new birth and a new identity. And it perhaps depends on the way this need is satisfied whether the process of change runs smoothly or is attended with convulsions and explosions.

It is of interest to have a quick look at the means employed by changeless primitive societies to tackle the one critical change no society can avoid: the change from childhood to manhood. In the Congo, boys at the age of fifteen are declared dead, taken into the forest, and there subjected to purification, flagellation, and intoxication with palm wine resulting in anesthesia. The priest-magician (nġanga) who is in charge teaches them a special language and gives them special food. Finally come the rites of reintegration, in which the novices "pretend not to know how to walk or eat and, in general, act as if they were newly born and must relearn all the gestures of ordinary life."[1] In several Australian tribes the boy is taken violently from his mother, who weeps for him. He is subjected to physical and mental weakening to simulate death and is finally resurrected and taught to live as a man.

The interest of these rites is in their motif of rebirth rather than in any bearing they may have on change in a civilized society. In the modern world change overtakes a whole population, and the denouement is not a return to an immemorial way of life. Here the sense of rebirth and a new identity is created by mass movements, mass migrations, or by a plunge into the perpetual becoming of sheer action and hustling. One becomes a member of a glorious Germany, a glorious Japan, a nation of heroic warriors

[1] Arnold van Gennep, *The Rites of Passage* (Chicago: Phoenix Books, University of Chicago Press, 1960), p. 81.

destined to conquer the world; or one joins a revolutionary or religious movement which envisages a new life and sees oneself as one of the elect marching in the van of mankind; or one actually emigrates to a new country and becomes a new man. Thus a time of drastic change is likely to become a time of wild dreams, extravagant fairy tales, gigantic masquerades, preposterous pretensions, marching multitudes with banners waving and drums beating, messiahs bringing glad tidings, and mass migrations to promised lands.

The tale of Moses and the Exodus is a luminous example of the difficulties encountered, and the outlandish means that have to be employed, in the realization of drastic change. Moses wanted to accomplish a relatively simple thing: he wanted to transform the enslaved Hebrews into free men. But, being a genuine leader, Moses knew that the task of endowing liberated slaves with a new identity and immersing them in a new life was not at all simple and required the employment of extravagant means. The Exodus from Egypt was the first step. But more vital was the idea of a chosen people led by a mighty Jehovah to a promised land—the kind of milieu essential for a drastic human transformation.

Now, the human transformation which took place during the last hundred years was not the turning of slaves into free men but drastic changes brought about by the Industrial Revolution; yet here, too, the sense of rebirth and a new life was generated by exoduses (mass migrations), the fiction of a chosen people (nationalism), and the vision of a promised land (revolutionary movements). It is fascinating to see how in Europe during the second half of the nineteenth century the wholesale transformation of peasants into industrial workers gave rise not only to nationalist and revolutionary movements, bringing the promise of a new life, but also to mass rushes to the New World, particularly the United States, where the European peasant was literally processed into a new man—made to learn a new language and adopt a new mode of dress, a new diet, and often a new name. One has the impression that emigration to a foreign country was more effective in adjusting the European peasant to a new life than migration to the industrial cities of his native country. Internal migration cannot impart a sense of rebirth and a new identity. Even now, the turning of Italian and Spanish peasants into industrial workers is probably realized more smoothly by emigration to Germany and France than by transference to Milan and Barcelona. So, too, the Negro who comes to New York from the West Indies adjusts himself more readily and smoothly to the new life than the Negro who comes from the South.

3

The juvenile, then, is the archetypal man in transition. When people of whatever age group and condition are subjected to drastic change, they recapitulate to some degree the adolescent's passage from childhood to manhood. Even the old when they undergo the abrupt change of retirement may display juvenile impulses, inclinations, and attitudes. This is particularly true in this country, where leisure is not an accepted component of the active life. Thus retired shopkeepers and farmers have made southern California a breeding ground of juvenile cults, utopias, and wild schemes. The John Birch Society with its unmistakable flavor of juvenile delinquency was initiated by a retired candy maker and is sustained by retired business executives, generals, and admirals.

The significant point is that juvenilization inevitably results in some degree of primitivization. We are up against the great paradox of the twentieth century: that a breakneck technological advance has gone hand in hand with a return to tribalism, charismatic leaders, medicine men, credulity, and tribal wars. The tendency has been to blame the machine. There is a considerable literature on the barbarizing and dehumanizing effects of the machine: how it turns us into robots and slaves, stifles our individuality, and dwarfs our lives. Most of these indictments come of course from writers, poets, philosophers, and scholars—men of words—who have no first-hand experience of working and living with machines. It should also be noted that long before the advent of the machine age the typical intellectual looked upon common people who did the world's work as soulless robots and automated ghouls. It is true that in the early decades of the Industrial Revolution, when men, women, and children had to be dovetailed with iron and steam, the factories were agencies of dehumanization. But we of the present know that communion with machines does not blunt our sensibilities or stifle our individuality. We know that machines can be as temperamental and willful as any living thing. The proficient mechanic is an alert and intuitive human being. On the waterfront one can see how the ability to make a forklift or a winch do one's bidding with precision and finesse generates a peculiar exhilaration, so that the skilled lift driver and winch driver are as a rule of good cheer and work as if at play. Even if it were proven beyond a doubt that the assembly line makes robots of workers, it still affects only a small fraction of the population and cannot be held responsible for the nature of a whole society.

No, it is not the machine as such but drastic change which produces this social primitivism. The rapid urbanization of untold millions scooped off the land has been the central experience of our age, and the need of these uprooted millions for a new identity has generated and shaped the temper of our time. Whatever the means employed to satisfy this need, the result will be some degree of primitivization. Where a new identity is found by embracing a mass movement the reason is obvious: a mass movement absorbs and assimilates the individual into its corporate body, and does so by stripping the individual of his own opinions, tastes, and values. He is thereby reduced to an infantile state. This is what a new birth really means: to become like a child, and children are primitive beings—they are credulous, follow a leader, and readily become members of a pack. Immigration produces a similar reaction. Like a child, the immigrant has to learn to speak and how to act and assert himself. Finally, primitivization also follows when the search for a new identity prompts people to be eternally on the way by plunging into ceaseless action and hustling. It takes leisure to mature. People in a hurry can neither grow nor decay; they are preserved in a state of perpetual puerility.

But is social primitivization a fortuitous, unfortunate by-product, or does it have some sort of a function in the process of change? What is it that a society needs above all when it has to adjust itself to wholly new conditions? It needs utmost flexibility, a high degree of human plasticity. Now, a population juvenilized and primitivized, whether by a mass movement, mass migration, or immersion in ceaseless hustling, tends to become a homogeneous, plastic mass. We who have lived through the Stalin-Hitler era know that one of the most striking functions of a mass movement is the inducement of boundless human plasticity—the creation of a population that will go through breathtaking somersaults at a word of command and can be made, in the words of Boris Pasternak, "to hate what it loves and love what it hates."

The true believer is, then, a plastic human type thrown up by a century of ceaseless change. The adaptation to change has also produced the American hustler, a type as juvenile, primitive, and plastic as the true believer but functioning without ideology and the magic of communion. The immigrant, too, having been stripped of his traditions and habits, is easily molded. Finally, there is the plastic type of the warrior. All through history, conquerors have learned more willingly and readily from the conquered than the other way around. The conqueror does not see imitation as an act of submission and proof of his inadequacy. It is a fact that nations with a warrior tradition, such as the Japanese and the inheritors of Genghis Khan in Outer Mongolia, find the transition of modernization less difficult than nations of subjected peasants such as Russia and China. There is thus a kernel of practicalness in the preposterous tendency of an Indonesia or an Egypt to cast its people in the role of warriors. It is also plausible that the defeat of forty million Arabs by tiny Israel is rendering modernization of the Arab world more difficult and painful.

The throes of the machine age stem, then, not from the machine as such but from the social dislocation caused by the rapid urbanization of millions of peasants. It was this abrupt change in the life of the European masses in the second half of the nineteenth century which released the nationalist, revolutionary, and racialist movements that are still with us. A similar change in the backward countries of Asia, Africa, and Latin America is now setting off the social tremors that keep our world in a state of perpetual shock.

Where large-scale urbanization of peasants has taken place without industrialization, the social consequences have been equally explosive, as we have seen in recent decades in Latin America. In largely nonindustrial Argentina, Chile, Cuba, Uruguay, and Venezuela, townsmen already outnumber countrymen. Here, rapid industrialization when it comes will find masses of urbanized peasants ready to be processed into factory workers, and the result is more likely to be an easing of social unrest than revolution.

The curious thing is that with the spread of automation we may see something like the present Latin-American pattern emerging in the advanced industrialized countries. The banishing of workers by automation from factories, warehouses, and docks will fill the cities with millions of unemployed workers waiting for something to happen. Condemned to inaction and deprived of a sense of usefulness and worth, they will become receptive to extremism and to political and racial intolerance. Thus it seems that in our present world problems come and go but the by-products remain the same, and the end of the Time of Juveniles is nowhere in sight.

4   CHANGE AND AUTHORITY

THE PEOPLE WHO CLAMOR for drastic change are mostly hostile toward authority, whether in government, family, school, factory, or even in the armed forces. It seems to them logical that the flow of change would be less impeded in a permissive society. However, in human affairs the logic of events does not always correspond to the logic of the mind, and it is a fact that during the past hundred years drastic changes have been realized in more or less authoritarian atmospheres.

The changes experienced by Japan during the last third of the nineteenth century were more drastic and rapid than any the world had seen. In a few decades Japan went through an evolution for which the Occident needed centuries, yet in every department of life authority remained unquestioned or was even enhanced. The Japanese discarded overnight many of their most cherished values, illusions, and skills without losing an atom of their confidence and self-righteousness. This seems incredible to us who have seen the failure of nerve of adults when drastic change disintegrated accepted values and made skills and experience obsolete.

Germany after 1870 is another instance of a country undergoing drastic change within an authoritarian framework. One has the feeling that in both Japan and Germany the men who engi-

---

From *In Our Time*.

neered the programs of drastic change were aware of the need for vigorous authority.

In the Western democracies, until recently, change in one field seemed compatible with stubborn conservatism in other fields. England managed to preserve social stability and continuity during the upheaval of the Industrial Revolution. In this country the vast economic changes after the Civil War were realized in an atmosphere of political and cultural conservatism. In France, hectic political change went hand in hand with a stubborn resistance to change in the economy, the family, and the school. Finally, the smoothest racial integration we have seen in this country took place in the army during the Truman administration when the old discipline was still in force.

It should be obvious that a society undergoing drastic change needs a strong framework of authority to hold it together and an anchor of continuity to preserve its identity. Morever, a drastic change is likely to be attended by unforeseen, explosive side effects which only a vigorous authority can prevent from vitiating and perverting the intended end result.

It is remarkable how little thought social scientists have given to the role of authority in the realization of change. Two men who have touched briefly upon the problem come to mind. De Tocqueville, in *Democracy in America,* said that only a despot could solve America's racial problem, while Plato went to the extreme of maintaining that tyranny is the government under which change is easiest and most rapid.

IV

THE TRUE BELIEVER

MAN *would fain be great and sees that he is little; would fain be happy and sees that he is miserable; would fain be perfect and sees that he is full of imperfections; would fain be the object of the love and esteem of men, and sees that his faults merit only their aversion and contempt. The embarrassment wherein he finds himself produces in him the most unjust and criminal passions imaginable, for he conceives a mortal hatred against that truth which blames him and convinces him of his faults.*
—Pascal, *Pensées*

Σ

And slime had they for mortar.
—Genesis 11

This essay deals with some peculiarities common to all mass movements, be they religious movements, social revolutions, or nationalist movements. It does not maintain that all movements are identical, but that they share certain essential characteristics which give them a family likeness.

All mass movements generate in their adherents a readiness to die and a proclivity for united action; all of them, irrespective of the doctrine they preach and the program they project, breed fanaticism, enthusiasm, fervent hope, hatred, and intolerance; all of them are capable of releasing a powerful flow of activity in certain departments of life; all of them demand blind faith and single-hearted allegiance.

All movements, however different in doctrine and aspiration, draw their early adherents from the same types of humanity; they all appeal to the same types of mind.

Though there are obvious differences between the fanatical Christian, the fanatical Muslim, the fanatical nationalist, the fanatical Communist, and the fanatical Nazi, it is yet true that the fanaticism which animates them may be viewed and treated as one. The same is true of the force which drives them on to expansion and world dominion. There is a certain uniformity in all types of dedication, of faith, of pursuit of power, of unity, and of self-sacrifice. There are vast differences in the contents of holy causes and doctrines, but a certain uniformity in the factors which make them effective. He who, like Pascal, finds precise reasons for the effectiveness of Christian doctrine has also found the reasons for the effectiveness of Communist, Nazi, and nationalist doctrine. However different the causes people die for, they perhaps die basically for the same thing.

This essay concerns itself chiefly with the active, revivalist phase of mass movements. This phase is dominated by the true believer—the man of fanatical faith who is ready to sacrifice his life for a holy cause—and an attempt is made to trace his genesis and outline his nature. As an aid in this effort, use is made of a working hypothesis. Starting out from the fact that the frustrated[1] predominate among the early adherents of all mass movements and that they usually join of their own accord, it is assumed (1) that frustration of itself, without any proselytizing prompting from the outside, can generate most of the peculiar characteristics of the true believer, and (2) that an effective technique of conversion consists basically in the inculcation and fixation of proclivities and responses indigenous to the frustrated mind.

To test the validity of these assumptions, it was necessary to inquire into the ills that afflict the frustrated, how they react against them, the degree to which these reactions correspond to the responses of the true believer, and, finally, the manner in which these reactions can facilitate the rise and spread of a mass

---

[1] The word "frustrated" is not used as a clinical term. It denotes here people who, for one reason or another, feel that their lives are spoiled or wasted.

movement. It was also necessary to examine the practices of contemporary movements, where successful techniques of conversion had been perfected and applied, in order to discover whether they corroborate the view that a proselytizing mass movement deliberately fosters in its adherents a frustrated state of mind, and that it automatically advances its interest when it seconds the propensities of the frustrated.

It is necessary for most of us these days to have some insight into the motives and responses of the true believer. For though ours is a godless age, it is the very opposite of irreligious. The true believer is everywhere on the march, and both by converting and antagonizing he is shaping the world in his own image. And whether we are to line up with him or against him, it is well that we should know all we can concerning his nature and potentialities.

It is perhaps not superfluous to add a word of caution. When we speak of the family likeness of mass movements, we use the word "family" in a taxonomical sense. The tomato and the nightshade are of the same family, the Solanaceae. Though the one is nutritious and the other poisonous, they have many morphological, anatomical, and physiological traits in common so that even the non-botanist senses a family likeness. The assumption that mass movements have many traits in common does not imply that all movements are equally beneficent or poisonous. This essay passes no judgments and expresses no preferences. It merely tries to explain, and the explanations—all of them theories—are in the nature of suggestions and arguments even when they are stated in what seems a categorical tone. I can do no better than quote Montaigne: "All I say is by way of discourse, and nothing by way of advice. I should not speak so boldly if it were my due to be believed."

1 THE APPEAL OF

MASS MOVEMENTS

Iт is a truism that many who join a rising revolutionary movement are attracted by the prospect of sudden and spectacular
change in their conditions of life. A revolutionary movement is a
conspicuous instrument of change.

Not so obvious is the fact that religious and nationalist movements too can be vehicles of change. Some kind of widespread
enthusiasm or excitement is apparently needed for the realization
of vast and rapid change, and it does not seem to matter whether
the exhilaration is derived from an expectation of untold riches or
is generated by an active mass movement. In this country the
spectacular changes since the Civil War were enacted in an atmosphere charged with the enthusiasm born of fabulous opportunities for self-advancement. Where self-advancement cannot, or is
not allowed to, serve as a driving force, other sources of enthusiasm have to be found if momentous changes, such as the awakening and renovation of a stagnant society or radical reforms in the
character and pattern of life of a community, are to be realized
and perpetuated. Religious, revolutionary, and nationalist movements are such generating plants of general enthusiasm.

In the past, religious movements were the conspicuous vehicles
of change. The conservatism of a religion—its orthodoxy—is the
inert coagulum of a once highly reactive sap. A rising religious
movement is all change and experiment, open to new views and
techniques from all quarters. Islam when it emerged was an organizing and modernizing medium. Christianity was a civilizing and

modernizing influence among the savage tribes of Europe. The Crusades and the Reformation both were crucial factors in shaking the Western world from the stagnation of the Middle Ages.

In modern times, the mass movements involved in the realization of vast and rapid change are revolutionary and nationalist— singly or in combination. Peter the Great was probably the equal, in dedication, power, and ruthlessness, of many of the most successful revolutionary or nationalist leaders. Yet he failed in his chief purpose, which was to turn Russia into a Western nation. And the reason he failed was that he did not infuse the Russian masses with some soul-stirring enthusiasm. He either did not think it necessary or did not know how to make of his purpose a holy cause. It is not strange that the Bolshevik revolutionaries who wiped out the last of the czars and Romanovs should have a sense of kinship with Peter—a czar and a Romanov. For his purpose is now theirs, and they hope to succeed where he failed. The Bolshevik revolution may figure in history as much an attempt to modernize a sixth of the world's surface as an attempt to build a Communist economy.

The fact that both the French and the Russian revolutions turned into nationalist movements seems to indicate that in modern times nationalism is the most copious and durable source of mass enthusiasm, and that nationalist fervor must be tapped if the drastic changes projected and initiated by revolutionary enthusiam are to be consummated. One wonders whether the difficulties encountered by the Labour government in instituting socialism in postwar Britain were not partly due to the fact that the attempt to change the economy of the country and the way of life of 49 million people was initiated in an atmosphere singularly free from fervor, exaltation, and wild hope. The revulsion from the ugly patterns developed by most contemporary mass movements kept the civilized and decent leaders of the Labour party shy of revolutionary enthusiasm.

The phenomenal modernization of Japan would probably not have been possible without the revivalist spirit of Japanese nationalism. It is perhaps also true that the rapid modernization of some European countries (Germany in particular) was facilitated to some extent by the upsurge and thorough diffusion of nationalist fervor. Judged by present indications, the renascence of Asia will

Dicipline, Prayer, fasting, Study, Exercise

be brought about through the instrumentality of nationalist movements rather than by other mediums. It was the rise of a genuine nationalist movement which enabled Kemal Atatürk to modernize Turkey almost overnight. In Egypt, untouched by a mass movement, modernization is slow and faltering, though its rulers, from the day of Mehemet Ali, have welcomed Western ideas, and its contacts with the West have been many and intimate. Zionism is an instrument for the renovation of a backward country and the transformation of shopkeepers and brain workers into farmers, laborers, and soldiers. Had Chiang Kai-shek known how to set in motion a genuine mass movement, or at least sustain the nationalist enthusiasm kindled by the Japanese invasion, he, not Mao Tsetung, might have been the leader of modern China. Since he did not know how, he was easily shoved aside by the masters of the art of "religiofication"—the art of turning practical purposes into holy causes. It is not difficult to see why the United States and Britain (or any Western democracy) could not play a direct and leading role in rousing the Asian countries from their backwardness and stagnation after the Second World War: the democracies were neither inclined nor perhaps able to kindle a revivalist spirit in Asia's millions. The contribution of the Western democracies to the awakening of the East has been indirect and certainly unintended. They have kindled an enthusiasm of resentment against the West; and it is this anti-Western fervor which has roused the Orient.

Though the desire for change is not infrequently a superficial motive, it is worth finding out whether a probing of this desire might not shed some light on the inner working of mass movements. We shall inquire therefore into the nature of the desire for change.

THE DESIRE FOR CHANGE

There is in us a tendency to locate the shaping forces of our existence outside ourselves. Success and failure are unavoidably related in our minds with the state of things around us. Hence it is that people with a sense of fulfillment think it a good world and would like to conserve it as it is, while the frustrated favor radical change. The tendency to look for all causes outside ourselves persists even when it is clear that our state of being is the product of personal qualities such as ability, character, appearance, health, and so on. "If anything ail a man," says Thoreau, "so that he does not perform his functions, if he have a pain in his bowels even . . . he forthwith sets about reforming—the world."

It is understandable that those who fail should incline to blame the world for their failure. The remarkable thing is that the successful, too, however much they pride themselves on their forsight, fortitude, thrift, and other "sterling qualities," are at bottom convinced that their success is the result of a fortuitous combination of circumstances. The self-confidence of even the consistently successful is never absolute. They are never sure that they know all the ingredients which go into the making of their success. The outside world seems to them a precariously balanced mechanism, and so long as it ticks in their favor they are afraid to tinker with it. Thus the resistance to change and the ardent desire for it spring from the same conviction, and the one can be as vehement as the other.

2

Discontent by itself does not invariably create a desire for change. Other factors have to be present before discontent turns into disaffection. One of these is a sense of power. *How?, When? q Wg?*

Those who are awed by their surroundings do not think of change, no matter how miserable their condition. When our mode of life is so precarious as to make it patent that we cannot control the circumstances of our existence, we tend to stick to the proven and the familiar. We counteract a deep feeling of insecurity by making of our existence a fixed routine. We hereby acquire the illusion that we have tamed the unpredictable. Fisherfolk, nomads, and farmers who have to contend with the willful elements, the creative worker who depends on inspiration, the savage awed by his surroundings—they all fear change. They face the world as they would an all-powerful jury. The abjectly poor, too, stand in awe of the world around them and are not hospitable to change. It is a dangerous life we live when hunger and cold are at our heels. There is thus a conservatism of the destitute as profound as the conservatism of the privileged, and the former is as much a factor in the perpetuation of a social order as the latter. Amen

The men who rush into undertakings of vast change usually feel they are in possession of some irresistible power. The generation that made the French Revolution had an extravagant conception of the omnipotence of man's reason and the boundless range of his intelligence. Never, says De Tocqueville, had humanity been prouder of itself, nor had it ever so much faith in its own omnipotence. And joined with this exaggerated self-confidence was a universal thirst for change which came unbidden to every mind. Lenin and the Bolsheviks who plunged recklessly into the chaos of the creation of a new world had blind faith in the omnipotence of Marxist doctrine. The Nazis had nothing as potent as that doctrine, but they had faith in an infallible leader and also faith in a new technique. For it is doubtful whether National Socialism would have made such rapid progress if it had not been for the electrifying conviction that the new techniques of blitzkrieg and propaganda made Germany irresistible.

Even the sober desire for progress is sustained by faith—faith in the intrinsic goodness of human nature and in the omnipotence of science. It is a defiant and blasphemous faith, not unlike that held by the men who set out to build "a city and a tower, whose top may reach unto heaven" and who believed that "nothing will be restrained from them, which they have imagined to do."

3

Offhand one would expect that the mere possession of power would automatically result in a cocky attitude toward the world and a receptivity to change. But it is not always so. The powerful can be as timid as the weak. What seems to count more than possession of instruments of power is faith in the future. Where power is not joined with faith in the future, it is used mainly to ward off the new and preserve the status quo. On the other hand, extravagant hope, even when not backed by actual power, is likely to generate a most reckless daring. For the hopeful can draw strength from the most ridiculous sources of power—a slogan, a word, a button. No faith is potent unless it is also faith in the future, unless it has a millennial component. So, too, an effective doctrine: as well as being a source of power, it must also claim to be a key to the door of the future.

Those who would transform a nation or the world cannot do so by breeding and captaining discontent or by demonstrating the reasonableness and desirability of the intended changes or by coercing people into a new way of life. They must know how to kindle and fan an extravagant hope. It matters not whether it be hope of a heavenly kingdom, of heaven on earth, of plunder and untold riches, or fabulous achievement, or of world dominion. If the Communists win the world, it will not be because they know how to stir up discontent or how to infect people with hatred, but because they know how to preach hope.

4

Thus the differences between the conservative and the radical seem to spring mainly from their attitude toward the future. Fear of the future causes us to lean against and cling to the present, while faith in the future renders us receptive to change. Both the rich and the poor, the strong and the weak, they who have achieved much or little can be afraid of the future. When the present seems so good that the most we can expect is its continuation in the future, change can only mean deterioration. Hence men of outstanding achievement and those who live full, happy lives usually set their faces against drastic innovation. The conservatism of invalids and people past middle age stems, too, from fear of the future. They are on the lookout for signs of decay and feel that any change is more likely to be for the worse than for the better. The abjectly poor also are without faith in the future. The future seems to them a booby trap buried on the road ahead. One must step gingerly. To change things is to ask for trouble.

As for the hopeful: it does not seem to make any difference who it is that is seized with a wild hope—whether it be an enthusiastic intellectual, a land-hungry farmer, a get-rich-quick speculator, a sober merchant or industrialist, a plain workingman, or a noble lord—they all proceed recklessly with the present, wreck it if necessary, and create a new world. There can thus be revolutions by the privileged as well as by the underprivileged. The movement of enclosure in sixteenth- and seventeenth-century

England was a revolution by the rich. The woolen industry rose to high prosperity, and grazing became more profitable than cropping. The landowners drove off their tenants, enclosed the commons, and wrought profound changes in the social and economic texture of the country. "The lords and nobles were upsetting the social order, breaking down ancient law and custom, sometimes by means of violence, often by pressure and intimidation."[1] Another English revolution by the rich occurred at the end of the eighteenth and the beginning of the nineteenth century. It was the Industrial Revolution. The breathtaking potentialities of mechanization set the minds of manufacturers and merchants on fire. They began a revolution "as extreme and radical as ever inflamed the minds of sectarians,"[2] and in a relatively short time these respectable, God-fearing citizens changed the face of England beyond recognition.

When hopes and dreams are loose in the streets, it is well for the timid to lock doors, shutter windows, and lie low until the wrath has passed. For there is often a monstrous incongruity between the hopes, however noble and tender, and the action which follows them. It is as if ivied maidens and garlanded youths were to herald the four horsemen of the apocalypse.

5

For men to plunge headlong into an undertaking of vast change, they must be intensely discontented yet not destitute, and they must have the feeling that by the possession of some potent doctrine, infallible leader, or new technique they have access to a source of irresistible power. They must also have an extravagant conception of the prospects and potentialities of the future. Finally, they must be wholly ignorant of the difficulties involved in their vast undertaking. Experience is a handicap. The men who started the French Revolution were wholly without political experience. The same is true of the Bolsheviks, the Nazis, and the revolutionaries in Asia and Africa. The experienced man of affairs is a latecomer. He enters the movement when it is already a going

[1] Karl Polanyi, *The Great Transformation* (New York: Farrar and Rinehart, Inc., 1944), p. 35.
[2] Ibid., p. 40.

concern. It is perhaps the Englishman's political experience that keeps him shy of mass movements.

THE DESIRE FOR SUBSTITUTES

There is a fundamental difference between the appeal of a mass movement and the appeal of a practical organization. The practical organization offers opportunities for self-advancement, and its appeal is mainly to self-interest. A mass movement, on the other hand, particularly in its active, revivalist phase, appeals not to those intent on bolstering and advancing a cherished self but to those who crave to be rid of an unwanted self. A mass movement attracts and holds a following not because it can satisfy the desire for self-advancement, but because it can satisfy the passion for self-renunciation.

People who see their lives as irremediably spoiled cannot find a worthwhile purpose in self-advancement. The prospect of an individual career cannot stir them to a mighty effort, nor can it evoke in them faith and a single-minded dedication. They look on self-interest as on something tainted and evil, something unclean and unlucky. Anything undertaken under the auspices of the self seems to them foredoomed. Nothing that has its roots and reasons in the self can be good and noble. Their innermost craving is for a new life—a rebirth—or, failing this, a chance to acquire new elements of pride, confidence, hope, a sense of purpose, and worth by an identification with a holy cause. An active mass movement offers them opportunities for both. If they join the movement as full converts they are reborn to a new life in its close-knit collective body, or if attracted as sympathizers they find elements of pride, confidence, and purpose by identifying themselves with the efforts, achievements, and prospects of the movement.

To the frustrated a mass movement offers substitutes either for the whole self or for the elements which make life bearable and which they cannot evoke out of their individual resources.

It is true that among the early adherents of a mass movement there are also adventurers who join in the hope that the movement will give a spin to their wheel of fortune and whirl them to fame and power. On the other hand, a degree of selfless dedication is sometimes displayed by those who join corporations, orthodox political parties, and other practical organizations. Still, the fact remains that a practical concern cannot endure unless it can appeal to and satisfy self-interest, while the vigor and growth of a rising mass movement depend on its capacity to evoke and satisfy the passion for self-renunciation. When a mass movement begins to attract people who are interested in their individual careers, it is a sign that it has passed its vigorous stage; it is no longer engaged in molding a new world but in possessing and preserving the present. It ceases then to be a movement and becomes an enterprise. According to Hitler, the more "posts and offices a movement has to hand out, the more inferior stuff it will attract, and in the end these political hangers-on overwhelm a successful party in such number that the honest fighter of former days no longer recognizes the old movement. . . . When this happens, the 'mission' of such a movement is done for."

2

Faith in a holy cause is to a considerable extent a substitute for the lost faith in ourselves.

The less justified a man is in claiming excellence for his own self, the more ready is he to claim all excellence for his nation, his religion, his race, or his cause.

A man is likely to mind his own business when it is worth minding. When it is not, he takes his mind off his own meaningless affairs by minding other people's business.

This minding of other people's business expresses itself in gossip, snooping, and meddling and also in feverish interest in communal, national, and racial affairs. In running away from ourselves we either fall on our neighbor's shoulder or fly at his throat.

The burning conviction that we have a holy duty toward others is often a way of attaching our drowning selves to a passing raft. What looks like giving a hand is often a holding on for dear life. Take away our holy duties and you leave our lives puny and meaningless. There is no doubt that in exchanging a self-centered for a selfless life we gain enormously in self-esteem. The vanity of the selfless, even those who practice utmost humility, is boundless.

3

One of the most potent attractions of a mass movement is its offering of a substitute for individual hope. This attraction is particularly effective in a society imbued with the idea of progress. For in the conception of progress, "tomorrow" looms large, and the frustration resulting from having nothing to look forward to is the more poignant. Hermann Rauschning says of pre-Hitlerian Germany that "The feeling of having come to the end of all things was one of the worst troubles we endured after the lost war." In a modern society, people can live without hope only when kept dazed and out of breath by incessant hustling. The despair brought by unemployment comes not only from the threat of destitution but from the sudden view of a vast nothingness ahead. The unemployed are more likely to follow the peddlers of hope than the handers-out of relief.

Mass movements are usually accused of doping their followers with hope of the future while cheating them on the enjoyment of the present. Yet to the frustrated the present is irremediably spoiled. Comforts and pleasures cannot make it whole. No real content or comfort can ever arise in their minds but from hope.

4

When our individual interests and prospects do not seem worth living for, we are in desperate need of something apart from us to live for. All forms of dedication, devotion, loyalty, and self-surrender are in essence a desperate clinging to something which might give worth and meaning to our futile, spoiled lives. Hence the embracing of a substitute will necessarily be passionate and extreme. We can have qualified confidence in ourselves, but the faith we have in our nation, religion, race, or cause has to be extravagant and uncompromising. A substitute embraced in moderation cannot supplant and efface the self we want to forget. We cannot be sure that we have something worth living for unless we are ready to die for it. This readiness to die is evidence to ourselves and others that what we had to take as a substitute for an irrevocably missed or spoiled first choice is indeed the best there ever was.

THE INTERCHANGEABILITY
OF MASS MOVEMENTS

When people are ripe for a mass movement, they are usually ripe for any effective movement, and not solely for one with a particular doctrine or program. In pre-Hitlerian Germany it was often a toss-up whether a restless youth would join the Communists or the Nazis. In the overcrowded pale of czarist Russia, the simmering Jewish population was ripe both for revolution and Zionism. In the same family, one member would join the revolutionaries and the other the Zionists. Chaim Weizmann quotes a saying of his mother in those days: "Whatever happens, I shall be well off. If Shemuel [the revolutionary son] is right, we shall all be happy in Russia; and if Chaim [the Zionist] is right, then I shall go to live in Palestine."

This receptivity to all movements does not always cease even after the potential true believer has become the ardent convert of a specific one. Where mass movements are in violent competition with each other, there are not infrequent instances of converts—even the most zealous—shifting their allegiance from one to the other. A Saul turning into Paul is neither a rarity nor a miracle. In our day, each proselytizing mass movement seems to regard the zealous adherents of its antagonist as its own potential converts. Hitler looked on the German Communists as potential National Socialists: "The *petit bourgeois* Social-Democrat and the trade-union boss will never make a National Socialist, but the Communist always will." Captain Röhm boasted that he could turn the reddest Communist into a glowing nationalist in four weeks. On the other hand, Karl Radek looked on the Nazi Brownshirts (SA) as a reserve for future Communist recruits.

Since all mass movements draw their adherents from the same types of humanity and appeal to the same types of mind, it follows that (1) all mass movements are competitive, and the gain of one in adherents is the loss of all the others; and (2) all mass movements are interchangeable. One mass movement readily transforms itself into another. A religious movement may develop into a social revolution or a nationalist movement; a social revolution into militant nationalism or a religious movement; a nationalist movement into a social revolution or a religious movement.

2

It is rare for a mass movement to be wholly of one character. Usually it displays some facets of other types of movement, and sometimes it is two or three movements in one. The exodus of the Hebrews from Egypt was a slave revolt, a religious movement, and a nationalist movement. The militant nationalism of the Japanese is essentially religious. The French Revolution was a new religion. It had "its dogmas, the sacred principles of the Revolution—*Liberté et sainte égalité*. It had its form of worship, an adaptation of Catholic ceremonial, which was elaborated in connection with civic *fêtes*. It had its saints, the heroes and martyrs of liberty."[3] At the same time, the French Revolution was also a nationalist movement. The legislative assembly decreed in 1792 that altars should be raised everywhere bearing the inscription "The citizen is born, lives, and dies for *la Patrie*."

The religious movements of the Reformation had a revolutionary aspect which expressed itself in peasant uprisings and were also nationalist movements. Said Luther, "In the eyes of the Italians we Germans are merely low Teutonic swine. They exploit us like charlatans and suck the country to the marrow. Wake up, Germany!"

The religious character of the Bolshevik and Nazi revolutions is generally recognized. The hammer and sickle and the swastika are in a class with the cross. The ceremonial of their parades is as the ceremonial of a religious procession. They have articles of faith, saints, martyrs, and holy sepulchers. The Bolshevik and Nazi revolutions are also full-blown nationalist movements. The Nazi revolution had been so from the beginning, while the nationalism of the Bolsheviks was a late development.

Zionism is a nationalist movement and a social revolution. To the orthodox Jew it is also a religious movement. Irish nationalism

[3]Carl L. Becker, *The Heavenly City of the Eighteenth-Century Philosophers* (New Haven: Yale University Press, 1932), p. 155.

has a deep religious tinge. The modern mass movements in Asia are both nationalist and revolutionary.

3

The problem of stopping a mass movement is often a matter of substituting one movement for another. A social revolution can be stopped by promoting a religious or nationalist movement. Thus in countries where Catholicism has recaptured its mass movement spirit, it counteracts the spread of communism. In Japan it was nationalism that canalized all movements of social protest. In our South, the movement of racial solidarity acted for many years as a preventive of social upheaveal. A similar situation may be observed among the French in Canada and among the Boers in South Africa.

This method of stopping one movement by substituting another is not always without danger, and it does not usually come cheap. It is well for those who hug the present, and want to preserve it as it is, not to play with mass movements. For it always fares ill with the present when a genuine mass movement is on the march. In prewar Italy and Germany, practical businessmen acted in an entirely "logical" manner when they encouraged a Fascist and a Nazi movement in order to stop communism. But in doing so, these practical and logical people promoted their own liquidation.

There are other safer substitutes for a mass movement. In general, any arrangement which either discourages atomistic individualism or facilitates self-forgetting or offers chances for action and new beginnings tends to counteract the rise and spread of mass movements. These subjects are dealt with in later sections. Here we shall touch upon one curious substitute for mass movements: emigration.

4

Emigration offers some of the things the frustrated hope to find when they join a mass movement: namely, change and a chance for a new beginning. The same types who swell the ranks of a rising mass movement are also likely to avail themselves of a chance to emigrate. Thus migration can serve as a substitute for a mass movement. It is plausible, for instance, that had the United States and the British Empire welcomed mass migration from Europe after the First World War, there might have been neither a Fascist nor a Názi revolution. In this country, free and easy migration over a vast continent contributed to our social stability.

However, because of the quality of their human material, mass migrations are fertile ground for the rise of genuine mass movements. It is sometimes difficult to tell where a mass migration ends and a mass movement begins and which came first. The migration of the Hebrews from Egypt developed into a religious and nationalist movement. The migrations of the barbarians in the declining days of the Roman Empire were more than mere shifts of population. The indications are that the barbarians were relatively few in number, but, once they invaded a country, they were joined by the oppressed and dissatisfied in all walks of life: "it was a social revolution started and masked by a superficial foreign conquest."[4]

Every mass movement is in a sense a migration, a movement toward a promised land; when feasible and expedient, an actual migration takes place. This happened, for example, in the case of the Puritans, Anabaptists, Mormons, Dukhobors, and Zionists. Migration, in the mass, strengthens the spirit and unity of a movement; and, whether in the form of foreign conquest, crusade, pilgrimage, or settlement of new land, it is practiced by most active mass movements.

[4] H. G. Wells, *The Outline of History* (New York: Macmillan Company, 1922), pp. 482–84.

2 THE POTENTIAL CONVERTS

There is a tendency to judge a race, a nation, or any distinct group by its least worthy members. Though manifestly unfair, this tendency has some justification. For the character and destiny of a group are often determined by its inferior elements.

The inert mass of a nation, for instance, is in its middle section. The decent, average people who do the nation's work in cities and on the land are worked upon and shaped by minorities at both ends—the best and the worst.[1]

The superior individual, whether in politics, literature, science, commerce, or industry, plays a large role in shaping a nation, but so do individuals at the other extreme—the failures, misfits, outcasts, criminals, and all those who have lost their footing, or never had one, in the ranks of the respectable. The game of history is usually played by the best and the worst over the heads of the majority in the middle.

The reason that the "inferior" elements of a nation can exert a marked influence on its course is that they are wholly without reverence toward the present. They see their lives and the present as spoiled beyond remedy, and they are ready to waste and wreck both: hence their recklessness and their will to chaos and anarchy. They also crave to dissolve their worthless, meaningless selves in

---

[1] A mild instance of the combined shaping by the best and worst is to be observed in the case of language. The respectable middle section of a nation sticks to the dictionary. Innovations come from the best—statesmen, poets, writers, scientists, specialists—and from the worst—slang makers.

some soul-stirring spectacular communal undertaking—hence their proclivity for united action. Thus they are among the early recruits of revolutions, of mass migrations, and of religious, racial, and chauvinist movements, and they imprint their mark upon those upheavals and movements which shape a nation's character and history.

The discarded and rejected are often the raw material of a nation's future. The stone the builders reject becomes the cornerstone of a new world. A nation without dregs and malcontents is orderly, decent, peaceful, and pleasant, but perhaps without the seed of things to come. It was not the irony of history that the undesired in the countries of Europe should have crossed an ocean to build a new world on this continent. Only they could do it.

Though the disaffected are found in all walks of life, they are most frequent in the following categories: the poor, misfits, out casts, adolescent youth, the inordinately selfish, the ambitious (whether facing insurmountable obstacles or unlimited opportunities), those in the grip of some vice or obsession, the impotent (in body or mind), minorities, the bored, the sinners.

The next sections deal with some of these types.

THE POOR

The New Poor

Not all who are poor are frustrated. Some of the poor stagnating in the slums of the cities are smug in their decay. They shudder at the thought of life outside their familiar cesspool. Even the respectable poor, when their poverty is of long standing, remain inert. They are awed by the immutability of the order of things. It takes a cataclysm—an invasion, a plague, or some other communal disaster—to open their eyes to the transitoriness of the "eternal order."

It is usually those whose poverty is relatively recent, the "new poor," who throb with the ferment of frustration. The memory of better things is as fire in their veins. They are the disinherited and dispossessed who respond to every rising mass movement. It was the new poor in seventeenth-century England who ensured the success of the Puritan Revolution. During the movement of enclosure, thousands of landlords drove off their tenants and turned their fields into pastures. "Strong and active peasants, enamored of the soil that nurtured them, were transformed into wageworkers or sturdy beggars; . . . city streets were filled with paupers."[2] It was this mass of the dispossessed who furnished the recruits for Cromwell's new-model army. In Germany and Italy the new poor coming from a ruined middle class formed the chief support of the Nazi and Fascist revolutions. The potential revolutionaries in post-imperial England were not the workers but the disinherited civil servants and businessmen. A class with a vivid memory of affluence and dominion is not likely to be easily reconciled to straitened conditions and political impotence.

There have been of late, both here and in other countries, enormous periodic increases of a new type of new poor, and their appearance undoubtedly has contributed to the rise and spread of contemporary mass movements. Until recently the new poor came mainly from the propertied classes, whether in cities or on the land, but lately, and perhaps for the first time in history, the plain workingman appears in this role.

So long as those who did the world's work lived on a level of bare subsistence, they were looked upon and felt themselves as the traditionally poor. They felt poor in good times and bad. Depressions, however severe, were not seen as aberrations and enormities. But with the wide diffusion of a high standard of living, depressions and the unemployment they bring assumed a new aspect. The present-day workingman in the Western world feels unemployment as a degradation. He sees himself disinherited and injured by an unjust order of things and is willing to listen to those who call for a new deal.

The Abjectly Poor

The poor on the borderline of starvation live purposeful lives. To be engaged in a desperate struggle for food and shelter is to be wholly free from a sense of futility. The goals are concrete and immediate. Every meal is a fulfillment; to go to sleep on a

[2] Charles A. and Mary R. Beard, *The Rise of American Civilization* (New York: Macmillan Company, 1939), Vol. I, p. 24.

full stomach is a triumph, and every windfall is a miracle. What need could they have for "an inspiring super individual goal which would give meaning and dignity to their lives?" They are immune to the appeal of a mass movement. Angelica Balabanoff describes the effect of abject poverty on the revolutionary ardor of famous radicals who flocked to Moscow in the early days of the Bolshevik revolution. "Here I saw men and women who had lived all their lives for ideas, who had voluntarily renounced material advantages, liberty, happiness, and family affection for the realisation of their ideals—completely absorbed by the problem of hunger and cold."

Where people toil from sunrise to sunset for a bare living, they nurse no grievances and dream no dreams. One of the reasons for the centuries-long unrebelliousness of the masses in China was the inordinate effort required there to scrape together the means of the scantiest subsistence. The intensified struggle for existence "is a static rather than a dynamic influence."[3]

2

Misery does not automatically generate discontent, nor is the intensity of discontent directly proportionate to the degree of misery.

Discontent is likely to be highest when misery is bearable; when conditions have so improved that an ideal state seems almost within reach. A grievance is most poignant when almost redressed. De Tocqueville in his researches into the state of society in France before the revolution was struck by the discovery that "in no one of the periods which have followed the Revolution of 1789 has the national prosperity of France augmented more rapidly than it did in the twenty years preceding that event." He was forced to conclude that "the French found their position the more intolerable the better it became." In both France and Russia the land-hungry peasants owned almost exactly one third of the agricultural land at the outbreak of revolution, and most of that land had been acquired during the generation or two preceding the revolution. It is not actual suffering but the taste of better things ✳

[3] Edward A. Ross, *The Changing Chinese* (New York: Century Company, 1911), p. 92.

which excites people to revolt. A popular upheaval in Soviet Russia is hardly likely before the people get a real taste of the good life. The most dangerous moment for the regime of the Politburo will be when a considerable improvement in the economic conditions of the Russian masses has been achieved and the iron totalitarian rule somewhat relaxed. It is of interest that the assassination, in December 1934, of Stalin's close friend Kirov happened not long after Stalin had announced the successful end of the first Five-Year Plan and the beginning of a new prosperous, joyous era.

The intensity of discontent seems to be in inverse proportion to the distance from the object fervently desired. This is true whether we move toward our goal or away from it. It is true both of those who have just come within sight of the promised land and of the disinherited who are still within sight of it; both of the about-to-be rich and free and of the new poor and those recently enslaved.

3

Our frustration is greater when we have much and want more than when we have nothing and want some. We are less dissatisfied when we lack many things than when we seem to lack but one thing.

We dare more when striving for superfluities than for necessities. Often when we renounce superfluities we end up lacking in necessities.

4

There is a hope that acts as an explosive, and a hope that disciplines and infuses patience. The difference is between the immediate hope and the distant hope.

A rising mass movement preaches the immediate hope. It is intent on stirring its followers to action, and it is the around-the-corner brand of hope that prompts people to act. Rising Christianity preached the immediate end of the world and the kingdom of heaven around the corner; Muhammad dangled loot and Paradise before the faithful; the Jacobins promised immediate liberty and equality; the early Bolsheviks promised bread and land; Hitler promised an immediate end to Versailles's bondage and work and action for all. Later, as the movement comes into possession of power, the emphasis is shifted to the distant hope—the dream and the vision. For an "arrived" mass movement is preoccupied with the preservation of the present, and it prizes obedience and patience above spontaneous action; when we "hope for that we see not, then do we with patience wait for it."

Every established mass movement has its distant hope, its brand of drug to dull the impatience of the masses and reconcile them with their lot in life. Stalinism is as much an opium of the people as are the established religions.

The Free Poor

Slaves are poor; yet where slavery is widespread and long-established, there is little likelihood of the rise of a mass movement. The absolute equality among the slaves, and the intimate communal life in slave quarters, preclude individual frustration. In a society with an institution of slavery, the troublemakers are the newly enslaved and the freed slaves. In the case of the latter it is the burden of freedom which is at the root of their discontent.

Freedom aggravates at least as much as it alleviates frustration. Freedom of choice places the whole blame of failure on the shoulders of the individual. And as freedom encourages a multiplicity of attempts, it unavoidably multiplies failure and frustration. Freedom alleviates frustration by making available the palliatives of action, movement, change, and protest.

Unless a man has the talents to make something of himself, freedom is an irksome burden. Of what avail is freedom to choose if the self be ineffectual? We join a mass movement to escape individual responsibility, or, in the words of one ardent young Nazi, "to be free from freedom." It was not sheer hypocrisy when the rank-and-file Nazis declared themselves not guilty of all the enormities they had committed. They considered themselves cheated and maligned when made to shoulder responsibility for obeying orders. Had they not joined the Nazi movement in order to be free from responsibility?

It would seem then that the most fertile ground for the propagation of a mass movement is a society with considerable freedom but lacking the palliatives of frustration. It was precisely because the peasants of eighteenth-century France, unlike the peasants of Germany and Austria, were no longer serfs and already owned land that they were receptive to the appeal of the French Revolution. Nor perhaps would there have been a Bolshevik revolution if the Russian peasant had not been free for a generation or more and had a taste of the private ownership of land.

2

Even the mass movements which rise in the name of freedom against an oppressive order do not realize individual liberty once they start rolling. So long as a movement is engaged in a desperate struggle with the prevailing order or must defend itself against enemies within or without, its chief preoccupation will be with unity and self-sacrifice, which require the surrender of the individual's will, judgment, and advantage. According to Robespierre, the revolutionary government was "the despotism of liberty against tyranny."

The important point is that the active mass movement, in forgetting or postponing individual liberty, does not run counter to the inclinations of a zealous following. Fanatics, says Renan, fear liberty more than they fear persecution. It is true that the adherents of a rising movement have a strong sense of liberation even though they live and breathe in an atmosphere of strict adherence to tenets and commands. This sense of liberation comes from having escaped the burdens, fears, and hopelessness of an untenable individual existence. It is this escape which they feel as a deliverance and redemption. The experience of vast change, too, conveys a sense of freedom, even though the changes are executed in a frame of strict discipline. It is only when the movement has passed its active stage and solidified into a pattern of stable institutions that individual liberty has a chance to emerge. The shorter the active phase, the more will it seem that the movement itself, rather than its termination, made possible the emergence of individual freedom. This impression will be the more pronounced the more tyrannical the dispensation which the mass movement overthrew and supplanted.

(3)

Those who see their lives as spoiled and wasted crave equality and fraternity more than they do freedom. If they clamor for freedom, it is but freedom to establish quality and uniformity. The passion for equality is partly a passion for anonymity: to be one thread of the many which make up a tunic, one thread not distinguishable from the others. No one can then point them out, measure them against others, and expose their inferiority.

They who clamor loudest for freedom are often the ones least likely to be happy in a free society. The frustrated, oppressed by their shortcomings, blame their failure on existing restraints. Actually their innermost desire is for an end to the free-for-all. They want to eliminate free competition and the ruthless testing to which the individual is continually subjected in a free society.

(4)

Where freedom is real, equality is the passion of the masses. Where equality is real, freedom is the passion of a small minority.

Equality without freedom creates a more stable social pattern than freedom without equality.

The Creative Poor

Poverty when coupled with creativeness is usually free of frustration. This is true of the poor artisan skilled in his trade and of the poor writer, artist, and scientist in the full possession of creative powers. Nothing so bolsters our self-confidence and reconciles us with ourselves as the continuous ability to create; to see things grow and develop under our hand, day in, day out. The decline of handicrafts in modern times is perhaps one of the causes for the rise of frustration and the increased susceptibility of the individual to mass movements.

It is impressive to observe how with a fading of the individual's creative powers there appears a pronounced inclination toward joining a mass movement. Here the connection between the escape from an ineffectual self and a responsiveness to mass movements is very clear. The slipping author, artist, scientist—slipping because of a drying up of the creative flow within—drifts sooner or later into the camps of ardent patriots, race mongers, uplift promoters, and champions of causes. Perhaps the sexually impotent are subject to the same impulse.

The Unified Poor

The poor who are members of a compact group—a tribe, a closely knit family, a compact racial or religious group—are relatively free of frustration and hence almost immune to the appeal of a proselytizing mass movement. The less a person sees himself as an autonomous individual capable of shaping his own course and solely responsible for his station in life, the less likely is he to see his poverty as evidence of his own inferiority. A member of a compact group has a higher "revolting point" than an autonomous individual. It requires more misery and personal humiliation to goad him to revolt. The cause of revolution in a totalitarian society is usually a weakening of the totalitarian framework rather than resentment against oppression and distress.

The strong family ties of the Chinese probably kept them for ages relatively immune to the appeal of mass movements. "The European who 'dies for his country' has behaved in a manner that is unintelligible to a Chinaman, because his family is not directly benefited—is, indeed, damaged by the loss of one of its members." On the other hand, he finds it understandable and honorable "when a Chinaman, in consideration of so much paid to his family, consents to be executed as a substitute for a condemned criminal."[4]

It is obvious that a proselytizing mass movement must break down all existing group ties if it is to win a considerable following. The ideal potential convert is the individual who stands alone, who has no collective body he can blend with and lose himself in and so mask the pettiness, meaninglessness, and shabbiness of his individual existence. Where a mass movement finds the corporate pattern of family, tribe, or country in a state of disruption and decay, it moves in and gathers the harvest. Where it finds the

[4] Arthur J. Hubbard, *The Fate of Empires* (New York: Longmans, Green & Company, 1913), p. 170.

corporate pattern in good repair, it must attack and disrupt. On the other hand, when as in Russia we see the Bolshevik movement bolstering family solidarity and encouraging national, racial, and religious cohesion, it is a sign that the movement has passed its dynamic phase, that it has already established its new pattern of life, and that its chief concern is to hold and preserve that which it has attained. In the rest of the world where communism is still a struggling movement, it does all it can to disrupt the family and discredit national, racial, and religious ties.

2

The attitude of rising mass movements toward the family is of considerable interest. Almost all our contemporary movements showed in their early stages a hostile attitude toward the family and did all they could to discredit and disrupt it. They did it by undermining the authority of the parents; by facilitating divorce; by taking over the responsibility for feeding, educating, and entertaining the children; and by encouraging illegitimacy. Crowded housing, exile, concentration camps, and terror also helped to weaken and break up the family. Still, not one of our contemporary movements was so outspoken in its antagonism toward the family as was early Christianity. Jesus minced no words: "For I am come to set a man at variance against his father, and the daughter against her mother, and the daughter in law against her mother in law. And a man's foes shall be they of his own household. He that loveth father or mother more than me is not worthy of me: and he that loveth son or daughter more than me is not worthy of me." When he was told that his mother and brothers were outside desiring to speak with him, he said, "Who is my mother? and who are my brethren? And he stretched forth his hand toward his disciples, and said, Behold my mother, and my brethren!" When one of his disciples asked leave to go and bury his father, Jesus said to him, "Follow me; and let the dead bury their dead." He seemed to sense the ugly family conflicts his movement was bound to provoke both by its proselytizing and by the fanatical hatred of its antagonists. "And the brother shall deliver up the brother to death, and the father the child: and the children shall rise up against their parents, and cause them to be

put to death." It is strange but true that he who preaches brotherly love also preaches against love of mother, father, brother, sister,
wife, and children. The Chinese sage Mo-Tzŭ, who advocated
brotherly love, was rightly condemned by the Confucianists, who
cherished the family above all. They argued that the principle of
universal love would dissolve the family and destroy society. The
proselytizer who comes and says "Follow me" is a family-wreck-
er, even though he is not conscious of any hostility toward the
family and has not the least intention of weakening its solidarity.
When Saint Bernard preached, his influence was such that "moth-
ers are said to have hid their sons from him, and wives their husbands, lest he should lure them away. He actually broke up so
many homes that the abandoned wives formed a nunnery."[5]

3

As one would expect, a disruption of the family, whatever
its causes, fosters automatically a collective spirit and creates a
responsiveness to the appeal of mass movements.

The Japanese invasion undoubtedly weakened the compact
family pattern of the Chinese and contributed to their increased
responsiveness to both nationalism and communism. In the industrialized Western world, the family is weakened and disrupted
mainly by economic factors. Economic independence for women
facilitates divorce. Economic independence for the young weakens parental authority and also hastens an early splitting up of the
family group. The drawing power of large industrial centers on
people living on farms and in small towns strains and breaks family ties. By weakening the family, these factors have contributed
to the growth of the collective spirit in modern times.

4

The discontent generated among Africans and Asians by
their contact with Western civilization is not primarily resentment
against exploitation by domineering foreigners. It is rather the result of a crumbling or weakening of tribal solidarity and communal life.

[5] Brooks Adams, *The Law of Civilization and Decay* (New York: Alfred A. Knopf,
Inc., 1943), p. 142.

The ideal of self-advancement which the West offers brings with it the plague of individual frustration. All the advantages brought by the West are ineffectual substitutes for the sheltering and soothing anonymity of a communal existence. Even when the Westernized Asian or African attains personal success—becomes rich or masters a respected profession—he is not happy. He feels naked and orphaned. The nationalist movements in the colonial countries are partly a striving after group existence and an escape from Western individualism.

The Western colonizing powers offer the gift of individual freedom and independence. They try to teach self-reliance. What it all actually amounts to is individual isolation. It means the cutting off of an immature and poorly furnished individual from the corporate whole and releasing him, in the words of the poet Khomiakov, "to the freedom of his own impotence." The feverish desire to band together and coalesce into marching masses so manifest both in our homelands and in the countries we colonize is the expression of a desperate effort to escape this ineffectual, purposeless individual existence. It is very possible, therefore, that modern nationalist movements may lead—even without Russian influence—to a more or less collectivist rather than democratic form of society.

The policy of an exploiting colonial power should be to encourage communal cohesion among the natives. It should foster equality and a feeling of brotherhood among them. For by how much the ruled blend and lose themselves into a compact whole, by so much is softened the poignancy of their individual futility; and the process which transmutes misery into frustration and revolt is checked at the source. The device of "divide and rule" is ineffective when it aims at a weakening of all forms of cohesion among the ruled. The breaking up of a village community, a tribe, or nation into autonomous individuals does not eliminate or stifle the spirit of rebellion against the ruling power. An effective division is one that fosters a multiplicity of compact bodies—racial, religious, or economic—vying with and suspicious of each other.

Even when a colonial power is wholly philanthropic and its sole aim is to bring prosperity and progress to a "backward" people, it must do all it can to preserve and reinforce the corporate pattern. It must not concentrate on the individual but inject the innovations and reforms into tribal or communal channels and let the tribe or the community progress as a whole. It is perhaps true that the successful modernization of a people can be brought about only within a strong framework of united action. The spectacular modernization of Japan was accomplished in an atmosphere charged with the fervor of united action and group consciousness.

Soviet Russia's advantage as a colonizing power—aside from her perceived lack of racial bias—is that it comes with a ready-made and effective pattern of united action. It can disregard, and indeed deliberately sweep away, all existing group ties without the risk of breeding individual discontent and eventual revolt. For the sovietized native is not left struggling alone in a hostile world. He begins his new life as a member of a closely knit group more compact and communal than his former clan or tribe.

The device of encouraging communal cohesion as a preventive of colonial unrest can also be used to prevent labor unrest in the industrialized countries.

The employer whose only purpose is to keep his workers at their task and get all he can out of them is not likely to attain his goal by dividing them—playing off one worker against the other. It is rather in his interest that the workers should feel themselves part of a whole, and preferably a whole which comprises the employer too. A vivid feeling of solidarity, whether racial, national, or religious, is undoubtedly an effective means of preventing labor unrest. Even when the type of solidarity is such that it cannot include the employer, it nevertheless tends to promote labor contentment and efficiency. Experience shows that production is at its best when the workers feel and act as members of a team. Any policy that disturbs and tears apart the team is bound to cause severe trouble. "Incentive wage plans that offer bonuses to individual workers do more harm than good.... Group incentive plans in which the bonus is based on the work of the whole team, including the foreman ... are much more likely to promote greater productivity and greater satisfaction on the part of the workers."[6]

[6] Peter F. Drucker, "The Way to Industrial Peace," *Harper's Magazine*, November 1946, p. 392.

5

A rising mass movement attracts and holds a following not by its doctrine and promises but by the refuge it offers from the anxieties, barrenness, and meaninglessness of an individual existence. It cures the poignantly frustrated not by conferring on them an absolute truth or by remedying the difficulties and abuses which made their lives miserable, but by freeing them from their ineffectual selves—and it does this by enfolding and absorbing them into a closely knit and exultant corporate whole.

It is obvious, therefore, that, in order to succeed, a mass movement must develop at the earliest moment a compact corporate organization and a capacity to absorb and integrate all comers. It is futile to judge the viability of a new movement by the truth of its doctrine and the feasibility of its promises. What has to be judged is its corporate organization for quick and total absorption of the frustrated. Where new creeds vie with each other for the allegiance of the populace, the one which comes with the most nearly perfected collective framework wins. Of all the cults and philosophies which competed in the Greco-Roman world, Christianity alone developed from its inception a compact organization. "No one of its rivals possessed so powerful and coherent a structure as did the church. No other gave its adherents quite the same feeling of coming into a closely knit community."[7] The Bolshevik movement outdistanced all other Marxist movements in the race for power because of its tight collective organization. The National Socialist movement, too, won out over all the other folkish movements which pullulated in the 1920s because of Hitler's early recognition that a rising mass movement can never go too far in advocating and promoting collective cohesion. He knew that the chief passion of the frustrated is "to belong," and that there cannot be too much cementing and binding to satisfy this passion.

6

The milieu most favorable for the rise and propagation of mass movements is one in which a once compact corporate struc-

[7] Kenneth Scott Latourette, *A History of the Expansion of Christianity* (New York: Harper & Brothers, 1937), vol. I, p. 164.

ture is, for one reason or another, in a state of disintegration. The age in which Christianity rose and spread "was one when large numbers of men were uprooted. The compact city-states had been partly merged into one vast empire . . . and the old social and political groupings had been weakened or dissolved."[8] Christianity made its greatest headway in the large cities where lived "thousands of deracinated individuals, some of them slaves, some freedmen, and some merchants, who had been separated by force or voluntarily from their hereditary milieu."[9] In the countryside where the communal pattern was least disturbed, the new religion found the ground less favorable. The villagers (*pagani*) and the heath-dwellers (heathen) clung longest to the ancient cults. A somewhat similar situation is to be observed in the rise of nationalist and socialist movements in the second half of the nineteenth century: "the extraordinary mobility and urbanization of the population served to create during those decades an extraordinary number of . . . persons uprooted from ancestral soil and local allegiance. Experiencing grave economic insecurity and psychological maladjustment, these were very susceptible to demagogic propaganda, socialist or nationalist or both."[10]

The general rule seems to be that as one pattern of corporate cohesion weakens, conditions become ripe for the rise of a mass movement and the eventual establishment of a new and more vigorous form of compact unity. When a church which was all-embracing relaxes its hold, new religious movements are likely to crystallize. H. G. Wells remarks that at the time of the Reformation people "objected not to the church's power, but to its weaknesses . . . Their movements against the church, within it and without, were movements not for release from a religious control, but for a fuller and more abundant religious control." If the religious mood is undermined by enlightenment, the rising movements will be socialist, nationalist, or racist. The French Revolution, which was also a nationalist movement, came as a reaction not against the vigorous tyranny of the Catholic Church and the ancient regime but against their weakness and ineffectuality.

[8] Latourette, op. cit., p. 23.
[9] Ibid., p. 163
[10] Carlton J. H. Hayes, *A Generation of Materialism* (New York: Harper & Brothers, 1941), p. 254.

When people revolt in a totalitarian society, they rise not against the wickedness of the regime but its weakness.

Where the corporate pattern is strong, it is difficult for a mass movement to find a footing. The communal compactness of the Jews, both in Palestine and the Diaspora, was probably one of the reasons that Christianity made so little headway among them. The destruction of the temple caused, if anything, a tightening of the communal bonds. The synagogue and the congregation received now much of the devotion which formerly flowed toward the temple and Jerusalem. Later, when the Christian church had the power to segregate the Jews in ghettos, it gave their communal compactness an additional reinforcement and thus, unintentionally, ensured the survival of Judaism intact through the ages. The coming of "enlightenment" undermined both orthodoxy and ghetto walls. Suddenly, and perhaps for the first time since the days of Job and Ecclesiastes, the Jew found himself an individual, terribly alone in a hostile world. There was no collective body he could blend with and lose himself in. The synagogue and the congregation had become shriveled lifeless things, while the traditions and prejudices of two thousand years prevented his complete integration with the Gentile corporate bodies. Thus the modern Jew became the most autonomous of individuals and inevitably, too, the most frustrated. It is not surprising, therefore, that the mass movements of modern times often found in him a ready convert. The Jew also crowded the roads leading to palliatives of frustration, such as hustling and migration. And he threw himself into a passionate effort to prove his individual worth by material achievements and creative work. There was, it is true, one speck of corporateness he could create around himself by his own efforts—the family—and he made the most of it. But in the case of the European Jew, Hitler chewed and scorched this only refuge in concentration camps and gas chambers. Thus now, more than ever before, the Jew, particularly in Europe, is the ideal potential convert. And it almost seems providential that Zionism should be on hand in the Jew's darkest hour to enfold him in its corporate embrace and cure him of his individual isolation. Israel is indeed a rare refuge: it is home and family, synagogue and congregation, nation and revolutionary party all in one.

The recent history of Germany also furnishes an interesting

example of the relation between corporate compactness and a receptivity to the appeal of mass movements. There was no likelihood of a genuine revolutionary movement arising in Wilhelmian Germany. The Germans were satisfied with the centralized, authoritarian Kaiser regime, and even defeat in the First World War did not impair their love for it. The revolution of 1918 was an artificial thing with little popular backing. The years of the Weimar Constitution which followed were for most Germans a time of irritation and frustration. Used as they were to commands from above and respect for authority, they found the loose, irreverent democratic order all confusion and chaos. They were shocked to realize "that they had to participate in government, choose a party, and pass judgment upon political matters."[11] They longed for a new corporate whole, more monolithic, all-embracing, and glorious to behold than even the regime of the Kaiser had been—and the Third Reich more than answered their prayer. Hitler's totalitarian regime, once established, was never in danger of mass revolt. So long as the ruling Nazi hierarchy was willing to shoulder all responsibilities and make all decisions, there was not the least chance for any popular antagonism to arise. A danger point could have been reached had Nazi discipline and its totalitarian control been relaxed. What De Tocqueville says of a tyrannical government is true of all totalitarian orders—their moment of greatest danger is when they begin to reform: that is to say, when they begin to show liberal tendencies.

Another and final illustration of the thesis that effective collective bodies are immune to the appeal of mass movements but that a crumbling collective pattern is the most favorable milieu for their rise is found in the relation between the collective body we know as an army and mass movements. There is hardly an instance of an intact army giving rise to a religious, revolutionary, or nationalist movement. On the other hand, a disintegrating army—whether by the orderly process of demobilization or by desertion due to demoralization—is fertile ground for a proselytizing movement. The man just out of the army is an ideal potential

[11] Theodore Abel, *Why Hitler Came into Power* (New York: Prentice-Hall, 1938), p. 150.

convert; we find him among the early adherents of all contemporary mass movements. He feels alone and lost in the free-for-all of civilian life. The responsibilities and uncertainties of an autonomous existence weigh and prey upon him. He longs for certitude, camaraderie, freedom from individual responsibility, and a vision of something altogether different from the competitive free society around him—and he finds all this in the brotherhood and the revivalist atmosphere of a rising movement.

MISFITS

The frustration of misfits can vary in intensity. There are first the temporary misfits: people who have not found their place in life but still hope to find it. Adolescent youth, unemployed college graduates, veterans, new immigrants, and the like are of this category. They are restless, dissatisfied, and haunted by the fear that their best years will be wasted before they reach their goal. They are receptive to the preaching of a proselytizing movement and yet do not always make staunch converts. For they are not irrevocably estranged from the self; they do not see it as irremediably spoiled. It is easy for them to conceive an autonomous existence that is purposeful and hopeful. The slightest evidence of progress and success reconciles them with the world and their selves.

The role of veterans in the rise of mass movements has just been touched upon. A prolonged war by national armies is likely to be followed by a period of social unrest for victors and vanquished alike. The reason is neither the unleashing of passions and the taste of violence during wartime nor the loss of faith in a social order that could not prevent so enormous and meaningless a waste of life and wealth; it is, rather, the prolonged break in the civilian routine of the millions enrolled in the national armies. The returning soldiers find it difficult to recapture the rhythm of their prewar lives. The readjustment to peace and home is slow and painful, and the country is flooded with temporary misfits.

Thus it seems that the passage from war to peace is more critical for an established order than the passage from peace to war.

2

The permanent misfits are those who because of a lack of talent or some irreparable defect in body or mind cannot do the one thing for which their whole being craves. No achievement, however spectacular, in other fields can give them a sense of fulfillment. Whatever they undertake becomes a passionate pursuit, but they never arrive, never pause. They demonstrate the fact that we can never have enough of that which we really do not want, and that we run fastest and farthest when we run from ourselves.

Permanent misfits can find salvation only in a complete separation from the self, and they usually find it by losing themselves in the compact collectivity of a mass movement. By renouncing individual will, judgment, and ambition and dedicating all their powers to the service of an eternal cause, they are at last lifted off the endless treadmill which can never lead them to fulfillment.

The most incurably frustrated—and, therefore, the most vehement—among the permanent misfits are those with an unfulfilled craving for creative work. Both those who try to write, paint, compose, and so on, and fail decisively and those who, after tasting the elation of creativeness, feel a drying up of the creative flow within and know that never again will they produce anything worthwhile are alike in the grip of a desperate passion. Neither fame nor power nor riches nor even monumental achievements in other fields can still their hunger. Even wholehearted dedication to a cause does not always cure them. Their unappeased hunger persists, and they are likely to become the most violent extremists in the service of their cause.

THE INORDINATELY SELFISH

The inordinately selfish are particularly susceptible to frustration. The more selfish a person, the more poignant his disappointments. It is the inordinately selfish, therefore, who are likely to be the most persuasive champions of selflessness.

The fiercest fanatics are often selfish people who were forced, by innate shortcomings or external circumstances, to lose faith in their own selves. They separate the excellent instrument of their selfishness from their ineffectual selves and attach it to the service of some cause. And though it be a faith of love and humility they adopt, they can be neither loving nor humble.

THE AMBITIOUS FACING UNLIMITED OPPORTUNITIES

Unlimited opportunities can be as potent a cause of frustration as a paucity or lack of opportunities. When opportunities are apparently unlimited, there is an inevitable deprecation of the present. The attitude is: "All that I am doing or possibly can do is chicken feed compared with what is left undone." Such is the frustration which broods over gold camps and haunts taut minds in boom times. Hence the remarkable fact that, joined with the ruthless self-seeking which seems to be the mainspring of gold-hunters, land-grabbers, and other get-rich-quick enthusiasts, there is an excessive readiness for self-sacrifice and united action. Patriotism, racial solidarity, and even the preaching of revolution find a more ready response among people who see limitless opportunities spread out before them than among those who move within the fixed limits of a familiar, orderly, and predictable pattern of existence.

MINORITIES

A minority is in a precarious position, however protected it be by law or force. The frustration engendered by the unavoidable sense of insecurity is less intense in a minority intent on preserving its identity than in one bent upon dissolving in and blending with the majority. A minority which preserves its identity is inevitably a compact whole which shelters the individual, gives him a sense of belonging, and immunizes him against frustration. On the other hand, in a minority bent on assimilation, the individual stands alone, pitted against prejudice and discrimination. He is also burdened with the sense of guilt, however vague, of a renegade.

Again, within a minority bent on assimilation, the least and most successful (economically and culturally) are likely to be more frustrated than those in between. The man who fails sees himself as an outsider; and, in the case of a member of a minority group who wants to blend with the majority, failure intensifies the feeling of not belonging. A similar feeling crops up at the other end of the economic or cultural scale. Those of a minority who attain fortune and fame often find it difficult to gain entrance to the exclusive circles of the majority. They are thus made conscious of their foreignness. Furthermore, having evidence of their individual superiority, they resent the admission of inferiority implied in the process of assimilation. Thus it is to be expected that the least and most successful of a minority bent on assimilation should be the most responsive to the appeal of a proselytizing mass movement. The least and most successful among the Italian Americans were the most ardent admirers of Mussolini's revolution; the least and most successful among the Irish Americans were the most responsive to De Valera's call; the least and most successful among the Jews are the most responsive to Zionism; the least and most successful among the Negroes are the most race conscious.

THE BORED

There is perhaps no more reliable indicator of a society's ripeness for a mass movement than the prevalence of unrelieved boredom. In almost all the descriptions of the periods preceding the rise of mass movements there is reference to vast ennui, and in their earliest stages mass movements are more likely to find sympathizers and support among the bored than among the exploited and oppressed. To a deliberate fomenter of mass upheavals, the report that people are bored stiff should be at least as encouraging as that they are suffering from intolerable economic or political abuses.

When people are bored, it is primarily with their own selves that they are bored. The consciousness of a barren, meaningless existence is the main fountainhead of boredom. People who are not conscious of their individual separateness, as is the case with those who are members of a compact tribe, church, or party, are not accessible to boredom. The differentiated individual is free of boredom only when he is engaged either in creative work or some absorbing occupation or when he is wholly engrossed in the struggle for existence. Pleasure-chasing and dissipation are ineffective palliatives. Where people live autonomous lives and are not badly off, yet are without abilities or opportunities for creative work or useful action, there is no telling to what desperate and fantastic shifts they might resort in order to give meaning and purpose to their lives.

Boredom probably accounts for the almost invariable presence of spinsters and middle-aged women at the birth of mass movements. Even in the case of Islam and the Nazi movement, which frowned upon female activity outside the home, we find women of a certain type playing an important role in the early stage of their development.

Marriage has had for women many equivalents of joining a mass movement. It has offered them a new purpose in life, a new future, and a new identity (a new name). The boredom of spinsters and of women who no longer find joy and fulfillment in marriage stems from an awareness of a barren, spoiled life. By embracing a cause and dedicating their energies and substance to its advancement, they find a new life of purpose and meaning. Hitler made full use of "the society ladies thirsting for adventure, sick of their empty lives, no longer getting a 'kick' out of love affairs."[12] He was financed by the wives of some of the great industrialists long before their husbands had heard of him. Miriam Beard tells of a similar role played by bored wives of businessmen before the French Revolution: "they were devastated with boredom and given to fits of the vapors. Restlessly, they applauded innovators."

THE SINNERS

The sardonic remark that patriotism is the last refuge of scoundrels has also a less derogatory meaning. Fervent patriotism as well as religious and revolutionary enthusiasm often serves as a refuge from a guilty conscience. It is a strange thing that both the injurer and the injured, the sinner and he who is sinned against,

---

[12] Hermann Rauschning, *Hitler Speaks* (New York: G. P. Putnam's Sons, 1940), p. 268.

should find in the mass movement an escape from a blemished life. Remorse and a sense of grievance seem to drive people in the same direction.

It sometimes seems that mass movements are custom-made to fit the needs of the criminal—not only for the catharsis of his soul but also for the exercise of his inclinations and talents. The technique of a proselytizing mass movement aims to evoke in the faithful the mood and frame of mind of a repentant criminal. Self-surrender, which is, as will be shown below, the source of a mass movement's unity and vigor, is a sacrifice, an act of atonement, and clearly no atonement is called for unless there is a poignant sense of sin. Here, as elsewhere, the technique of a mass movement aims to infect people with a malady and then offer the movement as a cure. "What a task confronts the American clergy," laments R. S. Aldrich, an American divine, "preaching the good news of a Savior to people who for the most part have no real sense of sin." An effective mass movement cultivates the idea of sin. It depicts the autonomous self not only as barren and helpless but also as vile. To confess and repent is to slough off one's individual distinctness and separateness, and salvation is found by losing oneself in the holy oneness of the congregation.

There is a tender spot for the criminal and an ardent wooing of him in all mass movements. Saint Bernard, the moving spirit of the Second Crusade, thus appealed for recruits: "For what is it but an exquisite and priceless chance of salvation due to God alone, that the omnipotent should deign to summon to his service, as though they were innocent, murderers, ravishers, adulterers, perjurers, and those guilty of every crime?" Revolutionary Russia too had a tender spot for the common criminal, though it was ruthless with the heretic—the ideological "deviationist." It is perhaps true that the criminal who embraces a holy cause is more ready to risk his life and go to extremes in its defense than people who are awed by the sanctity of life and property.

Crime is to some extent a substitute for a mass movement. Where public opinion and law enforcement are not too stringent, and poverty not absolute, the underground pressure of malcontents and misfits often leaks out in crime. It has been observed that in the exaltation of mass movements (whether patriotic, religious, or revolutionary) common crime declines.

3 UNITED ACTION

AND SELF-SACRIFICE

THE VIGOR OF A MASS MOVEMENT stems from the propensity of its followers for united action and self-sacrifice. When we ascribe the success of a movement to its faith, doctrine, propaganda, leadership, ruthlessness, and so on, we are but referring to instruments of unification and to means used to inculcate a readiness for self-sacrifice. It is perhaps impossible to understand the nature of mass movements unless it is recognized that their chief preoccupation is to foster, perfect, and perpetuate a facility for united action and self-sacrifice. To know the processes by which such a facility is engendered is to grasp the inner logic of most of the characteristic attitudes and practices of an active mass movement. With few exceptions, any group or organization which tries, for one reason or another, to create and maintain compact unity and a constant readiness for self-sacrifice usually manifests the peculiarities—both noble and base—of a mass movement. On the other hand, a mass movement is bound to lose much which distinguishes it from other types of organization when it relaxes its collective compactness and begins to countenance self-interest as a legitimate motive of activity. In times of peace and prosperity, a democratic nation is an institutionalized association of more or less free individuals. On the other hand, in time of crisis, when the nation's existence is threatened and it tries to reinforce its unity and generate in its people a readiness for self-sacrifice, it almost always assumes in some degree the character of a mass movement. The same is true of religious and revolutionary organizations: whether or not they develop into mass movements depends less on the doctrine they preach and the program they project than on the degree of their preoccupation with unity and the readiness for self-sacrifice.

The important point is that in the poignantly frustrated the propensities for united action and self-sacrifice arise spontaneously. It should be possible, therefore, to gain some clues concerning the nature of these propensities, and the technique to be employed for their deliberate inculcation, by tracing their spontaneous emergence in the frustrated mind. What ails the frustrated? It is the consciousness of an irremediably blemished self. Their chief desire is to escape that self—and it is this desire which manifests itself in a propensity for united action and self-sacrifice. The revulsion from an unwanted self, and the impulse to forget it, mask it, slough it off, and lose it, produce both a readiness to sacrifice the self and a willingness to dissolve it by losing one's individual distinctness in a compact collective whole. Moreover, the estrangement from the self is usually accompanied by a train of diverse and seemingly unrelated attitudes and impulses which a closer probing reveals to be essential factors in the process of unification and of self-sacrifice. In other words, frustration not only gives rise to the desire for unity and the readiness for self-sacrifice but also creates a mechanism for their realization. Such diverse phenomena as a deprecation of the present, a facility for make-believe, a proneness to hate, a readiness to imitate, credulity, a readiness to attempt the impossible, and many others which crowd the minds of the intensely frustrated are, as we shall see, unifying agents and prompters of recklessness.

Here an attempt will be made to show that when we set out to inculcate in people a facility for united action and self-sacrifice, we do all we can—whether we know it or not—to induce and encourage an estrangement from the self, and that we strive to evoke and cultivate in them many of the diverse attitudes and impulses which accompany the spontaneous estrangement from the self in the frustrated. In short, we shall try to show that the technique of an active mass movement consists basically in the inculcation and cultivation of proclivities and responses indigenous to the frustrated mind.

The reader is expected to quarrel with much that is said here. He is likely to feel that much has been exaggerated and much ignored. But this is not an authoritative text. It does not shy away from half-truths so long as they seem to hint at a new approach and help to formulate new questions. "To illustrate a principle," says Bagehot, "you must exaggerate much and you must omit much."

2

The capacities for united action and self-sacrifice seem almost always to go together. When we hear of a group that is particularly contemptuous of death, we are usually justified in concluding that the group is closely knit and thoroughly unified. On the other hand, when we face a member of a compact group, we are likely to find him contemptuous of death also. Both united action and self-sacrifice require self-diminution. In order to become part of a compact whole, the individual has to forego much. He has to give up privacy, individual judgment, and often individual possessions. To school a person for united action is, therefore, to ready him for acts of self-denial. On the other hand, the man who practices self-abnegation sloughs off the hard shell which keeps him apart from others and is thus made assimilable. Every unifying agent is, therefore, a promoter of self-sacrifice and vice versa. In the following sections, a division is made for the sake of convenience. But the dual function of each factor is always kept in mind.

FACTORS PROMOTING SELF-SACRIFICE

The technique of fostering a readiness to fight and to die consists in separating the individual from his flesh-and-blood self—in not allowing him to be his real self. This can be achieved by the thorough assimilation of the individual into a compact collective body; by endowing him with an imaginary self (make-believe); by implanting in him a deprecating attitude toward the present and riveting his interest on things that are not yet; by interposing a fact-proof screen between him and reality (doctrine); by preventing, through the injection of passions, the establishment of a stable equilibrium between the individual and his self (fanaticism).

Identification with a Collective Whole

To ripen a person for self-sacrifice he must be stripped of his individual identity and distinctness. He must cease to be George, Hans, Ivan, or Tadao—a human atom with an existence bounded by birth and death. The most drastic way to achieve this end is by the complete assimilation of the individual into a collective body. The fully assimilated individual does not see himself and others as human beings. When asked who he is, his automatic response is that he is a German, a Russian, a Japanese, a Christian, a Muslim, a member of a certain tribe or family. He has no purpose, worth, or destiny apart from his collective body; and as long as that body lives he cannot really die.

To a man utterly without a sense of belonging, mere life is all that matters. It is the only reality in an eternity of nothingness, and he clings to it with shameless despair. Dostoevski gave words to this state of mind in *Crime and Punishment*. The student Raskolnikov wanders about the streets of St. Petersburg in a delirious state. He has several days before murdered two old women with an ax. He feels cut off from mankind. As he passes through the red-light district near the Hay Market he muses, "If one had to live on some high rock on such a narrow ledge that he'd only room to stand, and the ocean, everlasting darkness, everlasting solitude, everlasting tempest around him, if he had to remain standing on a square yard of space all his life, a thousand years, eternity, it were better to live so than to die at once! Only to live, to live and live! Life whatever it may be!"

The effacement of individual separateness must be thorough. In every act, however trivial, the individual must by some ritual associate himself with the congregation, the tribe, the party, and so on. His joys and sorrows, his pride and confidence must spring from the fortunes and capacities of the group rather than from his individual prospects and abilities. Above all, he must never feel alone. Though stranded on a desert island, he must still feel that he is under the eyes of the group. To be cast out from the group should be equivalent to being cut off from life.

This is undoubtedly a primitive state of being, and its most perfect examples are found among primitive tribes. Mass movements strive to approximate this primitive perfection; we are not imagining things when the anti-individualist bias of contemporary mass movements strikes us as a throwback to the primitive.

2

The capacity to resist coercion stems partly from the individual's identification with a group. The people who stood up best in the Nazi concentration camps were those who felt themselves members of a compact party (the Communists), of a church (priests and ministers), or of a close-knit national group. The individualists, whatever their nationality, caved in. The Western European Jew proved to be the most defenseless. Spurned by Gentiles (even most of those within the concentration camps), and without vital ties with a Jewish community, he faced his tormentors alone—forsaken by the whole of humanity. One realizes now that the ghetto of the Middle Ages was for the Jews more a fortress than a prison. Without the sense of utmost unity and distinctness which the ghetto imposed upon them, they could not have endured with unbroken spirit the violence and abuse of those dark centuries. When the Middle Ages returned for a brief decade in our day, they caught the Jew without his ancient defenses and crushed him.

The unavoidable conclusion seems to be that when the individual faces torture or annihilation, he cannot rely on the resources of his own individuality. His only source of strength is in being not himself but part of something mighty, glorious, and indestructible. Faith here is primarily a process of identification, the process by which the individual ceases to be himself and becomes part of something eternal. Faith in humanity, in posterity, in the destiny of one's religion, nation, race, party, or family—what is it but the visualization of that eternal something to which we attach the self that is about to be annihilated?

It is somewhat terrifying to realize that the totalitarian leaders of our day, in recognizing this source of desperate courage, made use of it not only to steel the spirit of their followers but also to break the spirit of their opponents. In his purges of the old Bolshevik leaders, Stalin succeeded in turning proud and brave men into cringing cowards by depriving them of any possibility of identification with the party they had served all their lives and with the Russian masses. These old Bolsheviks had long before cut themselves off from people outside the Soviet Union. They had an unbounded contempt for the past and for history which could still be made by capitalistic humanity. They had renounced God. There was for them neither past nor future, neither memory nor glory outside the confines of Russia and the Communist party—and both these were now wholly and irrevocably in Stalin's hands. They felt themselves, in the words of Bukharin, "isolated from every thing that constitutes the essence of life." So they confessed. By humbling themselves before the congregation of the faithful, they broke out of their isolation. They renewed their communion with the eternal whole by reviling the self, accusing it of monstrous and spectacular crimes, and sloughing it off in public.

3

The same Russians who cringed and crawled before Stalin's secret police displayed unsurpassed courage when facing—singly or in a group—the invading Nazis. The reason for this contrasting behavior is not that Stalin's police were more ruthless than Hitler's armies, but that when facing Stalin's police the Russian felt a mere individual while, when facing the Germans, he saw himself a member of a mighty race, possessed of a glorious past and an even more glorious future.

Similarly, in the case of the Jews, their behavior in Palestine could not have been predicted from their behavior in Europe. The British colonial officials in Palestine followed a policy sound in logic but lacking in insight. They reasoned that since Hitler had managed to exterminate six million Jews without meeting serious resistance, it should not be too difficult to handle the 600,000 Jews in Palestine. Yet they found that the Jews in Palestine, however recently arrived, were a formidable enemy: reckless, stubborn, and resourceful. The Jew in Europe faced his enemies alone, an isolated individual, a speck of life floating in an eternity of nothingness. In Palestine he felt himself not a human atom but a member of an eternal race, with an immemorial past behind it and a breathtaking future ahead.

4

In order to maintain the submissiveness of the Russian masses, there must not be the least chance of an identification with any collective body outside Russia. The purpose of the Iron Curtain is perhaps more to prevent the Russian people from reaching out—even in thought—toward an outside world than to prevent the infiltration of spies and saboteurs. The curtain is both physical and psychological. The elimination of any chance of emigration blurs the awareness of outside humanity in Russian minds. One might as well dream and hope of escaping to another planet. The psychological barrier is equally important: the Kremlin's brazen propaganda strives to impress upon the Russians that there is nothing worthy and eternal, nothing deserving of admiration and reverence, nothing worth identifying oneself with, outside the confines of the Soviet Union.

Make-believe

Dying and killing seem easy when they are part of a ritual, ceremonial, dramatic performance, or game. There is need for some kind of make-believe in order to face death unflinchingly. To our real, naked selves there is not a thing on earth or in heaven worth dying for. It is only when we see ourselves as actors in a staged (and therefore unreal) performance that death loses its frightfulness and finality and becomes an act of make-believe and a theatrical gesture. It is one of the main tasks of a real leader to mask the grim reality of dying and killing by evoking in his followers the illusion that they are participating in a grandiose spectacle, a solemn or lighthearted dramatic performance.

Hitler dressed eighty million Germans in costumes and made them perform in a grandiose, heroic, and bloody opera. In Russia, where even the building of a latrine involved some self-sacrifice, life was an uninterrupted soul-stirring drama from the beginning of the revolution. The people of London acted heroically under a hail of bombs because Churchill cast them in the role of heroes. They played their heroic role before a vast audience—ancestors, contemporaries, and posterity—and on a stage lighted by a burning world city and to the music of barking guns and screaming bombs. It is doubtful whether in our contemporary world, with its widespread individual differentiation, any measure of general self-sacrifice can be realized without theatrical hocus-pocus and fireworks. It is difficult to see, therefore, how any Labour government in England could have fully realized a program of socialization, which demands some measure of self-sacrifice from every Briton, in the colorless and undramatic setting of a socialist Britain. The untheatricality of most British Socialist leaders was a mark of uprightness and intellectual integrity, but it handicapped the experiment of nationalization which was undoubtedly the central purpose of their lives.

2

The indispensability of play-acting in the grim business of dying and killing is particularly evident in the case of armies. Their uniforms, flags, emblems, parades, music, and elaborate etiquette and ritual are designed to separate the soldier from his flesh-and-blood self and mask the overwhelming reality of life and death. We speak of the "theater" of war and of battle "scenes." In their battle orders, army leaders invariably remind their soldiers that the eyes of the world are on them, that their ancestors are watching them, and that posterity shall hear of them. The great general knows how to conjure an audience out of the sands of the desert and the waves of the ocean.

Glory is largely a theatrical concept. There is no striving for glory without the vivid awareness of an audience—the knowledge that our mighty deeds will come to the ears of our contemporaries or "of those who are to be." We are ready to sacrifice our true, transitory self for the imaginary eternal self we are building up, by our heroic deeds, in the opinion and imagination of others.

In the practice of mass movements, make-believe plays perhaps a more enduring role than any other factor. When faith and the power to persuade or coerce are gone, make-believe lingers on. There is no doubt that in staging its processions, parades, rituals, and ceremonials, a mass movement touches a responsive chord in every heart. Even the most sober-minded are carried away by the sight of an impressive mass spectacle. There is an exhilaration and getting out of one's skin in both participants and spectators. It is possible that the frustrated are more responsive to the might and splendor of the mass than people who are self-sufficient. The desire to escape or camouflage their unsatisfactory selves develops in the frustrated a facility for pretending—for making a show— and also a readiness to identify themselves wholly with an imposing mass spectacle.

Deprecation of the Present

At its inception a mass movement seems to champion the present against the past. It sees in established institutions and privileges an encroachment of a vile, senile past on a virginal present. But, to pry loose the stranglehold of the past, there is need for utmost unity and unlimited self sacrifice. This means that the people called upon to attack the past in order to liberate the present must be willing to give up enthusiastically any chance of ever tasting or inheriting the present. The absurdity of the proposition is obvious. Hence the inevitable shift in emphasis once the movement starts rolling. The present—the original objective—is shoved off the stage and its place taken by posterity—the future. More still: the present is driven back as if it were an unclean thing and lumped with the detested past. The battle line is now drawn between things that are and have been, and the things that are not yet.

To lose one's life is but to lose the present; and, clearly, to lose a defiled, worthless present is not to lose much.

2

Not only does a mass movement depict the present as mean and miserable, it deliberately makes it so. It fashions a pattern of individual existence that is dour, hard, repressive, and dull. It decries pleasures and comforts and extols the rigorous life. It views ordinary enjoyment as trivial or even discreditable, and represents the pursuit of personal happiness as immoral. To enjoy oneself is to have truck with the enemy—the present. The prime objective of the ascetic ideal preached by most movements is to breed contempt for the present. The campaign against the appetites is an effort to pry loose tenacious tentacles holding on to the present. That this cheerless individual life runs its course against a colorful and dramatic background of collective pageantry serves to accentuate its worthlessness.

The very impracticability of many of the goals which a mass movement sets itself is part of the campaign against the present. All that is practicable, feasible, and possible is part of the present. To offer something practicable would be to increase the promise of the present and reconcile us with it. Faith in miracles, too, implies a rejection and a defiance of the present. When Tertullian proclaimed, "And He was buried and rose again; it is certain because it is impossible," he was snapping his fingers at the present. Finally, the mysticism of a movement is also a means of deprecating the present. It sees the present as the faded and distorted reflection of a vast unknown throbbing underneath and beyond us. The present is a shadow and an illusion.

3

There can be no genuine deprecation of the present without the assured hope of a better future. For however much we lament the baseness of our times, if the prospect offered by the future is that of advanced deterioration or even an unchanged continuation of the present, we are inevitably moved to reconcile ourselves with our existence—difficult and mean though it be.

All mass movements deprecate the present by depicting it as a mean preliminary to a glorious future, a mere doormat on the threshold of the millennium. To a religious movement the present is a place of exile, a vale of tears leading to the heavenly kingdom; to a social revolution it is a mean way station on the road to Utopia; to a nationalist movement it is an ignoble episode preceding the final triumph.

It is true of course that the hope released by a vivid visualization of a glorious future is a most potent source of daring and self-forgetting, more potent than the implied deprecation of the present. A mass movement has to center the hearts and minds of its followers on the future even when it is not engaged in a life-and-death struggle with established institutions and privileges. The self-sacrifice involved in mutual sharing and cooperative action is impossible without hope. When today is all there is, we grab all we can and hold on. We are afloat in an ocean of nothingness, and we hang on to any miserable piece of wreckage as if it were the tree of life. On the other hand, when everything is ahead and yet to come, we find it easy to share all we have and to forgo advantages within our grasp. The behavior of the members of the Donner party when they were buoyed by hope and, later, when hope was gone illustrates the dependence of cooperativeness and the communal spirit on hope. Those without hope are divided and driven to desperate self-seeking. Common suffering by itself, when not joined with hope, does not unite, nor does it evoke mutual generosity. The enslaved Hebrews in Egypt, "their lives made bitter with hard bondage," were a bickering, backbiting lot. Moses had to give them hope of a promised land before he could join them together. The thirty thousand hopeless people in the concentration camp of Buchenwald did not develop any form of united action, nor did they manifest any readiness for self-sacrifice. There was there more greed and ruthless selfishness than in the greediest and most corrupt of free societies. "Instead of studying the way in which they could best help each other they used all their ingenuity to dominate and oppress each other."[1]

4

A glorification of the past can serve as a means to belittle the present. But unless joined with sanguine expectations of the future, an exaggerated view of the past results in an attitude of caution and not in the reckless strivings of a mass movement. On the other hand, there is no more potent dwarfing of the present than by viewing it as a mere link between a glorious past and a glorious future. Thus, though a mass movement at first turns its back on the past, it eventually develops a vivid awareness, often specious, of a distant glorious past. Religious movements go back to the day of creation; social revolutions tell of a golden age when men were free, equal, and independent; nationalist movements

[1] Christopher Burney, *The Dungeon Democracy* (New York: Duell, Sloan & Pearce, 1946), p. 147. See also, on the same subject, Odd Nansen, *From Day To Day* (New York: G. P. Putnam's Sons, 1949), p. 335; also Arthur Koestler, *The Yogi and the Commissar* (New York: Macmillan Company, 1945), p. 178.

revive or invent memories of past greatness. This preoccupation with the past stems not only from a desire to demonstrate the legitimacy of the movement and the illegitimacy of the old order but also to show up the present as a mere interlude between past and future.

A historical awareness also imparts a sense of continuity. Possessed of a vivid vision of past and future, the true believer sees himself part of something that stretches endlessly backward and forward—something eternal. He can let go of the present (and of his own life) not only because it is a poor thing, hardly worth hanging on to, but also because it is not the beginning and the end of all things. Furthermore, a vivid awareness of past and future robs the present of its reality. It makes the present seem as a section in a procession or a parade. The followers of a mass movement see themselves on the march with drums beating and colors flying. They are participators in a soul-stirring drama played to a vast audience—generations gone and generations yet to come. They are made to feel that they are not their real selves but actors playing a role, and their doings a "performance" rather than the real thing. Dying, too, they see as a gesture, an act of make-believe.

5

A deprecating attitude toward the present fosters a capacity for prognostication. The well-adjusted make poor prophets. On the other hand, those who are at war with the present have an eye for the seeds of change and the potentialities of small beginnings.

A pleasant existence blinds us to the possibilities of drastic change. We cling to what we call our common sense, our practical point of view. Actually, these are but names for an all-absorbing familiarity with things as they are. The tangibility of a pleasant and secure existence is such that it makes other realities, however imminent, seem vague and visionary. Thus it happens that when the times become unhinged, it is the practical people who are caught unaware and are made to look like visionaries who cling to things that do not exist.

On the other hand, those who reject the present and fix their eyes and hearts on things to come have a faculty for detecting the embryo of future danger or advantage in the ripeness of their times. Hence the frustrated individual and the true believer make better prognosticators than those who have reason to want the preservation of the status quo. "It is often the fanatics, and not always the delicate spirits, that are found grasping the right thread of the solutions required by the future."[2]

6

It is of interest to compare here the attitudes toward present, future, and past shown by the conservative, the liberal, the skeptic, the radical, and the reactionary.

The conservative doubts that the present can be bettered, and he tries to shape the future in the image of the present. He goes to the past for reassurance about the present: "I wanted the sense of continuity, the assurance that our contemporary blunders were endemic in human nature, that our new fads were very ancient heresies, that beloved things which were threatened had rocked not less heavily in the past."[3] How, indeed, like the skeptic is the conservative! "Is there any thing whereof it may be said, See, this is new? it hath been already of old time, which was before us." To the skeptic the present is the sum of all that has been and shall be. "The thing that hath been, it is that which shall be; and that which is done is that which shall be done: and there is no new thing under the sun." The liberal sees the present as the legitimate offspring of the past and as constantly growing and developing toward an improved future: to damage the present is to maim the future. All three then cherish the present, and, as one would expect, they do not take willingly to the idea of self-sacrifice. Their attitude toward self-sacrifice is best expressed by the skeptic: "for a living dog is better than a dead lion. For the living know that they shall die: but the dead know not any thing . . . neither have they any more a portion for ever in any thing that is done under the sun."

The radical and the reactionary loathe the present. They see it as an aberration and a deformity. Both are ready to proceed ruth-

[2] Ernest Renan, *History of the People of Israel* (Boston: Little, Brown & Company, 1888–1896), vol. III, p. 416.
[3] John Buchan, *Pilgrim's Way* (Boston: Houghton Mifflin Company, 1940), p. 183.

lessly and recklessly with the present, and both are hospitable to the idea of self-sacrifice. Wherein do they differ? Primarily in their view of the malleability of man's nature. The radical has a passionate faith in the infinite perfectibility of human nature. He believes that by changing man's environment and by perfecting a technique of soul forming, a society can be wrought that is wholly new and unprecedented. The reactionary does not believe that man has unfathomed potentialities for good in him. If a stable and healthy society is to be established, it must be patterned after the proven models of the past. He sees the future as a glorious restoration rather than an unprecedented innovation.

In reality, the boundary line between radical and reactionary is not always distinct. The reactionary manifests radicalism when he comes to recreate his ideal past. His image of the past is based less on what it actually was than on what he wants the future to be. He innovates more than he reconstructs. A somewhat similar shift occurs in the case of the radical when he goes about building his new world. He feels the need for practical guidance, and since he has rejected and destroyed the present he is compelled to link the world with some point in the past. If he has to employ violence in shaping the new, his view of man's nature darkens and approaches closer to that of the reactionary.

The blending of the reactionary and the radical is particularly evident in those engaged in a nationalist revival. The followers of Gandhi in India and the Zionists in Palestine would revive a glorified past and simultaneously create an unprecedented Utopia. The prophets, too, were a blend of the reactionary and the radical. They preached a return to the ancient faith and also envisaged a new world and a new life.

7

That the deprecating attitude of a mass movement toward the present seconds the inclinations of the frustrated is obvious. What is surprising, when listening to the frustrated as they decry the present and all its works, is the enormous joy they derive from doing so. Such delight cannot come from the mere venting of a grievance. There must be something more—and there is. By expatiating upon the incurable baseness and vileness of the times, the frustrated soften their feeling of failure and isolation. It is as if they said, "Not only our blemished selves but the lives of all our contemporaries, even the most happy and successful, are worthless and wasted." Thus by deprecating the present they acquire a vague sense of equality.

The means, also, that a mass movement uses to make the present unpalatable strike a responsive chord in the frustrated. The self-mastery needed in overcoming the appetites gives them an illusion of strength. They feel that in mastering themselves they have mastered the world. The mass movement's advocacy of the impracticable and impossible also agrees with their taste. Those who fail in everyday affairs show a tendency to reach out for the impossible. It is a device to camouflage their shortcomings. For when we fail in attempting the possible, the blame is solely ours; but when we fail in attempting the impossible, we are justified in attributing it to the magnitude of the task. There is less risk in being discredited when trying the impossible than when trying the possible. It is thus that failure in everyday affairs often breeds an extravagant audacity.

One gains the impression that the frustrated derive as much satisfaction—if not more—from the means a mass movement uses as from the ends it advocates. The delight of the frustrated in chaos and in the downfall of the fortunate and prosperous does not spring from an ecstatic awareness that they are clearing the ground for the heavenly city. In their fanatical cry of "all or nothing at all" the second alternative echoes perhaps a more ardent wish than the first.

"Things Which Are Not"

One of the rules that emerges from a consideration of the factors that promote self-sacrifice is that we are less ready to die for what we have or are than for what we wish to have and to be. It is a perplexing and unpleasant truth that when men already have "something worth fighting for," they do not feel like fighting. People who live full, worthwhile lives are not usually ready to die for their own interests or for their country or for a cause.[4] Craving, not having, is the mother of a reckless giving of oneself.

"Things which are not" are indeed mightier than "things that are." In all ages men have fought most desperately for beautiful cities yet to be built and gardens yet to be planted. Satan did not digress to tell all he knew when he said, "All that a man hath will he give for his life." All he hath, yes. But he sooner dies than yield aught of that which he hath not yet.

It is strange, indeed, that those who hug the present and hang on to it with all their might should be the least capable of defending it. And that, on the other hand, those who spurn the present and dust their hands of it should have all its gifts and treasures showered on them unasked.

Dreams, visions, and wild hopes are mighty weapons and realistic tools. The practical-mindedness of a true leader consists in recognizing the practical value of these tools. Yet this recognition usually stems from a contempt of the present which can be traced to a natural ineptitude in practical affairs. The successful businessman is often a failure as a communal leader because his mind is attuned to the "things that are" and his heart set on that which can be accomplished "in our time." Failure in the management of practical affairs seems to be a qualification for success in the management of public affairs. And it is perhaps fortunate that some proud natures when suffering defeat in the practical world do not feel crushed but are suddenly fired with the apparently absurd conviction that they are eminently competent to direct the fortunes of the community and the nation.

2

It is not altogether absurd that people should be ready to die for a button, a flag, a word, an opinion, a myth, and so on. It is, on the contrary, the least reasonable thing to give one's life for something palpably worth having. For, surely, one's life is the most real of all things real, and without it there can be no having

[4] There is an echo of this disconcerting truth in a letter from Norway written at the time of the Nazi invasion: "The trouble with us is that we have been so favored in all ways that many of us have lost the true spirit of self-sacrifice. Life has been so pleasant to a great number of people that they are unwilling to risk it seriously." Quoted by J. D. Barry in the San Francisco *News*, June 22, 1940.

of things worth having. Self-sacrifice cannot be a manifestation of tangible self-interest. Even when we are ready to die in order not to get killed, the impulse to fight springs less from self-interest than from intangibles such as tradition, honor (a word), and, above all, hope. Where there is no hope, people either run or allow themselves to be killed without a fight. They will hang on to life as in a daze. How else explain the fact that millions of Europeans allowed themselves to be led into annihilation camps and gas chambers, knowing beyond doubt that they were being led to death? It was not the least of Hitler's formidable powers that he knew how to drain his opponents (at least in continental Europe) of all hope. His fanatical conviction that he was building a new order that would last a thousand years communicated itself both to followers and antagonists. To the former it gave the feeling that in fighting for the Third Reich they were in league with eternity, while the latter felt that to struggle against Hitler's new order was to defy inexorable fate.

We saw that the Jews who submitted to extermination in Hitler's Europe fought recklessly when transferred to Palestine. And though it is said that they fought in Palestine because they had no choice—they had to fight or have their throats cut by the Arabs— it is still true that their daring and reckless readiness for self-sacrifice sprang not from despair but from their fervent preoccupation with the revival of an ancient land and an ancient people. They, indeed, fought and died for cities yet to be built and gardens yet to be planted.

Doctrine

The readiness for self-sacrifice is contingent on an imperviousness to the realities of life. He who is free to draw conclusions from his individual experience and observation is not usually hospitable to the idea of martyrdom. For self-sacrifice is an unreasonable act. It cannot be the end product of a process of probing and deliberating. All active mass movements strive, therefore, to interpose a fact-proof screen between the faithful and the realities of the world. They do this by claiming that the ultimate and absolute truth is already embodied in their doctrine and that there is no truth or certitude outside it. The facts on which the true believer bases his conclusions must not be derived from his experience or observation but from holy writ. "So tenaciously should we cling to the word revealed by the Gospel, that were I to see all the Angels of Heaven coming down to me to tell me something different, not only would I not be tempted to doubt a single syllable, but I would shut my eyes and stop my ears, for they would not deserve to be either seen or heard."[5] To rely on the evidence of the senses and of reason is heresy and treason. It is startling to realize how much unbelief is necessary to make belief possible. What we know as blind faith is sustained by innumerable unbeliefs. The fanatical Japanese in Brazil refused to believe for years the evidence of Japan's defeat. The fanatical Communist refuses to believe any unfavorable report or evidence about Russia, nor will he be disillusioned by seeing with his own eyes the cruel misery inside the Soviet promised land.

It is the true believer's ability to shut his eyes and stop his ears to facts which do not deserve to be either seen or heard that is the source of his unequaled fortitude and constancy. He cannot be frightened by danger or disheartened by obstacle or baffled by contradictions because he denies their existence. Strength of faith, as Bergson pointed out, manifests itself not in moving mountains but in not seeing mountains to move. And it is the certitude of his infallible doctrine that renders the true believer impervious to the uncertainties, surprises, and unpleasant realities of the world around him.

Thus the effectiveness of a doctrine should not be judged by its profundity, its sublimity, or the validity of the truths it embodies, but by how thoroughly it insulates the individual from his self and the world as it is. What Pascal said of an effective religion is true of any effective doctrine: it must be "contrary to nature, to common sense, and to pleasure."

2

The effectiveness of a doctrine does not come from its meaning but from its certitude. No doctrine, however profound and sublime, will be effective unless it is presented as the embodi-

---

[5] Luther, "Table Talk, Number 1687." Quoted by Frantz Funck-Brentano, *Luther* (London: Jonathan Cape, Ltd., 1939), p. 246.

ment of the one and only truth. It must be the one word from which all things are and all things speak. Crude absurdities, trivial nonsense, and sublime truths are equally potent in readying people for self-sacrifice if they are accepted as the sole, eternal truth.

It is obvious, therefore, that in order to be effective a doctrine must not be understood but has to be believed in. We can be absolutely certain only about things we do not understand. A doctrine that is understood is shorn of its strength. Once we understand a thing, it is as if it had originated in us. And, clearly, those who are asked to renounce the self and sacrifice it cannot see eternal certitude in anything which originates in that self. The fact that they fully understand a thing impairs its validity and certitude in their eyes.

The devout are always urged to seek the absolute truth with their hearts and not their minds. "It is the heart which is conscious of God, not the reason," Pascal says. Rudolph Hess, when swearing in the entire Nazi party in 1934, exhorted his hearers, "Do not seek Adolph Hitler with your brains; all of you will find him with the strength of your hearts." When a movement begins to rationalize its doctrine and make it intelligible, it is a sign that its dynamic span is over; that it is primarily interested in stability. For, as will be shown, the stability of a regime requires the allegiance of the intellectuals, and it is to win them rather than to foster self-sacrifice in the masses that a doctrine is made intelligible.

If a doctrine is not unintelligible, it has to be vague; and if neither unintelligible nor vague, it has to be unverifiable. One has to get to heaven or the distant future to determine the truth of an effective doctrine. When some part of a doctrine is relatively simple, there is a tendency among the faithful to complicate and obscure it. Simple words are made pregnant with meaning and made to look like symbols in a secret message. There is thus an illiterate air about the most literate true believer. He seems to use words as if he were ignorant of their true meaning. Hence, too, his taste for quibbling, hairsplitting, and scholastic tortuousness.

3

To be in possession of an absolute truth is to have a net of familiarity spread over the whole of eternity. There are no surprises and no unknowns. All questions have already been answered, all decisions made, all eventualities foreseen. The true believer is without wonder and hesitation. In Pascal's words, "Who knows Jesus knows the reason of all things." The true doctrine is a master key to all the world's problems. With it the world can be taken apart and put together. The official history of the Communist party states: "The power of Marxist-Leninist theory lies in the fact that it enables the Party to find the right orientation in any situation, to understand the inner connection of current events, to foresee their course, and to perceive not only how and in what direction they are developing in the present but how and in what direction they are bound to develop in the future." The true believer is emboldened to attempt the unprecedented and the impossible not only because his doctrine gives him a sense of omnipotence but also because it gives him unqualified confidence in the future.

An active mass movement rejects the present and centers its interest on the future. It is from this attitude that it derives its strength, for it can proceed recklessly with the present—with the health, wealth, and lives of its followers. But it must act as if it had already read the book of the future to the last word. Its doctrine is proclaimed as a key to that book.

4

Are the frustrated more easily indoctrinated than the non-frustrated? Are they more credulous? Pascal was of the opinion that "one was well-minded to understand holy writ when one hated oneself." There is apparently some connection between dissatisfaction with oneself and a proneness to credulity. The urge to escape our real self is also an urge to escape the rational and the obvious. The refusal to see ourselves as we are develops a distaste for facts and cold logic. There is no hope for the frustrated in the actual and the possible. Salvation can come to them only from the miraculous, which seeps through a crack in the iron wall of inexorable reality. They ask to be deceived. What Stresemann said of the Germans is true of the frustrated in general: "[They] pray not only for [their] daily bread, but also for [their] daily illusion." The rule seems to be that those who find no difficulty in deceiving themselves are easily deceived by others. They are easily persuaded and led.

A peculiar side of credulity is that it is often joined with a proneness to imposture. The association of believing and lying is not characteristic solely of children. The inability or unwillingness to see things as they are promotes both gullibility and charlatanism.

Fanaticism

It was suggested in the first chapter that mass movements are often necessary for the realization of drastic and abrupt change. It seems strange that even practical and desirable changes, such as the renovation of stagnant societies, should require for their realization an atmosphere of intense passion and should have to be accompanied by all the faults and follies of an active mass movement. The surprise lessens when we realize that the chief preoccupation of an active mass movement is to instill in its followers a facility for united action and self-sacrifice, and that it achieves this facility by stripping each human entity of its distinctness and autonomy and turning it into an anonymous particle with no will and no judgment of its own. The result is not only a compact and fearless following but also a homogeneous plastic mass that can be kneaded at will. The human plasticity necessary for the realization of drastic and abrupt change seems, therefore, to be a by-product of the process of unification and of the inculcation of a readiness for self-sacrifice.

The important point is that the estrangement from the self, which is a precondition for both plasticity and conversion, almost always proceeds in an atmosphere of intense passion. For not only is the stirring of passion an effective means of upsetting an established equilibrium between a man and his self, it is also the inevitable by-product of such an upsetting. Passion is released even when the estrangement from the self is brought about by the most unemotional means. Only the individual who has come to terms with his self can have a dispassionate attitude toward the world. Once the harmony with the self is upset, and a man is impelled to reject, renounce, distrust, or forget his self, he turns into a highly reactive entity. Like an unstable chemical radical, he hungers to combine with whatever comes within his reach. He cannot stand apart, poised and self-sufficient, but has to attach himself wholeheartedly to one side or another.

By kindling and fanning violent passions in the hearts of their followers, mass movements prevent the settling of an inner balance. They also employ direct means to effect an enduring estrangement from the self They depict an autonomous self-sufficient existence not only as barren and meaningless but also as depraved and evil. Man on his own is a helpless, miserable, and sinful creature. His only salvation is in rejecting his self and in finding a new life in the bosom of a corporate body—be it a church, a nation, or a party. In its turn, this vilification of the self keeps passion at white heat.

2

The fanatic is perpetually incomplete and insecure. He cannot generate self-assurance out of his individual resources—out of his rejected self—but finds it only by clinging passionately to whatever support he happens to embrace. This passionate attachment is the essence of his blind devotion and religiosity, and he sees in it the source of all virtue and strength. Though his single-minded dedication is a holding on for dear life, he easily sees himself as the supporter and defender of the cause to which he clings. And he is ready to sacrifice his life to demonstrate to himself and others that such indeed is his role. He sacrifices his life to prove his worth.

It goes without saying that the fanatic is convinced that the cause he holds is monolithic and eternal—a rock of ages. Still, his sense of security is derived from his passionate attachment and not from the excellence of his cause. The fanatic is not really a stickler for principle. He embraces a cause not primarily because of its justness and holiness but because of his desperate need for something to hold on to. Often, indeed, it is his need for passionate attachment which turns every cause he embraces into a holy cause.

The fanatic cannot be weaned away from his cause by an appeal to his reason or moral sense. He fears compromise and cannot be persuaded to qualify the certitude and righteousness of his cause. But he finds no difficulty in swinging suddenly and wildly from one cause to another. He cannot be convinced but only converted. His passionate attachment is more vital than the quality of the cause to which he is attached.

3

Though they seem at opposite poles, fanatics of all kinds are actually crowded together at one end. It is the fanatic and the moderate who are poles apart and never meet. The fanatics of various hues eye each other with suspicion and are ready to fly at each other's throat. But they are neighbors and almost of one family. They hate each other with the hatred of brothers.

The opposite of the religious fanatic is not the fanatical atheist but the gentle cynic who cares not whether there is a God or not. The atheist is a religious person. He believes in atheism as though it were a new religion. He is an atheist with devoutness and unction. According to Renan, "The day after that on which the world should no longer believe in God, atheists would be the wretchedest of all men." So, too, the opposite of the chauvinist is not the traitor but the reasonable citizen who is in love with the present and has no taste for martyrdom and the heroic gesture. The traitor is usually a fanatic—radical or reactionary—who goes over to the enemy in order to hasten the downfall of a world he loathes. Most of the traitors in the Second World War came from the extreme right. "There seems to be a thin line between violent, extreme nationalism and treason."[6]

The kinship between the reactionary and the radical has been dealt with. All of us who lived through the Hitler decade know that the reactionary and the radical have more in common than either has with the liberal or the conservative.

4

It is doubtful whether the fanatic who deserts his holy cause or is suddenly left without one can ever adjust himself to an autonomous individual existence. He remains a homeless hitchhiker on the highways of the world, thumbing a ride on any eternal cause that rolls by. An individual existence, even when purposeful, seems to him trivial, futile, and sinful. To live without an ardent dedication is to be adrift and abandoned. He sees in toler-

[6] Harold Ettlinger, *The Axis on the Air* (Indianapolis: Bobbs-Merrill Company, 1943), p. 39.

ance a sign of weakness, frivolity, and ignorance. He hungers for the deep assurance which comes with total surrender—with the wholehearted clinging to a creed and a cause. What matters is not the contents of the cause but the total dedication and the communion with a congregation. He is even ready to take up arms against his former cause, but it must be a genuine crusade—uncompromising, intolerant, proclaiming the one and only truth.

Mass Movements and Armies

It is well at this point, before leaving the subject of self-sacrifice, to have a closer look at the similarities and differences between mass movements and armies.

The similarities are many: both mass movements and armies are collective bodies; both strip the individual of his separateness and distinctness; both demand self-sacrifice, unquestioning obedience, and single-hearted allegiance; both make extensive use of make-believe to promote daring and united action; and both can serve as a refuge for the frustrated who cannot endure an autonomous existence. A military body like the Foreign Legion attracts many of the types who usually rush to join a new movement. It is also true that the recruiting officer, the Communist agitator, and the missionary often fish simultaneously in the cesspools of skid row.

But the differences are fundamental: an army does not come to fulfill a need for a new way of life; it is not a road to salvation. It can be used as a stick in the hand of a coercer to impose a new way of life and force it down unwilling throats. But the army is mainly an instrument devised for the preservation or expansion of an established order—old or new. It is a temporary instrument that can be assembled and taken apart at will. The mass movement, on the other hand, seems an instrument of eternity, and those who join it do so for life. The ex-soldier is a veteran, even a hero; the ex–true believer is a renegade. The army is an instrument for bolstering, protecting, and expanding the present. The mass movement comes to destroy the present. Its preoccupation is with the future, and it derives its vigor and drive from this preoccupation. When a mass movement begins to be preoccupied with the present, it means that it has arrived. It ceases then to be a movement and becomes an institutionalized organization—an established church, a government, or an army (of soldiers or workers). The popular army, which is often an end product of a mass movement, retains many of the trappings of the movement—pious verbiage, slogans, holy symbols—but like any other army it is held together less by faith and enthusiasm than by the unimpassioned mechanism of drill, esprit de corps, and coercion. It soon loses the asceticism and unction of a holy congregation and displays the boisterousness and the taste for the joys of the present which is characteristic of all armies.

Being an instrument of the present, an army deals mainly with the possible. Its leaders do not rely on miracles. Even when animated by fervent faith, they are open to compromise. They reckon with the possibility of defeat and know how to surrender. On the other hand, the leader of a mass movement has an overwhelming contempt for the present—for all its stubborn facts and perplexities, even those of geography and the weather. He relies on miracles. His hatred of the present (his nihilism) comes to the fore when the situation becomes desperate. He destroys his country and his people rather than surrender.

The spirit of self-sacrifice within an army is fostered by devotion to duty, make-believe, esprit de corps, drill, faith in a leader, sportsmanship, the spirit of adventure, and the desire for glory. These factors, unlike those employed by a mass movement, do not spring from a deprecation of the present and a revulsion from an unwanted self. They can unfold therefore in a sober atmosphere. The fanatical soldier is usually a fanatic turned soldier rather than the other way around. An army's spirit of self-sacrifice is most nobly expressed in the words Sarpedon spoke to Glaucus as they stormed the Grecian wall: "O my friend, if we, leaving this war, could escape from age and death, I should not here be fighting in the van; but now, since many are the modes of death impending over us which no man can hope to shun, let us press on and give renown to other men, or win it for ourselves."

The most striking difference between mass movements and armies is in their attitude to the multitude and the rabble. De Tocqueville observed that soldiers are "the men who lose their heads most easily, and who generally show themselves weakest on days of revolution." To the typical general, the mass is something

his army would turn into if it were to fall apart. He is more aware
of the inconstancy of the mass and its will to anarchy than of its
readiness for self-sacrifice. He sees it as the poisonous end product
of a crumbling collective body rather than the raw material of a
new world. His attitude is a mixture of fear and contempt. He
knows how to suppress the mass but not how to win it. On the
other hand, the mass movement leader—from Moses to Hitler—
draws his inspiration from the sea of upturned faces, and the roar
of the mass is as the voice of God in his ears. He sees an irresistible
force within his reach, a force he alone can harness. And with this
force he will sweep away empires and armies and all the mighty
present. The face of the mass is as "the face of the deep" out of
which, like God on the day of creation, he will bring forth a new
world.

UNIFYING AGENTS

Hatred

Hatred is the most accessible and comprehensive of all unifying agents. It pulls and whirls the individual away from his own
self, makes him oblivious of his weal and future, frees him of
jealousies and self-seeking. He becomes an anonymous particle
quivering with a craving to fuse and coalesce with his like into
one flaming mass. Heine suggests that what Christian love cannot
do is effected by a common hatred.

Mass movements can rise and spread without belief in a God,
but never without belief in a devil. Usually the strength of a mass
movement is proportionate to the vividness and tangibility of its
devil. When Hitler was asked whether he thought the Jew must
be destroyed, he answered, "No. . . . We should have then to invent him. It is essential to have a tangible enemy, not merely an
abstract one." F. A. Voigt tells of a Japanese mission that arrived
in Berlin in 1932 to study the National Socialist movement. Voigt
asked a member of the mission what he thought of the movement.
He replied, "It is magnificent. I wish we could have something
like it in Japan, only we can't, because we haven't got any Jews."
It is perhaps true that the insight and shrewdness of the men who

know how to set a mass movement in motion, or how to keep one going, manifest themselves as much in knowing how to pick a worthy enemy as in knowing what doctrine to embrace and what program to adopt. The theoreticians of the Kremlin hardly waited for the guns of the Second World War to cool before they picked the democratic West, and particularly America, as the chosen enemy. It is doubtful whether any gesture of goodwill or any concession from our side would have reduced the volume and venom of vilification against us.

One of Chiang Kai-shek's most serious shortcomings was his failure to find an appropriate new devil once the Japanese enemy vanished from the scene. The ambitious but simple-minded general was perhaps too conceited to realize that it was not he but the Japanese devil who generated the enthusiasm, the unity, and the readiness for self-sacrifice of the Chinese masses during the war.

2

Common hatred unites the most heterogeneous elements. To share a common hatred, with an enemy even, is to infect him with a feeling of kinship and thus sap his powers of resistance. Hitler used anti-Semitism not only to unify his Germans but also to sap the resoluteness of Jew-hating Poland, Rumania, Hungary, and finally even France. He made a similar use of anticommunism.

3

It seems that, like the ideal deity, the ideal devil is one. We have it from Hitler—the foremost authority on devils—that the genius of a great leader consists in concentrating all hatred on a single foe, making "even adversaries far removed from one another seem to belong to a single category." When Hitler picked the Jew as his devil, he peopled practically the whole world outside Germany with Jews or those who worked for them. "Behind England stands Israel, and behind France, and behind the United States." Stalin, too, adhered to the monotheistic principle when picking a devil. Once this devil was a fascist; then he was an American plutocrat.

Again, like an ideal deity, the ideal devil is omnipotent and omnipresent. When Hitler was asked whether he was not attributing rather too much importance to the Jews, he exclaimed: "No, no, no! . . . It is impossible to exaggerate the formidable quality of the Jew as an enemy." Every difficulty and failure within the movement is the work of the devil, and every success is a triumph over his evil plotting.

Finally, it seems, the ideal devil is a foreigner. To qualify as a devil, a domestic enemy must be given a foreign ancestry. Hitler found it easy to brand the German Jews as foreigners. The Russian revolutionary agitators emphasized the foreign origin (Varangian, Tartar, Western) of the Russian aristocracy. In the French Revolution the aristocrats were seen as "descendants of barbarous Germans, while French commoners were descendants of civilized Gauls and Romans," and in the Puritan Revolution the royalists "were labeled 'Normans,' descendants of a group of foreign invaders."[7]

4

We do not usually look for allies when we love. Indeed, we often look on those who love with us as rivals and trespassers. But we always look for allies when we hate.

It is understandable that we should look for others to side with us when we have a just grievance and crave to retaliate against those who wronged us. The puzzling thing is that when our hatred does not spring from a visible grievance and does not seem justified, the desire for allies becomes more pressing. It is chiefly the unreasonable hatreds that drive us to merge with those who hate as we do, and it is this kind of hatred that serves as one of the most effective cementing agents.

Whence come these unreasonable hatreds, and why their unifying effect? They are an expression of a desperate effort to suppress an awareness of our inadequacy, worthlessness, guilt, and other shortcomings. Self-contempt is transmuted into hatred of others—and there is a most determined and persistent effort to mask the switch. Obviously, the most effective way of doing this

[7] Crane Brinton, *The Anatomy of Revolution* (New York: W. W. Norton & Company, Inc., 1938), p. 62.

is to find others, as many as possible, who hate as we do. Here more than anywhere else we need general consent, and much of our proselytizing consists perhaps in infecting others not with our brand of faith but with our particular brand of unreasonable hatred.

Even in the case of a just grievance, our hatred comes less from a wrong done to us than from the consciousness of our helplessness, inadequacy, and cowardice—in other words, from self-contempt. When we feel superior to our tormentors, we are likely to despise them, even pity them, but not hate them.[8] That the relation between grievance and hatred is not simple and direct is also seen from the fact that the released hatred is not always directed against those who wronged us. Often, when we are wronged by one person, we turn our hatred on a wholly unrelated person or group. Russians, bullied by Stalin's secret police, are easily inflamed against "capitalist warmongers"; Germans, aggrieved by the Versailles treaty, avenge themselves by exterminating Jews; Zulus, oppressed by Boers, butcher Hindus; poor whites, exploited by Dixiecrats, lynch Negroes.

Self-contempt, as Pascal said, produces in man "the most unjust and criminal passions imaginable, for he conceives a mortal hatred against that truth which blames him and convinces him of his faults."

5

That hatred springs more from self-contempt than from a legitimate grievance is seen in the intimate connection between hatred and a guilty conscience.

There is perhaps no surer way of infecting ourselves with virulent hatred toward a person than by doing him a grave injustice. That others have a just grievance against us is a more potent reason for hating them than that we have a just grievance against them. We do not make people humble and meek when we show them their guilt and cause them to be ashamed of themselves. We are more likely to stir their arrogance and rouse in them a reckless

[8] When John Huss saw an old woman dragging a fagot to add to his funeral pyre, he said, "O sancta simplicitas!" Quoted by Ernest Renan, *The Apostles* (Boston: Roberts Brothers, 1898), p. 43.

aggressiveness. Self-righteousness is a loud din raised to drown the voice of guilt within us.

There is a guilty conscience behind every brazen word and act and behind every manifestation of self-righteousness.

To wrong those we hate is to add fuel to our hatred. Conversely, to treat an enemy with magnanimity is to blunt our hatred for him.

The most effective way to silence our guilty conscience is to convince ourselves and others that those we have sinned against are indeed depraved creatures, deserving every punishment, even extermination. We cannot pity those we have wronged, nor can we be indifferent toward them. We must hate and persecute them or else leave the door open to self-contempt.

A sublime religion inevitably generates a strong feeling of guilt. There is an unavoidable contrast between loftiness of profession and imperfection of practice. And, as one would expect, the feeling of guilt promotes hate and brazenness. Thus it seems that the more sublime the faith the more virulent the hatred it breeds.

6

It is easier to hate an enemy with much good in him than one who is all bad. We cannot hate those we despise. The Japanese had an advantage over us in that they admired us more than we admired them. They could hate us more fervently than we could hate them. Modern Americans have been poor haters in international affairs because of their innate feeling of superiority over all foreigners. An American's hatred for a fellow American (for Hoover or Roosevelt) is far more virulent than any antipathy he can work up against foreigners. It is of interest that the long-backward South has shown more xenophobia than the rest of the country. Should Americans begin to hate foreigners wholeheartedly, it will be an indication that they have lost confidence in their own way of life.

The undercurrent of admiration in hatred manifests itself in the inclination to imitate those we hate. Thus every mass movement shapes itself after its specific devil. Christianity at its height realized the image of the antichrist. The Jacobins practiced all the evils of the tyranny they had risen against. Soviet Russia is realizing the purest and most colossal example of monopolistic capitalism. Hitler, who believed the forgery to be true, took the Protocols of the Elders of Zion for his guide and textbook; he followed them "down to the veriest detail."[9]

It is startling to see how the oppressed almost invariably shape themselves in the image of their hated oppressors. That the evil men do lives after them is partly because those who have reason to hate the evil most shape themselves after it and thus perpetuate it. It is obvious, therefore, that the influence of the fanatic is bound to be out of all proportion to his abilities. Both by converting and antagonizing, he shapes the world in his own image. Fanatic Christianity put its imprint upon the ancient world both by gaining adherents and by evoking in its pagan opponents a strange fervor and a new ruthlessness. Hitler imposed himself upon the world both by promoting Nazism and by forcing the democracies to become zealous, intolerant, and ruthless. Communist Russia shapes both its adherents and its opponents in its own image.

Thus, though hatred is a convenient instrument for mobilizing a community for defense, it does not, in the long run, come cheap. We pay for it by losing all or many of the values we have set out to defend.

Hitler, who sensed the undercurrent of admiration in hatred, drew a remarkable conclusion. It is of the utmost importance, he said, that the National Socialist should seek and deserve the violent hatred of his enemies. Such hatred would be proof of the superiority of the National Socialist faith. "The best yardstick for the value of his [the National Socialist's] attitude, for the sincerity of his conviction, and the force of his will is the hostility he receives from the . . . enemy."

7

It seems that when we are oppressed by the knowledge of our worthlessness we do not see ourselves as lower than some and higher than others, but as lower than the lowest of mankind. We hate then the whole world, and we would pour our wrath upon the whole of creation.

[9] Hermann Rauschning, *Hitler Speaks* (New York: G. P. Putnam's Sons, 1940), p. 235.

There is deep reassurance for the frustrated in witnessing the downfall of the fortunate and the disgrace of the righteous. They see in a general downfall an approach to the brotherhood of all. Chaos, like the grave, is a haven of equality. Their burning conviction that there must be a new life and a new order is fueled by the realization that the old will have to be razed before the new can be built. Their clamor for a millennium is shot through with a hatred for all that exists, and a craving for the end of the world.

8

Passionate hatred can give meaning and purpose to an empty life. Thus people haunted by the purposelessness of their lives try to find a new content not only by dedicating themselves to a cause but also by nursing a fanatical grievance. A mass movement offers them unlimited opportunities for both.

9

Whether it is true or not as Pascal says that "all men by nature hate each other," and that love and charity are only "a feint and a false image, for at bottom they are but hate," one cannot escape the impression that hatred is an all-pervading ingredient in the compounds and combinations of our inner life. All our enthusiasms, devotions, passions, and hopes, when they decompose, release hatred. On the other hand it is possible to synthesize an enthusiasm, a devotion, and a hope by activating hatred. Said Martin Luther, "When my heart is cold and I cannot pray as I should I scourge myself with the thought of the impiety and ingratitude of my enemies, the Pope and his accomplices and vermin, and Zwingli, so that my heart swells with righteous indignation and hatred and I can say with warmth and vehemence: 'Holy be Thy Name, Thy Kingdom come, Thy Will be done!' And the hotter I grow the more ardent do my prayers become."

10

Unity and self-sacrifice, of themselves, even when fostered by the most noble means, produce a facility for hating. Even

when men league themselves mightily together to promote tolerance and peace on earth, they are likely to be violently intolerant
toward those not of a like mind.

The estrangement from the self, without which there can be
neither selflessness nor a full assimilation of the individual into a
compact whole, produces, as already mentioned, a proclivity for
passionate attitudes, including passionate hatred. There are also
other factors which favor the growth of hatred in an atmosphere
of unity and selflessness. The act of self-denial seems to confer on
us the right to be harsh and merciless toward others. The impression somehow prevails that the true believer, particularly the religious individual, is a humble person. The truth is that the surren-
dering and humbling of the self breed pride and arrogance. The
true believer is apt to see himself as one of the chosen, the salt of
the earth, the light of the world, a prince disguised in meekness,
who is destined to inherit this earth and the kingdom of heaven
too. He who is not of his faith is evil; he who will not listen shall
perish.

There is also this: when we renounce the self and become part
of a compact whole, we not only renounce personal advantage but
are also rid of personal responsibility. There is no telling to what
extremes of cruelty and ruthlessness a man will go when he is
freed from the fears, hesitations, and doubts and the vague stirrings of decency that go with individual judgment. When we lose
our individual independence in the corporateness of a mass movement, we find a new freedom—freedom to hate, bully, lie, torture, murder, and betray without shame and remorse. Herein undoubtedly lies part of the attractiveness of a mass movement. We
find there the "right to dishonour," which according to Dostoevski
has an irresistible fascination. Hitler had a contemptuous opinion
of the brutality of the autonomous individual. "Any violence
which does not spring from a firm, spiritual base will be wavering
and uncertain. It lacks the stability which can only rest in a fanatical outlook."

Thus hatred is not only a means of unification but also its
product. Renan says that we have never, since the world began,
heard of a merciful nation. Nor, one may add, have we heard of a
merciful church or a merciful revolutionary party. The hatred
and cruelty which have their source in selfishness are ineffectual

things compared with the venom and ruthlessness born of selflessness.

When we see the bloodshed, terror, and destruction born of
such generous enthusiasms as the love of God, love of Christ, love
of a nation, compassion for the oppressed, and so on, we usually
blame this shameful perversion on a cynical, power-hungry leadership. Actually, it is the unification set in motion by these enthusiasms, rather than the manipulations of a scheming leadership,
that transmutes noble impulses into a reality of hatred and violence. The deindividualization which is a prerequisite for thorough integration and selfless dedication is also, to a considerable
extent, a process of dehumanization. The torture chamber is a
corporate institution.

Imitation

Imitation is an essential unifying agent. The development
of a close-knit group is inconceivable without a diffusion of uniformity. The one-mindedness and *Gleichschaltung* prized by every mass movement are achieved as much by imitation as by obedience. Obedience itself consists as much in the imitation of an
example as in the following of a precept.

Though the imitative capacity is present in all people, it can
be stronger in some than in others. The question is whether the
frustrated, who, as suggested earlier, not only have a propensity
for united action but are also equipped with a mechanism for its
realization, are particularly imitative. Is there a connection between frustration and the readiness to imitate? Is imitation in
some manner a means of escape from the ills that beset the frustrated?

The chief burden of the frustrated is the consciousness of a
blemished, ineffectual self, and their chief desire is to slough off
the unwanted self and begin a new life. They try to realize this
desire either by finding a new identity or by blurring and camouflaging their individual distinctness, and both these ends are
reached by imitation.

The less satisfaction we derive from being ourselves, the greater is our desire to be like others. We are therefore more ready to
imitate those who are different from us than those nearly like us,

and those we admire than those we despise. The imitativeness of the oppressed is notable.

As to the blurring and camouflaging of the self, it is achieved solely by imitation—by becoming as like others as possible. The desire to belong is partly a desire to lose oneself.

Finally, the lack of self-confidence characteristic of the frustrated also stimulates their imitativeness. The more we mistrust our judgment and luck, the more are we ready to follow the example of others.

2

Mere rejection of the self, even when not accompanied by a search for a new identity, can lead to increased imitativeness. The rejected self ceases to assert its claim to distinctness, and there is nothing to resist the propensity to copy. The situation is not unlike that observed in children and undifferentiated adults, where the lack of a distinct individuality leaves the mind without guards against the intrusion of influences from without.

3

A feeling of superiority counteracts imitation. Had the millions of immigrants who came to this country been superior people—the cream of the countries they came from—there would have been not one U.S.A. but a mosaic of lingual and cultural groups. It was because the majority of the immigrants were of the lowest and the poorest, the despised and the rejected, that the heterogeneous millions blended so rapidly and thoroughly. They came here with the ardent desire to shed their Old World identity and be reborn to a new life, and they were automatically equipped with an unbounded capacity to imitate and adopt the new. The strangeness of the new country attracted rather than repelled them. They craved a new identity and a new life—and the stranger the new world, the more it suited their inclination. Perhaps, to the non-Anglo-Saxons, the strangeness of the language was an added attraction. To have to learn to speak enhanced the illusion of being born anew.

4

Imitation is often a shortcut to a solution. We copy when we lack the inclination, the ability, or the time to work out an independent solution. People in a hurry will imitate more readily than people at leisure. Hustling thus tends to produce uniformity. And in the deliberate fusing of individuals into a compact group, incessant action will play a considerable role.

5

Unification of itself, whether brought about by persuasion, coercion, or spontaneous surrender, tends to intensify the imitative capacity. A civilian drafted into the army and made a member of a close-knit military unit becomes more imitative than he was in civilian life. The unified individual is without a distinct self; he is perennially incomplete and immature and therefore without resistance against influences from without. The marked imitativeness of primitive people is perhaps due less to their primitiveness than to the fact that they are usually members of compact clans or tribes.

The ready imitativeness of a unified following is both an advantage and a peril to a mass movement. The faithful are easily led and molded, but they are also particularly susceptible to foreign influences. One has the impression that a thoroughly unified group is easily seduced and corrupted. The preaching of all mass movements bristles with admonitions against copying foreign models and "doing after all their abominations." The imitation of outsiders is branded as treason and apostasy. "Whoever copies a foreigner is guilty of lèse-nation (an insult to the nation) like a spy who admits an enemy by a secret doorway."[10] Every device is used to cut off the faithful from intercourse with unbelievers. Some mass movements go to the extreme of leading their following into the wilderness in order to allow an undisturbed settling of the new pattern of life.

Contempt for the outside world is of course the most effective

---

[10] The Italian minister of education in 1926. Quoted by Julien Benda, *The Treason of the Intellectuals* (New York: William Morrow Company, 1928), p. 39.

defense against disruptive imitation. However, an active mass movement prizes hatred above passive contempt, and hatred does not stifle imitation but often stimulates it. Only in the case of small corporate bodies enclosed in a sea of foreignness, and intent solely on preserving their distinctness, is contempt employed as an insulator. It leads to an exclusiveness inhospitable to converts.

The imitativeness of its members gives a thoroughly unified group great flexibility and adaptability. It can adopt innovations and change its orientation with astounding ease. The rapid modernization of a united Japan or Turkey contrasts markedly with the slow and painful adaptation to new ways in China, Iran, and other countries not animated by a spirit of unity. A thoroughly unified Soviet Russia has a better chance of assimilating new methods and a new way of life than the loosely joined empire of the czars. It is also obvious that a primitive people with an intact collective framework can be more readily modernized than one with a crumbling tribal or communal pattern.

Persuasion and Coercion

We tend today to exaggerate the effectiveness of persuasion as a means of inculcating opinion and shaping behavior. We see in propaganda a formidable instrument. To its skillful use we attribute many of the startling successes of the mass movements of our time, and we have come to fear the word as much as the sword.

Actually the fabulous effects ascribed to propaganda have no greater foundation in fact than the fall of the walls of Jericho ascribed to the blast of Joshua's trumpets. Were propaganda by itself one tenth as potent as it is made out to be, the totalitarian regimes of Russia, Germany, Italy, and Spain would have been mild affairs. They would have been blatant and brazen but without the ghastly brutality of secret police, concentration camps, and mass extermination.

The truth seems to be that propaganda on its own cannot force its way into unwilling minds; neither can it inculcate something wholly new; nor can it keep people persuaded once they have ceased to believe. It penetrates only into minds already open, and rather than instill opinion it articulates and justifies opinions already present in the minds of its recipients. The gifted propagandist brings to a boil ideas and passions already simmering in the minds of his hearers. He echoes their innermost feelings. Where opinion is not coerced, people can be made to believe only in what they already "know."

Propaganda by itself succeeds mainly with the frustrated. Their throbbing fears, hopes, and passions crowd at the portals of their senses and get between them and the outside world. They cannot see but what they have already imagined, and it is the music of their own souls they hear in the impassioned words of the propagandist. Indeed, it is easier for the frustrated to detect their own imaginings and hear the echo of their own musings in impassioned double-talk and sonorous refrains than in precise words joined together with faultless logic.

Propaganda by itself, however skillful, cannot keep people persuaded once they have ceased to believe. To maintain itself, a mass movement has to order things so that when the people no longer believe, they can be made to believe by force.

As we shall see, words are an essential instrument in preparing the ground for a mass movement. But once the movement is realized, words, though still useful, cease to play a decisive role. So acknowledged a master of propaganda as Joseph Goebbels admitted in an unguarded moment that "A sharp sword must always stand behind propaganda if it is to be really effective." He also sounded apologetic when he claimed that "it cannot be denied that more can be done with good propaganda than by no propaganda at all."

2

Contrary to what one would expect, propaganda becomes more fervent and importunate when it operates in conjunction with coercion than when it has to rely solely on its own effectiveness.

Both they who convert and they who are converted by coercion need the fervent conviction that the faith they impose or are forced to adopt is the only true one. Without this conviction, the proselytizing terrorist, if he is not vicious to begin with, is likely to feel a criminal, and the coerced convert to see himself as a coward who prostituted his soul to live.

Propaganda thus serves more to justify ourselves than to convince others; and the more reason we have to feel guilty, the more fervent our propaganda.

3

It is probably as true that violence breeds fanaticism as that fanaticism begets violence. It is often impossible to tell which came first. Both those who employ violence and those subject to it are likely to develop a fanatical state of mind. Ferrero says of the terrorists of the French Revolution that the more blood they "shed the more they needed to believe in their principles as absolutes. Only the absolute might still absolve them in their own eyes and sustain their desperate energy. [They] did not spill all that blood because they believed in popular sovereignty as a religious truth; they tried to believe in popular sovereignty as a religious truth because their fear made them spill so much blood."[11] The practice of terror serves the true believer not only to cow and crush his opponents but also to invigorate and intensify his own faith. Every lynching in our South not only intimidated the Negro but also invigorated the fanatical conviction of white supremacy.

In the case of the coerced, too, violence can beget fanaticism. There is evidence that the coerced convert is often as fanatical in his adherence to the new faith as the persuaded convert, and sometimes even more so. It is not always true that "He who complies against his will is of his own opinion still." Islam imposed its faith by force, yet the coerced Muslims displayed a devotion to the new faith more ardent than that of the first Arabs engaged in the movement. According to Renan, Islam obtained from its coerced converts "a faith ever tending to grow stronger." Fanatical orthodoxy is in all movements a late development. It comes when the movement is in full possession of power and can impose its faith by force as well as by persuasion.

[11] Guglielmo Ferrero, *Principles of Power* (New York: G. P. Putnam's Sons, 1942), p. 100.

Thus coercion when implacable and persistent has an unequaled persuasiveness, and this not only with simple souls but also with those who pride themselves on the strength and integrity of their intellect. When an arbitrary decree from the Kremlin forces scientists, writers, and artists to recant their convictions and confess their errors, the chances are that such recantations and confessions represent genuine conversions rather than lip service. It needs fanatical faith to rationalize our cowardice.

4

There is hardly an example of a mass movement achieving vast proportions and a durable organization solely by persuasion. K. S. Latourette, a very Christian historian, has to admit that "However incompatible the spirit of Jesus and armed force may be, and however unpleasant it may be to acknowledge the fact, as a matter of plain history the latter has often made it possible for the former to survive."[12] It was the temporal sword that made Christianity a world religion. Conquest and conversion went hand in hand, the latter often serving as a justification and a tool for the former. Where Christianity failed to gain or retain the backing of state power, it achieved neither a wide nor a permanent hold. "In Persia . . . Christianity confronted a state religion sustained by the crown and never became the faith of more than a minority."[13] In the phenomenal spread of Islam, conquest was a primary factor and conversion a by-product. "The most flourishing periods for Mohammedanism have been at the times of its greatest political ascendancy; and it is at those times that it has received its largest accession from without."[14] The Reformation made headway only where it gained the backing of the ruling prince or the local government. Said Melanchthon, Luther's wisest lieutenant, "Without the intervention of the civil authority what would our precepts become?—Platonic laws." Where, as in France, the state power was against it, it was drowned in blood and never rose again. In

[12] Kenneth Scott Latourette, A History of the Expansion of Christianity (New York: Harper & Brothers, 1937), vol. I, p. 164.

[13] Kenneth Scott Latourette, The Unquenchable Light (New York: Harper & Brothers, 1941), p. 33.

[14] Charles Reginald Haines, Islam as a Missionary Religion (London: Society for Promoting Christian Knowledge, 1889), p. 206.

the case of the French Revolution, "It was the armies of the Revolution, not its ideas, that penetrated throughout the whole of Europe."[15] There was no question of intellectual contagion. Dumouriez protested that the French proclaimed the sacred law of liberty "like the Koran, sword in hand." The threat of communism in Europe does not come from the forcefulness of its preaching but from the fact that it is backed by one of the mightiest armies on earth.

It also seems that, where a mass movement can either persuade or coerce, it usually chooses the latter. Persuasion is clumsy and its results uncertain. Said the Spaniard Saint Dominic to the heretical Albigenses, "For many years I have exhorted you in vain, with gentleness, preaching, praying, and weeping. But according to the proverb of my country, 'Where blessing can accomplish nothing, blows may avail.' We shall rouse against you princes and prelates, who, alas, will arm nations and kingdoms against this land . . . and thus blows will avail where blessings and gentleness have been powerless."

5

The assertion that a mass movement cannot be stopped by force is not literally true. Force can stop and crush even the most vigorous movement. But to do so the force must be ruthless and persistent. And here is where faith enters as an indispensable factor. For a persecution that is ruthless and persistent can come only from fanatical conviction. "Any violence which does not spring from a firm, spiritual base, will be wavering and uncertain. It lacks the stability which can only rest in a fanatical outlook."[16] The terrorism which emanates from individual brutality neither goes far enough nor lasts long enough. It is spasmodic, subject to moods and hesitations. "But as soon as force wavers and alternates with forbearance, not only will the doctrine to be repressed recover again and again, but it will also be in a position to draw new benefit from every persecution."[17] The holy terror only knows no limit and never flags.

[15] Guglielmo Ferrero, *The Gamble* (Toronto: Oxford University Press, 1939), p. 297.
[16] Adolf Hitler, *Mein Kampf* (Boston: Houghton Mifflin Company, 1943), p. 171.
[17] Ibid.

Thus it seems that we need ardent faith not only to be able to resist coercion but also to be able to exercise it effectively.

6

Whence comes the impulse to proselytize?

Intensity of conviction is not the main factor which impels a movement to spread its faith to the four corners of the earth: "religions of great intensity often confine themselves to condemning, destroying, or at best pitying what is not themselves."[18] Nor is the impulse to proselytize an expression of an overabundance of power which as Bacon has it "is like a great flood, that will be sure to overflow." The missionary zeal seems rather an expression of some deep misgiving, some pressing feeling of insufficiency at the center. Proselytizing is more a passionate search for something not yet found than a desire to bestow upon the world something we already have. It is a search for a final and irrefutable demonstration that our absolute truth is indeed the one and only truth. The proselytizing fanatic strengthens his own faith by converting others. The creed whose legitimacy is most easily challenged is likely to develop the strongest proselytizing impulse. It is doubtful whether a movement which does not profess some preposterous and patently irrational dogma can be possessed of that zealous drive which "must either win men or destroy the world." It is also plausible that those movements with the greatest inner contradiction between profession and practice—that is to say, with a strong feeling of guilt—are likely to be the most fervent in imposing their faith on others. The more unworkable communism proves in Russia, and the more its leaders are compelled to compromise and adulterate the original creed, the more brazen and arrogant will be their attack on a nonbelieving world. The slaveholders of the South became the more aggressive in spreading their way of life the more it became patent that their position was untenable in a modern world. If free enterprise becomes a proselytizing holy cause, it will be a sign that its workability and advantages have ceased to be self-evident.

The passion for proselytizing and the passion for world domin-

[18] Jacob Burckhardt, *Force and Freedom* (New York: Pantheon Books, 1943), p. 129.

ion are both perhaps symptoms of some serious deficiency at the center. It is probably as true of a band of apostles or conquistadors as it is of a band of fugitives setting out for a distant land that they escape from an untenable situation at home. And how often indeed do the three meet, mingle, and exchange their parts.

Leadership

No matter how vital we think the role of leadership in the rise of a mass movement, there is no doubt that the leader cannot create the conditions which make the rise of a movement possible. He cannot conjure a movement out of the void. There has to be an eagerness to follow and obey, and an intense dissatisfaction with things as they are, before movement and leader can make their appearance. When conditions are not ripe, the potential leader, no matter how gifted, and his cause, no matter how potent, remain without a following. The First World War and its aftermath readied the ground for the rise of the Bolshevik, Fascist, and Nazi movements. Had the war been averted or postponed a decade or two, the fate of Lenin, Mussolini, and Hitler would not have been different from that of the brilliant plotters and agitators of the nineteenth century who never succeeded in ripening the frequent disorders and crises of their time into full-scale mass movements. Something was lacking. The European masses up to the cataclysmic events of the First World War had not utterly despaired of the present and were, therefore, not willing to sacrifice it for a new life and a new world. Even the nationalist leaders, who fared better than the revolutionists, did not succeed in making of nationalism the popular holy cause it has become since. Militant nationalism and militant revolutionism seem to be contemporaneous.

In Britain, too, the leader had to wait for the times to ripen before he could play his role. During the 1930s the potential leader, Churchill, was prominent in the eyes of the people and made himself heard, day in, day out. But the will to follow was not there. It was only when disaster shook the country to its foundation and made autonomous individual lives untenable and meaningless that the leader came into his own.

There is a period of waiting in the wings—often a very long

period—for all the great leaders whose entrance on the scene seems to us a most crucial point in the course of a mass movement. Accidents and the activities of other men have to set the stage for them before they can enter and start their performance. "The commanding man in a momentous day seems only to be the last accident in a series."[19]

2

Once the stage is set, the presence of an outstanding leader is indispensable. Without him there will be no movement. The ripeness of the time does not automatically produce a mass movement, nor can elections, laws, and administrative bureaus hatch one. It was Lenin who forced the flow of events into the channels of the Bolshevik revolution. Had he died in Switzerland, or on his way to Russia in 1917, it is almost certain that the other prominent Bolsheviks would have joined a coalition government. The result might have been a more or less liberal republic run chiefly by the bourgeoisie. In the case of Mussolini and Hitler the evidence is even more decisive: without them there would have been neither a Fascist nor a Nazi movement.

Events in England after the Second World War also demonstrate the indispensability of a gifted leader for the crystallization of a mass movement. A genuine leader (a Socialist Churchill) at the head of the Labour government would have initiated the drastic reforms of nationalization in the fervent atmosphere of a mass movement and not in the undramatic drabness of Socialist austerity. He would have cast the British worker in the role of a heroic producer and in that of a pioneer in truly scientific industrialism. He would have made the British feel that their chief task was to show the whole world, and America and Russia in particular, what a truly civilized nation could do with modern methods of production when free alike from the confusion, waste, and greed of capitalist management and from the byzantinism, barbarism, and ignorance of a Bolshevik bureaucracy. He would have known how to infuse the British people with the same pride and hope that sustained them in the darkest hours of the war.

[19] John Morley, *Notes on Politics and History* (New York: Macmillan Company, 1914), pp. 69–70.

It needs the iron will, daring, and vision of an exceptional leader to concert and mobilize existing attitudes and impulses into the collective drive of a mass movement. The leader personifies the certitude of the creed and the defiance and grandeur of power. He articulates and justifies the resentment dammed up in the souls of the frustrated. He kindles the vision of a breathtaking future so as to justify the sacrifice of a transitory present. He stages the world of make-believe so indispensable for the realization of self-sacrifice and united action. He evokes the enthusiasm of communion—the sense of liberation from a petty and meaningless individual existence.

What are the talents requisite for such a performance?

Exceptional intelligence, noble character, and originality seem neither indispensable nor perhaps desirable. The main requirements seem to be audacity and a joy in defiance, an iron will, a fanatical conviction that he is in possession of the one and only truth, faith in his destiny and luck, a capacity for passionate hatred, contempt for the present, a cunning estimate of human nature, a delight in symbols (spectacles and ceremonials), unbounded brazenness which finds expression in a disregard of consistency and fairness, a recognition that the innermost craving of a following is for communion and that there can never be too much of it, and a capacity for winning and holding the utmost loyalty of a group of able lieutenants. This last faculty is one of the most essential and elusive. The uncanny powers of a leader manifest themselves not so much in the hold he has on the masses as in his ability to dominate and almost bewitch a small group of able men. These men must be fearless, proud, intelligent, and capable of organizing and running large-scale undertakings, and yet they must submit wholly to the will of the leader, draw their inspiration and driving force from him, and glory in this submission.

Not all the qualities just enumerated are equally essential. The most decisive for the effectiveness of a mass movement leader seem to be audacity, fanatical faith in the cause, an awareness of the importance of a close-knit collectivity, and, above all, the ability to evoke fervent devotion in a group of able lieutenants. Trotsky's failure as a leader came from his neglect, or more probably his inability, to create a machine of able and loyal lieutenants. He did not attract personal sympathies, or if he did he could not keep

them. An additional shortcoming was his ineradicable respect for
the individual, particularly the creative individual. He was not
convinced of the sinfulness and ineffectuality of an autonomous
individual existence and did not grasp the overwhelming importance of communion to a mass movement. Sun Yat-sen "attracted
to himself . . . an extraordinary number of able and devoted followers, firing their imaginations with his visions of the new China
and compelling loyalty and self-sacrifice."[20] Unlike him, Chiang
Kai-shek seems to have lacked every essential quality of a mass
movement leader. On the other hand, De Gaulle was certainly a
man to watch. Those leaders of Communist parties outside Russia
who remain subservient to the Politburo cannot attain the status
of genuine leaders. They remain able lieutenants. For communism to become an effective mass movement in any Western
country, the local Communist party has to cut loose from Russia
and, after the manner of Tito, flaunt its defiance against both
capitalism and Stalinism. Had Lenin been the emissary of a leader
and a politburo sitting in some distant foreign land, it is doubtful
whether he could have exercised his fateful influence on the
course of events in Russia.

3

The crude ideas advanced by many of the successful mass
movement leaders of our time incline one to assume that a certain
coarseness and immaturity of mind is an asset to leadership. However, it was not the intellectual crudity of an Aimee McPherson or
a Hitler which won and held their following but the boundless
self-confidence which prompted these leaders to give full rein to
their preposterous ideas. A genuinely wise leader who dared to
follow out the course of his wisdom would have an equal chance
of success. The quality of ideas seems to play a minor role in mass
movement leadership. What counts is the arrogant gesture, the
complete disregard of the opinion of others, the single-handed defiance of the world.

Charlatanism of some degree is indispenable to effective leadership. There can be no mass movement without some deliberate

[20] Frank Wilson Price, "Sun Yat-sen," *Encyclopedia of the Social Sciences.*

misrepresentation of facts. No solid, tangible advantage can hold a following and make it zealous and loyal unto death. The leader has to be practical and a realist, yet must talk the language of the visionary and the idealist.

Originality is not a prerequisite of great mass movement leadership. One of the most striking traits of the successful mass movement leader is his readiness to imitate both friend and foe, both past and contemporary models. The daring which is essential to this type of leadership consists as much in the daring to imitate as in the daring to defy the world. Perhaps the clue to any heroic career is an unbounded capacity for imitation; a single-minded fashioning after a model. This excessive capacity for imitation indicates that the hero is without a fully developed and realized self. There is much in him that is rudimentary and suppressed. His strength lies in his blind spots and in plugging all outlets but one.

4

The total surrender of a distinct self is a prerequisite for the attainment of both unity and self-sacrifice, and there is probably no more direct way of realizing this surrender than by inculcating and extolling the habit of blind obedience. When Stalin forced scientists, writers, and artists to crawl on their bellies and deny their individual intelligence, sense of beauty, and moral sense, he was not indulging a sadistic impulse but was solemnizing, in a most impressive way, the supreme virtue of blind obedience. All mass movements rank obedience with the highest virtues and put it on a level with faith: "union of minds requires not only a perfect accord in the one Faith, but complete submission and obedience of will to the Church and the Roman Pontiff as to God Himself."[21] Obedience is not only the first law of God but also the first tenet of a revolutionary party and of fervent nationalism. "Not to reason why" is considered by all mass movements the mark of a strong and generous spirit.

The disorder, bloodshed, and destruction which mark the trail

[21] Leo XIII, *Sapientiae Christianae*. According to Luther, "Disobedience is a greater sin than murder, unchastity, theft, and dishonesty." Quoted by Jerome Frank, *Fate and Freedom* (New York: Simon and Schuster, Inc., 1945), p. 281.

of a rising mass movement lead us to think of the followers of the movement as being by nature rowdy and lawless. Actually, mass ferocity is not always the sum of individual lawlessness. Personal truculence militates against united action. It moves the individual to strike out for himself. It produces the pioneer, adventurer, and bandit. The true believer, no matter how rowdy and violent his acts, is basically an obedient and submissive person. The Christian converts who staged razzias against the University of Alexandria and lynched professors suspected of unorthodoxy were submissive members of a compact church. The Communist rioter is a servile member of a party. Both the Japanese and Nazi rowdies were the most disciplined people the world has seen. In this country, the American employer may find the racist fanatic—so given to mass violence—a respectful and docile factory hand. The army, too, finds him particularly amenable to discipline.

5

People whose lives are barren and insecure seem to show a greater willingness to obey than people who are self-sufficient and self-confident. To the frustrated, freedom from responsibility is more attractive than freedom from restraint. They are eager to barter their independence for relief from the burdens of willing, deciding, and being responsible for inevitable failure. They willingly abdicate the directing of their lives to those who want to plan, command, and shoulder all responsibility. Moreover, submission by all to a supreme leader is an approach to their ideal of equality.

In time of crisis, during floods, earthquakes, epidemics, depressions, and wars, separate individual effort is of no avail, and people of every condition are ready to obey and follow a leader. To obey is then the only firm point in a chaotic day-by-day existence.

6

The frustrated are also likely to be the most steadfast followers. It is remarkable that, in a cooperative effort, the least self-reliant are the least likely to be discouraged by defeat. For they join others in a common undertaking not so much to ensure the success of a cherished project as to avoid an individual shouldering of blame in case of failure. When the common undertaking fails, they are still spared the one thing they fear most: the showing up of their individual shortcomings. Their faith remains unimpaired, and they are eager to follow in a new attempt.

The frustrated follow a leader less because of their faith that he is leading them to a promised land than because of their immediate feeling that he is leading them away from their unwanted selves. Surrender to a leader is not a means to an end but a fulfillment. Whither they are led is of secondary importance.

7

There is probably a crucial difference between a mass movement leader and a leader in a free society. In a more or less free society, the leader can retain his hold on the people only when he has blind faith in their wisdom and goodness. A second-rate leader possessed of this faith will outlast a first-rate leader who is without it. This means that in a free society the leader follows the people even as he goes ahead. He must, as someone said, find out where the people are going so that he may lead them. When the leader in a free society becomes contemptuous of the people, he sooner or later proceeds on the false and fatal theory that all men are fools and eventually blunders into defeat. Things are different where the leader can employ ruthless coercion. Where, as in an active mass movement, the leader can exact blind obedience, he can operate on the sound theory that all men are cowards, treat them accordingly, and get results.

One of the reasons that Communist leaders lost out in our unions is that by following the line and adopting the tactics of the party, they assumed the attitude and used the tactics of a mass movement leader in organizations made up of free men.

Action

Action is a unifier. There is less individual distinctness in the genuine man of action—the builder, soldier, sportsman, and even the scientist—than in the thinker or in one whose creativeness flows from communion with the self. The go-getter and the hustler have much in them that is abortive and undifferentiated. One is never really stripped for action unless one is stripped of a distinct and differentiated self. An active people thus tends toward uniformity. It is doubtful whether without the vast action involved in the conquest of a continent, our nation of immigrants could have attained its amazing homogeneity in so short a time. Those who came to this country to act (to make money) were more quickly and thoroughly Americanized than those who came to realize some lofty ideal. The former felt an immediate kinship with the millions absorbed in the same pursuit. It was as if they were joining a brotherhood. They recognized early that in order to succeed they had to blend with their fellowmen, do as others do, learn the lingo, and play the game. Moreover, the mad rush in which they joined prevented the unfolding of their being, so that, without a distinct individuality, they could not, even if they had been so inclined, put up an effective resistance against the influence of their new environment. On the other hand, those who came to this country to realize an ideal (of freedom, justice, equality) measured the realities of the new land against their ideal and found them wanting. They felt superior and inevitably insulated themselves against the new environment.

2

Men of thought seldom work well together, whereas between men of action there is usually an easy camaraderie. Teamwork is rare in intellectual or artistic undertakings, but common and almost indispensable among men of action. The cry "Go to, let us build us a city and a tower" is always a call for united action. A Communist commissar of industry has probably more in common with a capitalist industrialist than with a Communist theoretician. The real International is that of men of action.

3

All mass movements avail themselves of action as a means of unification. The conflicts a mass movement seeks and incites serve not only to down its enemies but also to strip its followers of their distinct individuality and render them more soluble in the collective medium. Clearing of land, building of cities, exploration, and large-scale industrial undertakings serve a similar purpose. Even mere marching can serve as a unifier. The Nazis made vast use of this preposterous variant of action. Hermann Rauschning, who at first thought the eternal marching a senseless waste of time and energy, recognized later its subtle effect. "Marching diverts men's thoughts. Marching kills thought. Marching makes an end of individuality."

A mass movement's call for action evokes an eager response in the frustrated. For the frustrated see in action a cure for all that ails them. It brings self-forgetting, and it gives them a sense of purpose and worth. Indeed it seems that frustration stems chiefly from an inability to act, and that the most poignantly frustrated are those whose talents and temperament equip them ideally for a life of action but are condemned by circumstances to rust away in idleness. How else explain the surprising fact that the Lenins, Trotskys, Mussolinis, and Hitlers who spent the best part of their lives talking their heads off in cafés and meetings reveal themselves suddenly as the most able and tireless men of action of their time?

4

Faith organizes and equips man's soul for action. To be in possession of the one and only truth and never doubt one's righteousness; to feel that one is backed by a mysterious power, whether it be God, destiny, or the law of history; to be convinced that one's opponents are the incarnation of evil and must be crushed; to exult in self-denial and devotion to duty—these are admirable qualifications for resolute and ruthless actions in any field. Psalm-singing soldiers, pioneers, businessmen, and even sportsmen have proved themselves formidable. Revolutionary and nationalist enthusiasms have a similar effect: they, too, can turn spiritless and inert people into fighters and builders. Here, then, is another reason for the apparent indispensability of a mass movement in the modernization of backward and stagnant countries.

However, the exceptional fitness of the true believer for a life of action can be as much a danger as an aid to the prospects of a mass movement. By opening vast fields of feverish action, a mass movement may hasten its end. Successful action tends to become an end in itself. It drains all energies and fervors into its own channels. Faith and holy cause, instead of being the supreme purpose, become mere lubricants for the machine of action. The true believer who succeeds in all he does gains self-confidence and becomes reconciled with his self and the present. He no longer sees his only salvation in losing himself in the oneness of a corporate body and in becoming an anonymous particle with no will, judgment, and responsibility of his own. He seeks and finds his salvation in action, in proving his worth and in asserting his individual superiority. Action cannot lead him to self-realization, but he readily finds in it self-justification. If he still hangs on to his faith, it is but to bolster his confidence and legitimatize his success. Thus the taste of continuous successful action is fatal to the spirit of collectivity. A people steeped in action is likely to be the least religious, the least revolutionary, and the least chauvinist. The relative social stability and political and religious tolerance of the Anglo-Saxon peoples in modern times has been owing in part to the relative abundance among them of the will, skill, and opportunities for action. Action has served them as a substitute for a mass movement.

There is of course the constant danger that should the avenues of action be thoroughly blocked by a severe depression or defeat in war the resulting frustration would be so intense that almost any proselytizing mass movement would find the situation readymade for its propagation. The explosive situation in Germany after the First World War was partly a result of the inactivity forced upon a population that knew itself admirably equipped for action. Hitler gave them a mass movement. But what was probably more important, he opened before them unlimited opportunities for feverish, incessant, and spectacular action. No wonder they hailed him as their Savior.

Suspicion

We have seen that the acrid secretion of the frustrated mind, though composed chiefly of fear and ill will, acts yet as a marvelous slime to cement the embittered and disaffected into one compact whole. Suspicion too is an ingredient of this acrid slime, and it too can act as a unifying agent.

The awareness of their individual blemishes and shortcomings inclines the frustrated to detect ill will and meanness in their fellowmen. Self-contempt, however vague, sharpens our eyes for the imperfections of others. We usually strive to reveal in others the blemishes we hide in ourselves. Thus when the frustrated congregate in a mass movement, the air is heavy-laden with suspicion. There is prying and spying, tense watching, and a tense awareness of being watched. The surprising thing is that this pathological mistrust within the ranks leads not to dissension but to strict conformity. Knowing themselves continually watched, the faithful strive to escape suspicion by adhering zealously to prescribed behavior and opinion. Strict orthodoxy is as much the result of mutual suspicion as of ardent faith.

Mass movements make extensive use of suspicion in their machinery of domination. The rank-and-file within the Nazi party were made to feel that they were continually under observation and were kept in a permanent state of uneasy conscience and fear. Fear of one's neighbors, one's friends, and even one's relatives seems to be the rule within all mass movements. Now and then innocent people are deliberately accused and sacrificed in order to keep suspicion alive. Suspicion is given a sharp edge by associating all opposition within the ranks with the enemy threatening the movement from without. This enemy—the indispensable devil of every mass movement—is omnipresent. He plots both outside and inside the ranks of the faithful. It is his voice that speaks through the mouth of the dissenter, and the deviationists are his stooges. If anything goes wrong within the movement, it is his doing. It is the sacred duty of the true believer to be suspicious. He must be constantly on the lookout for saboteurs, spies, and traitors.

2

Collective unity is not the result of the brotherly love of the faithful for each other. The loyalty of the true believer is to the whole—church, party, or nation—and not to his fellow true believer. True loyalty between individuals is possible only in a loose and relatively free society. As Abraham was ready to sacrifice his only son to prove his devotion to Jehovah, so must the fanatical Nazi or Communist be ready to sacrifice relatives and friends to demonstrate his total surrender to the cause. The active mass movement sees in the personal ties of blood and friendship a diminution of its own corporate cohesion. Thus mutual suspicion within the ranks is not only compatible with corporate strength but, one might almost say, a precondition of it. "Men of strong convictions and strong passions, when leagued together, watch one another with suspicion, and find their strength in it; for mutual suspicion creates mutual dread, binds them as by an iron band, prevents desertion, and braces them against moments of weakness."[22]

It is part of the formidableness of a genuine mass movement that the self-sacrifice it promotes includes also a sacrifice of some of the moral sense which cramps and restrains our nature. In Montaigne's words, "Our zeal works wonders when it seconds our propensity to hatred, cruelty, ambition, avarice, detraction, rebellion."

The Effects of Unification

Thorough unification, whether brought about by spontaneous surrender, persuasion, coercion, necessity, or ingrained habit, or a combination of these, tends to intensify the inclinations and attitudes which promote unity. We have seen that unification intensifies the propensity to hatred and the imitative capacity. It is also true that the unified individual is more credulous and obedient than the potential true believer who is still an autonomous individual. Though it is true that the leadership of a collective body usually keeps hatred at a white heat, encourages imitation and credulity, and fosters obedience, the fact remains that unification by itself, even when not aided by the manipulations of the leadership, intensifies the reactions which function as unifying agents.

This at first sight is a surprising fact. We have seen that most unifying factors originate in the revulsion of the frustrated indi-

---

[22] Ernest Renan, *Antichrist* (Boston: Roberts Brothers, 1897), p. 381.

vidual from an unwanted self and an untenable existence. But the true believer who is wholly assimilated into a compact collective body is no longer frustrated. He has found a new identity and a new life. He is one of the chosen, bolstered and protected by invincible powers, and destined to inherit the earth. His is a state of mind the very opposite of that of the frustrated individual; yet he displays, with increased intensity, all the reactions which are symptomatic of inner tension and insecurity.

What happens to the unified individual?

Unification is more a process of diminution than of addition. In order to be assimilated into a collective medium, a person has to be stripped of his individual distinctness. He has to be deprived of free choice and independent judgment. Many of his natural bents and impulses have to be suppressed or blunted. All these are acts of diminution. The elements which are apparently added—faith, hope, pride, confidence—are negative in origin. The exaltation of the true believer does not flow from reserves of strength and wisdom but from a sense of deliverance; he has been delivered from the meaningless burdens of an autonomous existence. "We Germans are so happy. We are free from freedom," said a young Nazi. His happiness and fortitude come from his no longer being himself. Attacks against the self cannot touch him. His powers of endurance when at the mercy of an implacable enemy or when facing insupportable circumstances are superior to those of an autonomous individual. But this invincibility depends upon the lifeline which connects him with the collective whole. As long as he feels himself part of that whole and nothing else, he is indestructible and immortal. All his fervor and fanaticism are, therefore, clustered around this lifeline. His striving for utmost unity is more intense than the vague longing of the frustrated for an escape from an untenable self. The frustrated individual still has a choice: he can find a new life not only by becoming part of a corporate body but also by changing his environment or by throwing himself wholeheartedly into some absorbing undertaking. The unified individual, on the other hand, has no choice. He must cling to the collective body or, like a fallen leaf, wither and fade. It is doubtful whether the excommunicated priest, the expelled Communist, and the renegade chauvinist can ever find peace of mind as autonomous individuals. They cannot stand on their own but must embrace a new cause and attach themselves to a new group.

The true believer is eternally incomplete, eternally insecure.

2

It is of interest to note the means by which a mass movement accentuates and perpetuates the individual incompleteness of its adherents. By elevating dogma above reason, the individual's intelligence is prevented from becoming self-reliant. Economic dependence is maintained by centralizing economic power and by a deliberately created scarcity of the necessities of life. Social self-sufficiency is discouraged by crowded housing or communal quarters and by enforced daily participation in public functions. Ruthless censorship of literature, art, music, and science prevents even the creative few from living self-sufficient lives. The inculcated devotions to church, party, country, leader, and creed also perpetuate a state of incompleteness. For every devotion is a socket which demands the fitting in of a complementary part from without.

Thus people raised in the atmosphere of a mass movement are fashioned into incomplete and dependent human beings even when they have within themselves the making of self-sufficient entities. Though strangers to frustration and without a grievance, they will yet exhibit the peculiarities of people who crave to lose themselves and be rid of an existence that is irrevocably spoiled.

Mass movements do not usually rise until the prevailing order
has been discredited. The discrediting is not an automatic result of
the blunders and abuses of those in power, but the deliberate
work of men of words with a grievance. Where the articulate are
absent or without a grievance, the prevailing dispensation, though
incompetent and corrupt, may continue in power until it falls and
crumbles of itself. On the other hand, a dispensation of undoubted
merit and vigor may be swept away if it fails to win the allegiance of the articulate minority.

As pointed out in the section on persuasion and coercion, the
realization and perpetuation of a mass movement depend on
force. A full-blown mass movement is a ruthless affair, and its
management is in the hands of ruthless fanatics who use words
only to give an appearance of spontaneity to a consent obtained
by coercion. But these fanatics can move in and take charge only
after the prevailing order has been discredited and has lost the
allegiance of the masses. The preliminary work of undermining
existing institutions, of familiarizing the masses with the idea of
change, and of creating a receptivity to a new faith can be done
only by men who are, first and foremost, talkers or writers and
are recognized as such by all. As long as the existing order functions in a more or less orderly fashion, the masses remain basically
conservative. They can think of reform but not of total innovation. The fanatical extremist, no matter how eloquent, strikes
them as dangerous, traitorous, impractical, or even insane. They

will not listen to him. Lenin himself recognized that where the ground is not ready for them the Communists "find it hard to approach the masses . . . and even get them to listen to them." Moreover, the authorities, even when feeble or tolerant, are likely to react violently against the activist tactics of the fanatic and may gain from his activities, as it were, a new vigor.

Things are different in the case of the typical man of words. The masses listen to him because they know that his words, however urgent, cannot have immediate results. The authorities either ignore him or use mild methods to muzzle him. Thus imperceptibly the man of words undermines established institutions, discredits those in power, weakens prevailing beliefs and loyalties, and sets the stage for the rise of a mass movement.

The division between men of words, fanatics, and practical men of action, as outlined in the following sections, is not meant to be categorical. Men like Gandhi and Trotsky start out as apparently ineffectual men of words and later display exceptional talents as administrators or generals. A man like Muhammad starts out as a man of words, develops into an implacable fanatic, and finally reveals a superb practical sense. A fanatic like Lenin is a master of the spoken word and unequaled as a man of action. What the classification attempts to suggest is that the readying of the ground for a mass movement is done best by men whose chief claim to excellence is their skill in the use of the spoken or written word, that the hatching of an actual movement requires the temperament and the talents of the fanatic, and that the final consolidation of the movement is largely the work of practical men of action.

The emergence of an articulate minority where there was none before is a potential revolutionary step. The Western powers were indirect and unknowing fomenters of mass movements in Asia not only by kindling resentment but also by creating articulate minorities through educational work which was largely philanthropic. Many of the revolutionary leaders in India, China, and Indonesia received their training in conservative Western institutions. The American college at Beirut, which is directed and supported by God-fearing, conservative Americans, was a school for revolutionaries in the illiterate Arabic world. Nor is there any doubt that the God-fearing missionary schoolteachers in China were unknowingly among those who prepared the ground for the Chinese revolution.

THE MEN OF WORDS

The men of words are of diverse types. They can be priests, scribes, prophets, writers, artists, professors, students, and intellectuals in general. Where, as in China, reading and writing is a difficult art, mere literacy can give one the status of a man of words. A similar situation prevailed in ancient Egypt, where the art of picture writing was the monopoly of a minority.

Whatever the type, there is a deep-seated craving common to almost all men of words which determines their attitude to the prevailing order. It is a craving for recognition, a craving for a clearly marked status above the common run of humanity. "Vanity," said Napoleon, "made the Revolution; liberty was only a pretext." There is apparently an irremediable insecurity at the core of every intellectual, be he noncreative or creative. Even the most gifted and prolific seem to live a life of eternal self-doubting and have to prove their worth anew each day. What Charles de Rémusat said of Thiers is perhaps true of most men of words: "He has much more vanity than ambition; and he prefers consideration to obedience, and the appearance of power to power itself. Consult him constantly, and then do just as you please. He will take more notice of your deference to him than of your actions."

There is a moment in the career of almost every fault-finding man of words when a deferential or conciliatory gesture from those in power may win him over to their side. Although it is true that once the man of words formulates a philosophy and a program, he is likely to stand by them and be immune to blandishments and enticements, at a certain stage most men of words are ready to become timeservers and courtiers. Jesus himself might not have preached a new gospel had the dominant Pharisees taken him into the fold, called him rabbi, and listened to him with deference. A bishopric conferred on Luther at the right moment might have cooled his ardor for a Reformation. The young Karl

Marx could perhaps have been won over to Prussiandom by the bestowal of a title and an important government job; and Lassalle, by a title and a court uniform.

However much the protesting man of words sees himself as the champion of the downtrodden and injured, the grievance which animates him is, with very few exceptions, private and personal. His pity is usually hatched out of his hatred for the powers that be. "It is only a few rare and exceptional men who have that kind of love toward mankind at large that makes them unable to endure patiently the general mass of evil and suffering, regardless of any relation it may have to their own lives."[1] Thoreau states the fact with fierce extravagance: "I believe that what so saddens the reformer is not his sympathy with his fellows in distress, but, though he be the holiest son of God, is his private ail. Let this be righted . . . and he will forsake his generous companions without apology." When his superior status is suitably acknowledged by those in power, the man of words usually finds all kinds of lofty reasons for siding with the strong against the weak. A Luther, who, when first defying the established church, spoke feelingly of "the poor, simple, common folk," proclaimed later, when allied with the German princelings, that "God would prefer to suffer the government to exist no matter how evil, rather than to allow the rabble to riot, no matter how justified they are in doing so." A Burke patronized by lords and nobles spoke of the "swinish multitude" and recommended to the poor "patience, labor, sobriety, frugality, and religion." The pampered and flattered men of words in Nazi Germany felt no impulse to side with the persecuted and terrorized against the ruthless leaders and their secret police.

2

Whenever we find a dispensation enduring beyond its span of competence, there is either an entire absence of an educated class or an intimate alliance between those in power and the men of words. Where all learned men are clergymen, the church is unassailable. Where all learned men are bureaucrats or where

[1] Bertrand Russell, *Proposed Roads to Freedom* (New York: Blue Ribbon Books, 1931). Introduction, p. viii.

education gives a man an acknowledged superior status, the prevailing order is likely to be free from movements of protest.

The Catholic Church sank to its lowest level in the tenth century, at the time of Pope John XII. It was then far more corrupt and ineffectual than at the time of the Reformation. But in the tenth century all learned men were priests, whereas in the fifteenth century, as the result of the introduction of printing and paper, learning had ceased to be the monopoly of the church. It was the nonclerical humanists who formed the vanguard of the Reformation. Those of the scholars affiliated with the church or who, as in Italy, enjoyed the patronage of the Popes "showed a tolerant spirit on the whole toward existing institutions, including the ecclesiastical abuses, and, in general, cared little how long the vulgar herd was left in superstitious darkness which befitted their state"[2]

The stability of imperial China, like that of ancient Egypt, was due to an intimate alliance between the bureaucracy and the literati. It is of interest that the Tai-ping rebellion, the only effective Chinese mass movement while the Empire was still a going concern, was started by a scholar who failed again and again in the state examination for the highest mandarin caste.

The long endurance of the Roman Empire resulted in some degree from the wholehearted partnership between the Roman rulers and the Greek men of words. The conquered Greeks felt that they gave laws and civilization to the conquerors. It is disconcerting to read how the deformed and depraved Nero, who was extravagant in his admiration of Hellas, was welcomed hysterically by the Greeks on his visit in A.D. 67. They took him to their hearts as a fellow intellectual and artist. "To gratify him, all the games had been crowded into a single year. All the cities sent him the prizes of their contests. Committees were continually waiting on him, to beg him to go and sing at every place."[3] And he in turn loaded them with privileges and proclaimed the freedom of Greece at the Isthmian games.

In *A Study of History*, A. J. Toynbee quotes the Latin hexameters that Claudian of Alexandria wrote in praise of Rome almost five hundred years after Caesar set foot on Egyptian soil; he adds

[2] "Reformation," *Encyclopaedia Britannica*.
[3] Ernest Renan, *Antichrist* (Boston: Roberts Brothers, 1897), p. 245.

ruefully, "It would be easy to prove that the British Raj had been in many respects a more benevolent and also perhaps a more beneficent institution than the Roman Empire, but it would be hard to find a Claudian in any of the Alexandrias of Hindustan." Now it is not altogether farfetched to assume that, had the British in India, instead of cultivating the nizams, maharajas, nawabs, gekawars, and so on, made an effort to win the Indian intellectual; had they treated him as an equal, encouraged him in his work, and allowed him a share of the fleshpots, they could perhaps have maintained their rule there indefinitely. As it was, the British who ruled India were of a type altogether lacking in the aptitude for getting along with intellectuals in any land, and least of all in India. They were men of action imbued with a faith in the innate superiority of the British. For the most part they scorned the Indian intellectual both as a man of words and as an Indian. The British in India tried to preserve the realm of action for themselves. They did not to any real extent encourage Indians to become engineers, agronomists, or technicians. The educational institutions they established produced "impractical" men of words; and it is an irony of fate that this system, instead of safeguarding British rule, hastened its end.

Britain's failure in Palestine was also due in part to the lack of rapport between the typical British colonial official and men of words. The majority of the Palestinian Jews, although steeped in action, were by upbringing and tradition men of words, and thin-skinned to a fault. They smarted under the contemptuous attitude of the British official, who looked on the Jews as on a pack of unmanly and ungrateful quibblers—an easy prey for the warlike Arabs once Britain withdrew its protective hand. The Palestinian Jews also resented the tutelage of mediocre officials, their inferiors in both experience and intelligence. Britons of the caliber of Julian Huxley, Harold Nicolson, or Richard Crossman just possibly might have saved Palestine for the Empire.

In both the Bolshevik and the Nazi regimes there is evident an acute awareness of the fateful relation between men of words and the state. In Russia, men of letters, artists, and scholars share the privileges of the ruling group. They are all superior civil servants. And though made to toe the party line, they are but subject to the same discipline imposed on the rest of the elite. In the case of Hitler, there was a diabolical realism in his plan to make all learning the monopoly of the elite who were to rule his envisioned world empire and keep the anonymous masses barely literate.

3

The men of letters of eighteenth-century France are the most familiar example of intellectuals pioneering a mass movement. A somewhat similar pattern may be detected in the periods preceding the rise of most movements. The ground for the Reformation was prepared by the men who satirized and denounced the clergy in popular pamphlets, and by men of letters like Johann Reuchlin, who fought and discredited the Roman curia. The rapid spread of Christianity in the Roman world was partly owing to the fact that the pagan cults it sought to supplant were already thoroughly discredited. The discrediting was done, before and after the birth of Christianity, by the Greek philosophers, who were bored with the puerility of the cults and denounced and ridiculed them in schools and city streets. Christianity made little headway against Judaism because the Jewish religion had the ardent allegiance of the Jewish men of words. The rabbis and their disciples enjoyed an exalted status in the Jewish life of that day, where the school and the book supplanted the temple and the fatherland. In any social order where men of words reign supreme, no opposition can develop within and no foreign mass movement can gain a foothold.

The mass movements of modern time, whether socialist or nationalist, were invariably pioneered by poets, writers, historians, scholars, philosophers, and the like. The connection between intellectual theoreticians and revolutionary movements needs no emphasis. But it is equally true that all nationalist movements—from the cult of *la patrie* in revolutionary France to the latest nationalist risings—have been conceived not by men of action but by fault-finding intellectuals. German intellectuals were the originators of German nationalism, just as Jewish intellectuals were the originators of Zionism. The generals, industrialists, landowners, and businessmen who are considered pillars of patriotism are late-

comers who join the movement after it has become a going concern. The most strenuous effort of the early phase of every nationalist movement consists in convincing and winning over these
future pillars of patriotism. The Czech historian Palacký said that
if the ceiling of a room in which he and a handful of friends were
dining one night had collapsed, there would have been no Czech
nationalist movement.

It is the deep-seated craving of the man of words for an exalted status which makes him particularly sensitive to any humiliation imposed on the class or community (racial, lingual, or religious) to which he belongs, however loosely. It was Napoleon's
humiliation of the Germans, particularly the Prussians, which
drove Fichte and the German intellectuals to call on the German
masses to unite into a mighty nation which would dominate Europe. Theodor Herzl and the Jewish intellectuals were driven to
Zionism by the humiliations heaped upon millions of Jews in Russia and by the calumnies to which the Jews in the rest of continental Europe were subjected toward the end of the nineteenth century. To a degree the nationalist movement which forced the
British out of India had its inception in the humiliation of a
scrawny and bespectacled Indian man of words in South Africa.

4

It is easy to see how the fault-finding man of words, by
persistent ridicule and denunciation, shakes prevailing beliefs and
loyalties and familiarizes the masses with the idea of change.
What is not so obvious is the process by which the discrediting of
existing beliefs and institutions makes possible the rise of a new
fanatical faith. For it is a remarkable fact that the militant man of
words, who in Pascal's words "sounds the established order to its
source to mark its want of authority and justice," often prepares
the ground not for a society of freethinking individuals but for a
corporate society that cherishes utmost unity and blind faith. A
wide diffusion of doubt and irreverence thus leads often to unexpected results. The irreverence of the Renaissance was a prelude
to the new fanaticism of Reformation and Counter Reformation.
The Frenchmen of the Enlightenment who debunked church and

crown and preached reason and tolerance released a burst of revolutionary and nationalist fanaticism which has not abated yet. Marx and his followers discredited religion, nationalism, and the passionate pursuit of business and brought into being the new fanaticism of socialism, communism, and Stalinist nationalism.

When we debunk a fanatical faith or prejudice, we do not strike at the root of fanaticism. We merely prevent its leaking out at a certain point, with the likely result that it will leak out at some other point. Thus by denigrating prevailing beliefs and loyalties, the militant man of words unwittingly creates in the disillusioned masses a hunger for faith. For the majority of people cannot endure the barrenness and futility of their lives unless they have some ardent dedication or some passionate pursuit in which they can lose themselves. Thus, in spite of himself, the scoffing man of words becomes the precursor of a new faith.

The genuine man of words values the search for truth as much as truth itself. He delights in the clash of thought and in the give-and-take of controversy. If he formulates a philosophy and a doctrine, they are more an exhibition of brilliance and an exercise in dialectics than a program of action and the tenets of a faith. His vanity, it is true, often prompts him to defend his speculations with savagery and even venom, but his appeal is usually to reason. The fanatics and the faith-hungry masses, however, are likely to invest such speculations with the certitude of holy writ and make them the fountainhead of a new faith. Jesus was not a Christian, nor was Marx a Marxist.

To sum up, the militant man of words prepares the ground for the rise of a mass movement: (1) by discrediting prevailing creeds and institutions and detaching from them the allegiance of the people; (2) by indirectly creating a hunger for faith in the hearts of those who cannot live without it, so that when the new faith is preached it finds an eager response among the disillusioned masses; (3) by furnishing the doctrine and the slogans of the new faith; and (4) by undermining the convictions of the "better people"—those who can get along without faith—so that when the new fanaticism makes its appearance they are without the capacity to resist it. They see no sense in dying for convictions and principles, and yield to the new order without a fight.

Thus when the irreverent intellectual has done his work:

> The best lack all conviction, while the worst
> Are full of passionate intensity.
> Surely some revelation is at hand,
> Surely the Second Coming is at hand.[4]

The stage is now set for the fanatics.

5

The tragic figures in the history of a mass movement are often the intellectual precursors who live long enough to see the downfall of the old order by the action of the masses.

The impression that mass movements, and revolutions in particular, are born of the resolve of the masses to overthrow a corrupt and oppressive tyranny and win for themselves freedom of action, speech, and conscience has its origin in the din of words let loose by the intellectual originators of the movement in their skirmishes with the prevailing order. The fact that mass movements, as they arise, often manifest less individual freedom than the order they supplant is usually ascribed to the trickery of a power-hungry clique that kidnaps the movement at a critical stage and cheats the masses of the freedom about to dawn. Actually, the only people cheated in the process are the intellectual precursors. They rise against the established order, deride its irrationality and incompetence, denounce its illegitimacy and oppressiveness, and call for freedom of self-expression and self-realization. They take it for granted that the masses who respond to their call and range themselves behind them crave the same things. However, the freedom the masses crave is not freedom of self-expression and self-realization but freedom from the intolerable burden of an autonomous existence. They want freedom from what Dostoevski called "the fearful burden of free choice," freedom from the arduous responsibility of realizing their ineffectual selves and shouldering the blame for the blemished product. They do not want freedom of conscience but rather faith—blind, authoritarian faith. They sweep away the old order not to create a society of free and

---

[4] William Butler Yeats, "The Second Coming," *Collected Poems* (New York: Macmillan Company, 1933).

independent men but to establish uniformity, individual anonymity, and a new structure of perfect unity. It is not the wickedness of the old regime they rise against but its weakness; not its oppression but its failure to hammer them together into one solid, mighty whole. The persuasiveness of the intellectual demagogue consists not so much in convincing people of the vileness of the established order as in demonstrating its helpless incompetence. The immediate result of a mass movement usually corresponds to what the people want. They are not cheated in the process.

The reason for the tragic fate which almost always overtakes the intellectual midwives of a mass movement is that, no matter how much they preach and glorify the united effort, they remain essentially individualists. They believe in the possibility of individual happiness and the validity of individual opinion and initiative. But once a movement gets rolling, power falls into the hands of those who have neither faith in nor respect for the individual. And the reason they prevail is not so much that their disregard of the individual gives them a capacity for ruthlessness but that their attitude is in full accord with the ruling passion of the masses.

THE FANATICS

When the movement is ripe, only the fanatic can hatch a genuine mass movement. Without him the disaffection engendered by militant men of words remains undirected and can vent itself only in pointless and easily suppressed disorders. Without him the initiated reforms, even when drastic, leave the old way of life unchanged, and any change in government usually amounts to no more than a transfer of power from one set of men of action to another. Without him there can perhaps be no new beginning.

When the old order begins to fall apart, many of the vociferous men of words, who prayed so long for the day, are in a funk. The first glimpse of the face of anarchy frightens them out of their wits. They forget all they said about the "poor simple folk" and run for help to strong men of action—princes, generals, administrators, bankers, landowners—who know how to deal with the rabble and how to stem the tide of chaos.

Not so the fanatic. Chaos is his element. When the old order begins to crack, he wades in with all his might and recklessness to blow the whole hated present to high heaven. He glories in the sight of a world coming to a sudden end. To hell with reforms! All that already exists is rubbish, and there is no sense in reforming rubbish. He justifies his will to anarchy with the plausible assertion that there can be no new beginning so long as the old clutters the landscape. He shoves aside the frightened men of words, if they are still around, though he continues to extol their doctrines and mouth their slogans. He alone knows the innermost craving of the masses in action: the craving for communion, for the mustering of the host, for the dissolution of cursed individuality in the majesty and grandeur of a mighty whole. Posterity is king; and woe to those, inside and outside the movement, who hug and hang on to the present.

2

Whence come the fanatics? Mostly from the ranks of the noncreative men of words. The most significant division among men of words is between those who can find fulfillment in creative work and those who cannot. The creative man of words, no matter how bitterly he may criticize and deride the existing order, is actually attached to the present. His passion is to reform, not to destroy. When the mass movement remains wholly in his keeping, he turns it into a mild affair. The reforms he initiates are of the surface, and life flows on without a sudden break. But such a development is possible only when the anarchic action of the masses does not come into play, either because the old order abdicates without a struggle or because the man of words allies himself with strong men of action the moment chaos threatens to break loose. When the struggle with the old order is bitter and chaotic and victory can be won only by utmost unity and self-sacrifice, the creative man of words is usually shoved aside and the management of affairs falls into the hands of the noncreative men of words—the eternal misfits and the fanatical contemners of the present.

The man who wants to write a great book, paint a great picture, create an architectural masterpiece, become a great scientist, and knows that never in all eternity will he be able to realize this,

his innermost desire, can find no peace in a stable social order, old or new. He sees his life as irrevocably spoiled and the world perpetually out of joint. He feels at home only in a state of chaos. Even when he submits to or imposes an iron discipline, he is but submitting to or shaping the indispensable instrument for attaining a state of eternal flux, eternal becoming. Only when engaged in change does he have a sense of freedom and the feeling that he is growing and developing. It is because he can never be reconciled with his self that he fears finality and a fixed order of things. Marat, Robespierre, Lenin, Mussolini, and Hitler are outstanding examples of fanatics arising from the ranks of noncreative men of words. Peter Viereck points out that most of the Nazi bigwigs had artistic and literary ambitions which they could not realize. Hitler tried painting and architecture; Goebbels, drama, the novel, and poetry; Rosenberg, architecture and philosophy; Von Shirach, poetry; Funk, music; Streicher, painting. "Almost all were failures, not only by the usual vulgar criterion of success but by their own artistic criteria." Their artistic and literary ambitions "were originally far deeper than political ambitions: and were integral parts of their personalities."

The creative man of words is ill at ease in the atmosphere of an active movement. He feels that its whirl and passion sap his creative energies. So long as he is conscious of the creative flow within him, he will not find fulfillment in leading millions and in winning victories. The result is that, once the movement starts rolling, he either retires voluntarily or is pushed aside. Moreover, since the genuine man of words can never wholeheartedly and for long suppress his critical faculty, he is inevitably cast in the role of the heretic. Thus unless the creative man of words stifles the newborn movement by allying himself with practical men of action or unless he dies at the right moment, he is likely to end up either a shunned recluse or in exile or facing a firing squad.

3

The danger of the fanatic to the development of a movement is that he cannot settle down. Once victory has been won and the new order begins to crystallize, the fanatic becomes an element of strain and disruption. The taste for strong feeling drives him on to search for mysteries yet to be revealed and secret doors yet to be opened. He keeps groping for extremes. Thus on the morrow of victory most mass movements find themselves in the grip of dissension. The ardor which yesterday found an outlet in a life-and-death struggle with external enemies now vents itself in violent disputes and clash of factions. Hatred has become a habit. With no more outside enemies to destroy, the fanatics make enemies of one another. Hitler—himself a fanatic—could diagnose with precision the state of mind of the fanatics who plotted against him within the ranks of the National Socialist party. In his order to the newly appointed chief of the SA after the purge of Röhm in 1934, he speaks of those who will not settle down: "without realizing it, [they] have found in nihilism their ultimate confession of faith . . . their unrest and disquietude can find satisfaction only in some conspiratorial activity of the mind, in perpetually plotting the disintegration of whatever the set-up of the moment happens to be." As was often the case with Hitler, his accusations against antagonists (inside and outside the Reich) were a self-revelation. He, too, particularly in his last days, found in nihilism his "ultimate philosophy and valediction."[5]

If allowed to have their way, the fanatics may split a movement into schism and heresies which threaten its existence. Even when the fanatics do not breed dissension, they can still wreck the movement by driving it to attempt the impossible. Only the entrance of a practical man of action can save the achievements of the movement.

THE PRACTICAL MEN OF ACTION

A movement is pioneered by men of words, materialized by fanatics, and consolidated by men of action.

It is usually an advantage to a movement, and perhaps a prerequisite for its endurance, that these roles should be played by different men succeeding each other as conditions require. When the same person or persons (or the same type of person) leads a movement from its inception to maturity, it usually ends in disas-

[5] H. R. Trevor-Roper, The Last Days of Hitler (New York: Macmillan Company, 1947), p. 4.

ter. The Fascist and Nazi movements were without a successive change in leadership, and both ended in disaster. It was Hitler's fanaticism, his inability to settle down and play the role of a practical man of action, which brought ruin.

There is, of course, the possibility of a change in character. A man of words might change into a genuine fanatic or into a practical man of action. Yet the evidence suggests that such metamorphoses are usually temporary, and that sooner or later there is a reversion to the original type. Trotsky was essentially a man of words—vain, brilliant, and an individualist to the core. The cataclysmic collapse of an empire and Lenin's overpowering will brought him into the camp of the fanatics. In the civil war he displayed unequaled talents as an organizer and general. But the moment the strain lessened at the end of the civil war, he was a man of words again, without ruthlessness and dark suspicions, putting his trust in words rather than in relentless force, and allowed himself to be pushed aside by the crafty Stalin.

Stalin himself was a combination of fanatic and man of action, with the fanatical tinge predominating. His disastrous blunders— the senseless liquidation of the kulaks and their offspring, the terror of the purges, the pact with Hitler, the clumsy meddling with the creative work of writers, artists, and scientists—were the blunders of a fanatic. There was small chance that the Russians would taste the joys of the present while Stalin the fanatic was in power.

Hitler, too, was primarily a fanatic, and his fanaticism vitiated his remarkable achievements as a man of action.

There are, of course, rare leaders such as Lincoln, Gandhi, even FDR, Churchill, and Nehru. They do not hesitate to harness man's hungers and fears to weld a following and make it zealous unto death in the service of a holy cause; but unlike a Hitler, a Stalin, or even a Luther and a Calvin,[6] they are not tempted to use the slime of frustrated souls as mortar in the building of a new world. The self-confidence of these rare leaders is derived from and blended with their faith in humanity, for they know that no one can be honorable unless he honors mankind.

[6] Both Luther and Calvin "aimed to set up a new church authority which would be more powerful, more dictatorial and exacting, and far more diligent in persecuting heretics than the Catholic Church." Jerome Frank, *Fate and Freedom* (New York: Simon and Schuster, 1945), p. 283.

2

The man of action saves the moment from the suicidal dissensions and the recklessness of the fanatics. But his appearance usually marks the end of the dynamic phase of the movement. The war with the present is over. The genuine man of action is intent not on renovating the world but on possessing it. Whereas the life breath of the dynamic phase was protest and a desire for drastic change, the final phase is chiefly preoccupied with administering and perpetuating the power won.

With the appearance of the man of action, the explosive vigor of the movement is embalmed and sealed in sanctified institutions. A religious movement crystallizes in a hierarchy and a ritual; a revolutionary movement, in organs of vigilance and administration; a nationalist movement, in governmental and patriotic institutions. The establishment of a church marks the end of the revivalist spirit; the organs of a triumphant revolution liquidate the revolutionary mentality and technique; the governmental institutions of a new or revived nation put an end to chauvinistic belligerence. The institutions freeze a pattern of united action. The members of the institutionalized collective body are expected to act as one man, yet they must represent a loose aggregation rather than a spontaneous coalescence. They must be unified only through their unquestioning loyalty to the institutions. Spontaneity is suspect, and duty is prized above devotion.

3

The chief preoccupation of a man of action when he takes over an "arrived" movement is to fix and perpetuate its unity and readiness for self-sacrifice. His ideal is a compact, invincible whole that functions automatically. To achieve this he cannot rely on enthusiasm, for enthusiasm is ephemeral. Persuasion, too, is unpredictable. He inclines, therefore, to rely mainly on drill and coercion. He finds the assertion that all men are cowards less debatable than that all men are fools, and, in the words of Sir John Maynard, inclines to found the new order on the necks of the people rather than in their hearts. The genuine man of action is not a man of faith but a man of law.

Still, he cannot help being awed by the tremendous achievements of faith and spontaneity in the early days of the movement when a mighty instrument of power was conjured out of the void. The memory of it is still vivid. He therefore takes great care to preserve in the new institutions an impressive façade of faith and maintains an incessant flow of fervent propaganda, though he relies mainly on the persuasiveness of force. His orders are worded in pious vocabulary, and the old formulas and slogans are continually on his lips. The symbols of faith are carried high and given reverence. The men of words and the fanatics of the early period are canonized. Though the steel fingers of coercion make themselves felt everywhere and great emphasis is placed on mechanical drill, the pious phrases and the fervent propaganda give to coercion a semblance of persuasion, and to habit a semblance of spontaneity. No effort is spared to present the new order as the glorious consummation of the hopes and struggles of the early days.

The man of action is eclectic in the methods he uses to endow the new order with stability and permanence. He borrows from near and far and from friend and foe. He even goes back to the old order which preceded the movement and appropriates from it many techniques of stability, thus unintentionally establishing continuity with the past. The institution of an absolute dictator which is characteristic of this stage is as much the deliberate employment of a device as the manifestation of a sheer hunger for power. Byzantinism is likely to be conspicuous both at the birth and the decline of an organization. It is the expression of a desire for a stable pattern, and it can be used either to give shape to the as yet amorphous, or to hold together that which seems to be falling apart. The infallibility of the bishop of Rome was propounded by Irenaeus (second century) in the earliest days of the papacy, and by Pius IX in 1870, when the papacy seemed to be on the brink of extinction.

Thus the order evolved by a man of action is a patchwork. Stalin's Russia was a patchwork of Bolshevisim, czarism, nationalism, pan-Slavism, dictatorship and borrowings from Hitler, and monopolistic capitalism. Hitler's Third Reich was a conglomerate of nationalism, racialism, Prussianism, dictatorship, and borrowings from fascism, Bolshevism, Shintoism, Catholicism, and the ancient Hebrews. Christianity, too, when after the conflicts and dissensions of the first few centuries it crystallized into an authoritarian church, was a patchwork of old and new and of borrowings from friend and foe. It patterned its hierarchy after the bureaucracy of the Roman Empire, adopted portions of the antique ritual, developed the institution of an absolute leader, and used every means to absorb all existent elements of life and power.

4

In the hands of a man of action, the mass movement ceases to be a refuge from the agonies and burdens of an individual existence and becomes a means of self-realization for the ambitious. The irresistible attraction which the movement now exerts on those preoccupied with their individual careers is a clear-cut indication of the drastic change in its character and of its reconciliation with the present. It is also clear that the influx of these career men accelerates the transformation of the movement into an enterprise. Hitler, who had a distinct vision of the whole course of a movement even while he was nursing his infant National Socialism, warned that a movement retains its vigor only so long as it can offer nothing in the present—only "honor and fame in the eyes of posterity," and that when it is invaded by those who want to make the most of the present, "the 'mission' of such a movement is done for."

The movement at this stage still concerns itself with the frustrated—not to harness their discontent in a deadly struggle with the present but to reconcile them with it, to make them patient and meek. To them it offers the distant hope, the dream, and the vision. Thus at the end of its vigorous span the movement is an instrument of power for the successful and an opiate for the frustrated.

GOOD AND BAD MASS MOVEMENTS

The Unattractiveness and Sterility of the Active Phase

This essay concerns itself chiefly with the active phase of mass movements—the phase molded and dominated by the true believer. It is in this phase that mass movements of all types often

manifest the common traits we have tried to outline. Now it seems
to be true that no matter how noble the original purpose of a
movement and however beneficent the end result, its active phase
is bound to strike us as unpleasant, if not evil. The fanatic who
personifies this phase is usually an unattractive human type. He is
ruthless, self-righteous, credulous, disputatious, petty, and rude.
He is often ready to sacrifice relatives and friends for his holy
cause. The absolute unity and the readiness for self-sacrifice
which give an active movement its irresistible drive and enable it
to undertake the impossible are usually achieved at a sacrifice of
much that is pleasant and precious in the autonomous individual.
No mass movement, however sublime its faith and worthy its purpose, can be good if its active phase is overlong, and, particularly,
if it is continued after the movement is in undisputed possession
of power. Such mass movements as we consider more or less beneficent—the Reformation, the Puritan, French, and American
revolutions, and many of the nationalist movements of the past
hundred years—had active phases which were relatively short,
though while they lasted they bore, to a greater or lesser degree,
the imprint of the fanatic. The mass movement leader who benefits his people and humanity knows not only how to start a movement but, like Gandhi, when to end its active phase.

Where a mass movement preserves for generations the pattern
shaped by its active phase (as in the case of the militant church
through the Middle Ages), or where by a successive accession of
fanatical proselytes its orthodoxy is continually strengthened (as in
the case of Islam), the result is an era of stagnation—a dark age.
Whenever we find a period of genuine creativeness associated
with a mass movement, it is almost always a period which either
precedes or, more often, follows the active phase. Provided the
active phase of the movement is not too long and does not involve
excessive bloodletting and destruction, its termination, particularly when it is abrupt, often releases a burst of creativeness. This
seems to be true both when the movement ends in triumph (as in
the case of the Dutch Rebellion) or when it ends in defeat (as in
the case of the Puritan Revolution). It is not the idealism and the
fervor of the movement which are the cause of any cultural renascence which may follow it, but rather the abrupt relaxation of
collective discipline and the liberation of the individual from the

stifling atmosphere of blind faith and the disdain of his self and the present. Sometimes the craving to fill the void left by the lost or deserted cause becomes a creative impulse.[7]

The active phase itself is sterile. Trotsky knew that "Periods of high tension and social passions leave little room for contemplation and reflection. All the muses—even the plebeian muse of journalism in spite of her sturdy hips—have hard sledding in times of revolution." On the other hand, Napoleon and Hitler were mortified by the anemic quality of the literature and art produced in their heroic age and clamored for masterpieces which would be worthy of the mighty deeds of the times. They had not an inkling that the atmosphere of an active movement cripples or stifles the creative spirit. Milton, who in 1640 was a poet of great promise, with a draft of *Paradise Lost* in his pocket, spent twenty sterile years of pamphlet writing while he was up to his neck in the "sea of noises and hoarse disputes"[8] which was the Puritan Revolution. With the revolution dead and himself in disgrace, he produced *Paradise Lost, Paradise Regained*, and *Samson Agonistes*.

2

The interference of an active mass movement with the creative process is deep-reaching and manifold: (1) The fervor it generates drains the energies which would have flowed into creative work. Fervor has the same effect on creativeness as dissipation. (2) It subordinates creative work to the advancement of the movement. Literature, art, and science must be propagandistic and "practical." The true-believing writer, artist, or scientist does not create to express himself, or to save his soul, or to discover the true and the beautiful. His task, as he sees it, is to warn, to advise, to urge, to glorify, and to denounce. (3) Where a mass movement opens vast fields of action (war, colonization, industrialization), there is an additional drain of creative energy. (4) The fanatical state of mind by itself can stifle all forms of creative work. The fanatic's disdain for the present blinds him to the complexity and uniqueness of life. The things which stir the creative worker seem

[7] For example, review the careers of Milton and Bunyan, Koestler and Silone.
[8] "John Milton," *Encyclopaedia Britannica*.

to him either trivial or corrupt. "Our writers must march in serried ranks, and he who steps off the road to pick flowers is like a deserter." These words of Konstantin Simonov echo the thought and the very words of fanatics through the ages. Said Rabbi Jacob (first century A.D.): "He who walks in the way . . . and interrupts his study [of the Torah] saying: 'How beautiful is this tree' [or] 'How beautiful is this plowed field' . . . [has] made himself guilty against his own soul." Saint Bernard of Clairvaux could walk all day by the lake of Geneva and never see the water. In *Refinement of the Arts,* David Hume tells of the monk "who, because the windows of his cell opened upon a noble prospect, made a covenant with his eyes never to turn that way." The blindness of the fanatic is a source of strength (he sees no obstacles), but it is the cause of intellectual sterility and emotional monotony.

The fanatic is also mentally cocky, and hence barren of new beginnings. At the root of his cockiness is the conviction that life and the universe conform to a simple formula—his formula. He is thus without the fruitful intervals of groping, when the mind is as it were in solution—ready for all manner of new reactions, new combinations, and new beginnings.

3

When an active mass movement displays originality, it is usually an originality of application and of scale. The principles, methods, techniques, and so on which a mass movement applies and exploits are usually the product of a creativeness which was or still is active outside the sphere of the movement. All active mass movements have that unabashed imitativeness which we have come to associate with the Japanese. Even in the field of propaganda, the Nazis and the Communists imitate more than they originate. They sell their brand of holy cause the way the capitalist advertiser sells his brand of soap or cigarettes. Much that strikes us as new in the methods of the Nazis and Communists stems from the fact that they are running (or trying to run) vast territorial empires the way a Ford or a du Pont runs his industrial empire. It is perhaps true that the success of the Communist experiment will always depend on the unfettered creativeness proceeding in the outside non-Communist world. The brazen men in the Kremlin think it a magnanimous concession when they say that communism and capitalism can continue for long side by side. Actually, if there were no free societies outside the Communist orbit, they might have found it necessary to establish them by ukase.

Some Factors Which Determine the Length of the Active Phase

A mass movement with a concrete, limited objective is likely to have a shorter active phase than a movement with a nebulous, indefinite objective. The vague objective is perhaps indispensable for the development of chronic extremism. Said Oliver Cromwell, "A man never goes so far as when he does not know whither he is going."

When a mass movement is set in motion to free a nation from tyranny, either domestic or foreign, or to resist an aggressor, or to renovate a backward society, there is a natural point of termination once the struggle with the enemy is over or the process of reorganization is nearing completion. On the other hand, when the objective is an ideal society of perfect unity and selflessness—whether it be the City of God, a Communist heaven on earth, or Hitler's warrior state—the active phase is without an automatic end. Where unity and self-sacrifice are indispensable for the normal functioning of a society, everyday life is likely to be either religiofied (common tasks turned into holy causes) or militarized. In either case, the pattern developed by the active phase is likely to be fixed and perpetuated. Jacob Burckhardt and Ernest Renan were among the very few in the hopeful second half of the nineteenth century who sensed the ominous implications lurking in the coming millennium. Burckhardt saw the militarized society: "I have a premonition which sounds like utter folly, and yet which positively will not leave me: the military state must become one great factory. . . . What must logically come is a definite and supervised stint of misery, with promotions and in uniform, daily begun and ended to the sound of drums." Renan's insight went deeper. He felt that socialism was the coming religion of the Occident and that being a secular religion it would lead to a religiofication of politics and economics. He also feared a revival of Catholicism as a reaction against the new religion: "Let us tremble.

At this very moment, perchance, the religion of the future is in the making; and we have no part in it! . . . Credulity has deep roots. Socialism may bring back by the complicity of Catholicism a new Middle Age, with barbarians, churches, eclipses of liberty and individuality—in a word, of civilization."

2

There is perhaps some hope to be derived from the fact that, in most instances where an attempt to realize an ideal society gave birth to the ugliness and violence of a prolonged active mass movement, the experiment was made on a vast scale and with a heterogeneous population. Such was the case in the rise of Christianity and Islam, and in the French, Russian, and Nazi revolutions. The promising communal settlements in the small state of Israel and the successful programs of socialization in the small Scandinavian states indicate perhaps that when the attempt to realize an ideal society is undertaken by a small nation with a more or less homogeneous population, it can proceed and succeed in an atmosphere which is neither hectic nor coercive. The horror a small nation has of wasting its precious human material, its urgent need for internal harmony and cohesion as a safeguard against aggression from without, and, finally, the feeling of its people that they are all of one family make it possible to foster a readiness for utmost cooperation without recourse to either religiofication or militarization. It would probably be fortunate for the Occident if the working out of all extreme social experiments were left wholly to small states with homogeneous, civilized populations. The principle of a pilot plant, practiced in the large mass-production industries, could thus perhaps be employed in the realization of social progress. That the small nations should give the Occident the blueprint of a hopeful future would in itself be part of a long-established pattern. For the small states of the Middle East, Greece, and Italy have given us our religion and the essential elements of our culture and civilization.

There is one other connection between the quality of the masses and the nature and duration of an active mass movement. The fact is that the Japanese, Russians, and Germans, who allowed the interminable continuation of an active mass movement without a show of opposition, were inured to submissiveness or iron discipline for generations before the rise of their respective modern mass movements. Lenin was aware of the enormous advantage the submissiveness of the Russian masses gave him: "How can you compare [he exclaimed] the masses of Western Europe with our people—so patient, so accustomed to privation?" Whoever reads what Madame de Staël said of the Germans over a century ago cannot but realize what ideal material they were for an interminable mass movement: "The Germans," she said, "are vigorously submissive. They employ philosophical reasonings to explain what is the least philosophic thing in the world, respect for force and the fear which transforms that respect into admiration."

One cannot maintain with certitude that it would be impossible for a Hitler or a Stalin to rise in a country with an established tradition of freedom. What can be asserted with some plausibility is that in a traditionally free country a Hitler or a Stalin might find it not too difficult to gain power but extremely hard to maintain himself indefinitely. Any marked improvement in economic conditions would almost certainly activate the tradition of freedom, which is a tradition of revolt. In Russia, as pointed out in chapter 3, the individual who pitted himself against Stalin had nothing to identify himself with, and his capacity to resist coercion was nil. But in a traditionally free country the individual who pits himself against coercion does not feel an isolated human atom but one of a mighty race—his rebellious ancestors.

3

The personality of the leader is probably a crucial factor in determining the nature and duration of a mass movement. Such rare leaders as Lincoln and Gandhi not only try to curb the evil inherent in a mass movement but are willing to put an end to the movement when its objective is more or less realized. They are of the very few in whom "power [has] developed a grandeur and generosity of the soul."[9] Stalin's medieval mind and his tribal ruthlessness were chief factors in the prolonged dynamism of the Communist movement. It is futile to speculate on what the Rus-

[9] John Maynard, *Russia in Flux* (London: Victor Gollancz, 1941), p. 29.

sian Revolution might have been like had Lenin lived a decade or two longer. One has the impression that he was without that barbarism of the soul so evident in Hitler and Stalin, which, as Heraclitus said, makes our eyes and ears "evil witnesses to the doings of men." Cromwell's death brought the end of the Puritan Revolution, while the death of Robespierre marked the end of the active phase of the French Revolution. Had Hitler died in the middle of the 1930s, Nazism would probably have shown, under the leadership of a Goering, a fundamental change in its course, and the Second World War might have been averted. Yet the sepulcher of Hitler, the founder of a Nazi religion, might perhaps have been a greater evil than all the atrocities, bloodshed, and destruction of Hitler's war.

4

The manner in which a mass movement starts out can also have some effect on the duration and mode of termination of its active phase. When we see the Reformation, the Puritan, American, and French revolutions, and many of the nationalist uprisings terminate, after a relatively short active phase, in a social order marked by increased individual liberty, we are witnessing the realization of moods and examples which characterized the earliest days of these movements. All of them started out by defying and overthrowing a long-established authority. The more clear-cut this initial act of defiance and the more vivid its memory in the minds of the people, the more likely is the eventual emergence of individual liberty. There was no such clear-cut act of defiance in the rise of Christianity. It did not start by overthrowing a king, a hierarchy, a state, or a church. Martyrs there were, but not individuals shaking their fists under the nose of proud authority and defying it in the view of the whole world. Hence perhaps the fact that the authoritarian order ushered in by Christianity endured almost unchallenged for fifteen hundred years. The eventual emancipation of the Christian mind at the time of the Renaissance in Italy drew its inspiration not from the history of early Christianity but from the stirring examples of individual independence and defiance in the Greco-Roman past. There was a similar lack of a dramatic act of defiance at the birth of Islam and of the

Japanese collective body. German nationalism, too, unlike the nationalism of most Western countries, did not start with a spectacular act of defiance against established authority. It was taken under the wing from its beginning by the Prussian army.[10] The seed of individual liberty in Germany is in its Protestantism, not its nationalism. The Reformation, the American, French, and Russian revolutions, and most of the nationalist movements opened with a grandiose overture of individual defiance, and the memory of it is kept green.

By this test, the eventual emergence of individual liberty in Russia is perhaps not impossible.

Useful Mass Movements

In the eyes of the true believer, people who have no holy cause are without backbone and character—pushovers for men of faith. On the other hand, the true believers of various hues, though they view each other with mortal hatred and are ready to fly at each other's throat, recognize and respect each other's strength. Hitler looked on the Bolsheviks as his equals and gave orders that former Communists should be admitted to the Nazi party at once. Stalin in his turn saw in the Nazis and the Japanese the only nations worthy of respect. Even the religious fanatic and the militant atheist are not without respect for each other. Dostoevski puts the following words in Bishop Tihon's mouth: "outright atheism is more to be respected than worldly indifference . . . the complete atheist stands on the penultimate step to most perfect faith . . . but the indifferent person has no faith whatever except a bad fear."

All the true believers of our time—whether Communist, Nazi, or Fascist, nationalist or religious—have declaimed volubly on the decadence of the Western democracies. The burden of their talk is that in the democracies people are too soft, too pleasure-loving, and too selfish to die for a nation, a God, or a holy cause. This lack of a readiness to die, we are told, is indicative of an inner rot—a moral and biological decay. The democracies are old, corrupt, and decadent. They are no match for the virile congregations of the faithful who are about to inherit the earth.

[10] Said Hardenberg to the King of Prussia after the defeat at Jena, "Your Majesty, we must do from above what the French have done from below."

There is a grain of sense and more than a grain of nonsense in these declamations. The readiness for united action and self-sacrifice is, as indicated in chapter 3, a mass movement phenomenon. In normal times a democratic nation is an institutionalized association of more or less free individuals. When its existence is threatened and it has to unify its people and generate in them a spirit of utmost self-sacrifice, the democratic nation must transform itself into something akin to a militant church or a revolutionary party. This process of religiofication, though often difficult and slow, does not involve deep-reaching changes. The true believers themselves imply that the "decadence" they declaim about so volubly is not an organic decay. According to the Nazis, Germany was decadent in the 1920s and wholly virile in the 1930s. Surely a decade is too short a time to work significant biological or even cultural changes in a population of millions.

It is nevertheless true that in times like the Hitler decade the ability to produce a mass movement in short order is of vital importance to a nation. The mastery of the art of religiofication is an essential requirement in the leader of a democratic nation, even though the need to practice it might not arise. And it is perhaps true that extreme intellectual fastidiousness or a businessman's practical-mindedness disqualifies a man for national leadership. There are also perhaps certain qualities in the normal life of a democratic nation which can facilitate the process of religiofication in time of crisis and are therefore the elements of a potential national virility. The measure of a nation's potential virility is as the reservoir of its longing. The saying of Heraclitus that "it would not be better for mankind if they were given their desires" is true of nations as well as of individuals. When a nation ceases to want things fervently or directs its desires toward an ideal that is concrete and limited, its potential virility is impaired. Only a goal which lends itself to continued perfection can keep a nation potentially virile even though its desires are continually fulfilled. The goal need not be sublime. The gross ideal of an ever-rising standard of living has kept the United States fairly virile. Modern England's ideal of the country gentleman and France's ideal of the retired rentier are concrete and limited. This definiteness of their national ideal has perhaps something to do with the lessened drive of the two nations. In America and Russia the ideal is indefinite and unlimited.

2

As indicated at the start, mass movements are often a factor in the awakening and renovation of stagnant societies. Though it cannot be maintained that mass movements are the only effective instrument of renascence, it seems yet to be true that in large and heterogeneous social bodies such as Russia, India, China, the Arabic world, and even Spain, the process of awakening and renovation depends on the presence of some widespread fervent enthusiasm which perhaps only a mass movement can generate and maintain. When the process of renovation has to be realized in short order, mass movements may be indispensable even in small homogeneous societies. The inability to produce a full-fledged mass movement can be, therefore, a grave handicap to a social body. Ortega y Gasset was of the opinion that the inability of a country to produce a genuine mass movement indicates some ethnological defect. He said of his own Spain that its "ethnological intelligence has always been an atrophied function and has never had a normal development."

It is probably better for a country that when its government begins to show signs of chronic incompetence it should be overthrown by a mighty mass upheaval—even though such overthrow involves a considerable waste of life and wealth—than that it should be allowed to fall and crumble of itself. A genuine popular upheaval is often an invigorating, renovating, and integrating process. Where governments are allowed to die a lingering death, the result is often stagnation and decay—perhaps irremediable decay. And since men of words usually play a crucial role in the rise of mass movements, it is obvious that the presence of an educated and articulate minority is probably indispensable for the continued vigor of a social body. It is necessary, of course, that the men of words should not be in intimate alliance with the established government. The long social stagnation of the Orient had many causes, but there is no doubt that one of the most important is the fact that for centuries the educated were not only few but almost always part of the government—either as officials or priests.

The revolutionary effect of the educational work done by Western colonizing powers has already been mentioned. One wonders whether India's capacity to produce a Gandhi and a

Nehru is not due less to rare elements in Indian culture than to the long presence of the British Raj. Foreign influence seems to be a prevailing factor in the process of social renascence. Jewish and Christian influences were active in the awakening of Arabia at the time of Muhammad. In the awakening of Europe from the stagnation of the Middle Ages we also find foreign influences—Greco-Roman and Arabic. Western influences were active in the awakening of Russia, Japan, and several Asiatic countries. The important point is that the foreign influence does not act in a direct way. It is not the introduction of foreign fashions, manners, speech, and ways of thinking and doing things which shakes a social body out of its stagnation. The foreign influence acts mainly by creating an educated minority where there was none before or by alienating an existing articulate minority from the prevailing dispensation; and it is this articulate minority which accomplishes the work of renascence by setting in motion a mass movement. In other words, the foreign influence is merely the first link in a chain of processes, the last link of which is usually a mass movement; and it is the mass movement which shakes the social body out of its stagnation. In the case of Arabia, the foreign influences alienated the man of words, Muhammad, from the prevailing dispensation in Mecca. Muhammad started a mass movement (Islam) which shook and integrated Arabia for a time. In the time of the Renaissance, the foreign influences (Greco-Roman and Arabic) facilitated the emergence of men of words who had no connection with the church, and also alienated many traditional men of words from the prevailing Catholic dispensation. The resulting movement of the Reformation shook Europe out of its torpor. In Russia, European influence (including Marxism) detached the allegiance of the intelligentsia from the Romanovs, and the eventual Bolshevik revolution is still at work. In Japan, the foreign influence acted not on men of words but on a rare group of men of action which included Emperor Meiji. These practical men had the vision which Peter the Great, also a man of action, lacked, and they succeeded where he failed. They knew that the mere introduction of foreign customs and foreign methods would not stir Japan to life, nor could it drive it to make good in decades the backwardness of centuries. They recognized that the art of religiofication is an indispensable factor in so unprecedented a task.

They set in motion one of the most effective mass movements of modern times. The evils of this movement are well known. Yet it is doubtful whether any other agency of whatever nature could have brought about the phenomenal feat of renovation which was accomplished in Japan. In Turkey, too, the foreign influence reacted on a man of action, Kemal Atatürk, and the last link in the chain was a mass movement.

J. B. S. Haldane counts fanaticism among the only four really important inventions made between 3000 B.C. and A.D. 1400. It was a Judaic-Christian invention. It is strange to think that in receiving this malady of the soul, the world also received a miraculous instrument for raising societies and nations from the dead— an instrument of resurrection.

V

THE SPIRIT
OF AN AGE

IT IS REMARKABLE that after a century of upheavals the paths of change have not become smooth and easy. On the contrary, our world seems to be getting less and less suitable for people who undergo change. Never before has the passage from boyhood to manhood been so painful and so beset with explosions. The passage from backwardness to modernity which in the nineteenth century seemed a natural process is now straining a large part of the world to the breaking point. The hoped-for moves from poverty to affluence, from subjection to freedom, from work to leisure do not enhance social stability but threaten social dissolution. However noble the intentions and however wholehearted the efforts of those who initiate change, the results are often the opposite of that which was reasonable to expect. Social chemistry has gone awry: no matter what ingredients are placed in the retort, the end product is more often than not an explosive.

Σ

War, nationalism, and scarcity are sources of social cohesion and discipline. We tend to forget that social bodies were, to begin with, organs of struggle: struggle with external enemies, and struggle to wrest a livelihood from grudging nature. Hence in a time like ours, when the possibility of abundance goes hand in hand with an absence of external threats, social cohesion is bound to diminish. It is a paradox of the human condition that the longed for end of war and of want should bring societies to the brink of anarchy.

Σ

One hundred years ago, our whole nation was up to its nose in a morass of corruption. Not only the robber barons but people in every walk of life wallowed in crookedness. Crooks on a grand scale were folk heroes, and anecdotes about them pushed out of currency the earlier myths of Franklin, Washington, and the founding fathers. Charles Francis Adams described the mood in his autobiography: "Failure seems to be regarded as the one unpardonable crime, success as the all-redeeming virtue, the acquisition of wealth as the single worthy aim of life. The hair-raising revelations of skulduggery and grand-scale thievery merely incite others to surpass by yet bolder outrages and more corrupt combinations." Nevertheless, the wholesale depravity did not have lasting effects. There was something that kept corruption from harming the social fiber. What was it? Hope. The air was tense with hope, with unbounded faith in the future. What one did in the present did not matter because the present was a mere mat on the doorstep of the future, something that would be thrown away and forgotten. Hope immunizes a society against degeneration and decay. Where there is no hope, even the moral equivalent of sniffles may prove fatal.

Σ

We are living in an epoch of great disillusionment. We are beginning to suspect that to fulfill a hope is to defeat it, and to make a dream come true is to turn it into a nightmare. For a moment it seemed to us that we had arrived, that we had solved all material problems and could sit back and enjoy an eternal sabbath. But we are discovering that the more triumphant our technology, the less does society function automatically. In a time of widespread automation nothing happens automatically. You have to push and pull, threaten and beg, if you want anything done. It seems that by mastering matter we have drained material factors of their potency to shape events.

Σ

It was a shock to a materialistic civilization to discover that the most important facts about a human entity are its illusions, its fictions, its unfounded convictions. A society without illusions is without vigor and without order and continuity. It took a triumphant technology to demonstrate that "things which are not are mightier than things that are."

Σ

In the past not only were illusions long-lived, but the fading of one illusion automatically heightened the receptivity to a new one. But right now in the Western world illusions no longer have the power to lure people to strenuous effort. Life is no longer as visibly miserable as it was in the past, and the opportunities for full-bodied fun easily outbid the appeal of a distant hope. The question is how a population wholly oriented toward the present can be induced to submit to the self-denial indispensable for social cohesion and discipline. Is there a substitute for illusion?

Σ

If one were to pick the chief trait which characterizes the temper of our time, it would be impatience. Tomorrow has become a dirty word. The future is now, and hope has turned into desire. The adolescent cannot see why he should wait to become a man before he has a say in the ordering of domestic and foreign affairs. The backward, also, panting to catch up tomorrow with our yesterdays, want to act as pathfinders in the van of mankind. Everywhere you look you see countries leaping. There is no time to grow. New countries want to bloom and bear fruit even as they sprout, and many have decked themselves out with artificial flowers.

Σ

Some generations have patience and some are without it. This is one of the most crucial differences between eras. There is a time when the word "eventually" has the soothing effect of a promise, and a time when the word evokes in us a bitterness and scorn.

Σ

There has been a gradual narrowing of the range of predictability during the past five hundred years. In the heyday of Christianity, predictability reached the utmost limit—the life beyond. In the idea of progress, which took the place of millennial prognostication, the range of predictability was narrowed to a century or so. With the end of the First World War, predictability shrank further: the craving for security took the place of hope, and people were satisfied if they could foresee the course of a single lifetime. If the shrinking continues, we shall be satisfied if we can predict in the evening the eventualities of next morning. This has already happened in some totalitarian countries, where a man considers himself fortunate if he can be certain that he will not be imprisoned, exiled, or liquidated between going to bed and getting up.

In the past, societies with a vivid conception of a life beyond were indifferent to divination and prophecy. The ancient Egyptians, who expended much treasure and effort in preparing for a hereafter, did not develop any sort of astrology, while the Babylonians, who had no faith in a life beyond, cultivated divination. Hebrew prophecy was at its height when resurrection was not as yet an article of faith. In Europe, astrology came into prominence during the Renaissance when millennial Christianity was losing its hold on the educated.

It is a paradox that in our time of rapid, drastic change, when the future is in our midst, devouring the present before our eyes, we have never been less certain about what is ahead of us. Our need for predictability is far more urgent than in times past, and we are addicted to forecasters and pollsters. Even when the forecasts are wrong we go on asking for them. We watch our experts read their graphs the way the ancients watched their soothsayers read the entrails of a chicken.

Σ

It is a most puzzling fact of our age that at a time when the management of men has become a central task, managers everywhere are ineffectual and unimpressive.

Great leaders are likely to appear where there are abundant opportunities for savoring and exercising power. We savor power when our commands are obeyed, when we have plenty amidst scarcity, and when we can foresee and shape the future. Right now, all such opportunities are scarce. We are witnessing the culmination of a movement of disobedience which, according to Guglielmo Ferrero, had its start at the emergence of the modern

Occident. In no department of life can obedience be taken for granted. Even in armies obedience is no longer automatic. Nor can the possession of plenty give a sense of power where advanced technology promises the end of scarcity. Finally, in a world dominated by the human factor, unpredictability is so innate that it is impossible to savor power by foreseeing, let alone shaping, the future.

Σ

The tendency is to see America's phenomenal conformity as a curse. Actually, the fact that we are shaped by example more readily than other countries may be an advantage in a world that for some mysterious reason cannot produce outstanding leaders. In this country, impressive acts of courage and dedication staged by relatively small groups will find millions of emulators. Such groups can do for us many of the things we expect from a great leader.

Σ

So evanescent are world situations that we cannot suit our actions to facts. The better part of statesmanship might be to know clearly and precisely what not to do and leave action to the improvisation of chance. It might be wise to wait for our enemies to defeat themselves, and heed Bacon's advice to treat friends as if they might one day become our enemies, and enemies as if they might one day become our friends.

Σ

It is evident that drastic change, no matter how desirable, is difficult and dangerous. We are discovering that broken habits can be more painful and crippling than broken bones, and that disintegrating values may have as deadly a fallout as disintegrating atoms.

Σ

We know that our time is more pregnant with meaning and has more lessons to teach than any era in the past. The belly of the world has been ripped open, and we have seen with our eyes things which past generations could only guess at. We need a new type of historian who would mine the present for clues about the past.

There are some who still believe that the historian's task is to write about the past rather than learn from the present. They do all they can to sew up the ripped belly so that they can resume guessing.

Σ

The contemporary explosion of avant-garde innovation in literature, art, and music is wholly unprecedented. The nearest thing that comes to mind is the outburst of sectarian innovation at the time of the Reformation when every yokel felt competent to start a new religion. Obviously, what our age has in common with the age of the Reformation is the fallout of disintegrating values. What needs explaining is the presence of a receptive audience. More significant than the fact that poets write abstrusely, painters paint abstractly, and composers compose unintelligible music is that people should admire what they cannot understand.

Σ

It is remarkable how little history can teach us at present. The past seems too remote and different to matter. We can obtain insights about the present not from books of history but from books dealing with the human condition. The post-industrial age will be dominated by psychological factors, and a meaningful history of our time must base itself on the assumption that man makes history.

Σ

About a hundred years ago, the historian Jacob Burckhardt had a premonition of impending chaos caused by the intrusion of the masses onto the stage of history. The masses, he thought, loathed stability and continuity; they wanted something to happen all the time, and their clamor for change would topple everything that was noble and precious. There were others, well into the twentieth century, who, like Burckhardt, saw the masses as the womb of anarchy. To Freud it seemed that "the individuals composing the masses support one another in giving free rein to their indiscipline." Not one of these learned people had an inkling that the coming anarchy would originate in tiny minorities, including a minority of the learned. Everything that has been said in the past about the anarchic propensity of the masses fits perfectly the activities of students, professors, writers, artists, and their hangers-on during the 1960s, whereas the masses are now the protagonists of stability, of continuity, and of law and order.

Ours is a golden age of minorities. At no time in the past have dissident minorities felt so much at home and had so much room to throw their weight around. They speak and act as if they were "the people," and what they abominate most is the dissent of the majority. The self-assertion of the majority, except on election day, is seen as a threat to freedom. It used to be that minorities looked over their shoulders wondering what the majority thought of them. Now it is the majority that wonders what the minorities think.

The trouble is that the intimidation of the majority is occurring at a time when traditional authority has lost its effectiveness.

Σ

The untalented are more at ease in a society that gives them valid alibis for not achieving than in one where opportunities are abundant. In an affluent society the alienated who clamor for change are largely untalented people who cannot make use of the unprecedented opportunities for self-realization and cannot face the confrontation with an ineffective self.

There is a spoiled-brat quality about the self-consciously alienated. Life has to have a meaning, history must have a goal, and everything must be in apple-pie order if they are to cease being alienated. Actually there is no alienation that a little power will not cure.

Σ

Everywhere we look at present we see something new trying to be born. A pregnant, swollen world is writhing in labor, and everywhere untrained quacks are officiating as obstetricians. These quacks say that the only way the new can be born is by cesarean operation. They lust to rip the belly of the world open.

Σ

The Americanization of the world is an unprecedented phenomenon. The penetration of a foreign influence has almost always depended on the hospitableness of the educated and the well-to-do. Yet the worldwide diffusion of American habits, fashions, and ways is proceeding in the teeth of the shrill opposition of the intellectuals and the hostility of the "better" people. The only analogy which comes to mind is the early spread of Christianity, with the difference that Americanization is not being pushed by apostles and missionaries but, like a chemical reagent, penetrates of its own accord and instantly combines with the common people and the young. "The American way of life," says a British observer, "has become the religion of the masses in five continents."

Σ

There is grandeur in the uniformity of the mass. When a fashion, a dance, a song, a slogan, or a joke sweeps like wildfire from one end of the continent to the other, and a hundred million people roar with laughter, sway their bodies in unison, hum one song, or break forth in anger and denunciations, there is the overpowering feeling that in this country we have come nearer the brotherhood of man than ever before.

Σ

Perhaps, as things are now, it may well be that the survival of the species will depend on the ability to foster a boundless capacity for compassion. Compassion seems to have its roots in the family. We think of those we love as easily bruised, and our love is shot through with imaginings of the hurts lying in wait for them. Parents overflow with compassion as they watch their children go out into a strange, cold world.

Can compassion be made to leak out into wider circles? Does the present weakening of the family in both free and nonfree countries increase the tendency to transfer family attitudes to other institutions—to schools, factories, offices, and various forms of associations? This would mean, of course, that the spread of compassion would cause a wide diffusion of esprit de corps, which is the creation of family ties between strangers.

Would the adoption of a tragic view of life be fruitful of a strong feeling for others? We feel close to each other when we see ourselves as strangers on this planet and when we see our planet as a tiny island of life in an immensity of nothingness. We also draw together when we become aware that night must close in on all living things, that we are condemned to death at birth, and life is a bus ride to the place of execution. All our squabbling and vying are about seats on the bus, and the ride is over before we know it.

1 THE SPIRIT
OF OUR AGE

Up to the end of the eighteenth century there was nowhere a vivid awareness of epochs and ages totally distinct from, and almost incomprehensible to, each other. Even in this country up to 1800, the quality of everyday life was not totally different from what it was, say, four thousand years ago in Mesopotamia and Egypt. Despite a succession of momentous historical events, of empires rising and falling, of new religions, conceptions, discoveries, and inventions, the first forty centuries or so of recorded history, even if not, in the words of Ibn-Khaldun, "as alike as two drops of water," had enough in common to make the idea of the spirit of an age meaningless. George Washington would have felt at home in Cheops's Egypt. Even Napoleon could have engaged in profitable discourse with any of the pharaohs, though if he had met a modern American president they would have had little to say to each other.

The feeling that the present is so novel and unprecedented that, living in it, one can only by an effort of the imagination understand the past came with the Industrial Revolution. Around 1850 the Occident was catapulted into a trajectory away from the ageless, rutted highway of history.

Does this mean that drastic differences in technology make ages incomprehensible to each other? Is the spirit of an age an emanation of technology?

From *First Things, Last Things.*

The eloquent Africanist Laurens Van der Post in his travels through Russia in 1963 was struck by the similarity between the patient, submissive humanity he saw in Russia and the primitive black crowds he had seen in African railroad stations and public offices. He saw "the same silent acceptance of their fate implicit in the expression and attitude of these waiting figures." Everywhere he went, the thought came to him unbidden that "for all its twentieth century trappings, its applied science, its protestation of being objective and rational, Russia was basically neither new nor modern but is a reversion to an exceedingly ancient and primitive state of spirit." He began to suspect that one could not have a real understanding of Russian behavior unless one saw in it an expression of "an archaic, religious and profoundly superstitious system."

Clearly, the technology of present-day Russia, not dissimilar from, and not too far behind, the technology of America, has not made of Russia a nation of our time, imbued with the spirit of our age.

2

Why has an advanced technology not made Russia a modern country?

Saint-Simon characterized the coming of the industrial age as a passage from the management of men to the administration of things. Now there is no doubt that in Russia the Communist party has poured enormous wealth and energies into "the administration of things," and its feats in mastering nature are among the outstanding achievements of the twentieth century. But it is also true that in Russia the central preoccupation has been and still is the management of men—the regimentation of people in every sphere of life. To a ruling Communist party, its role as initiator and director of activities in every field is more vital than the spontaneous flow of copious energies which is the hallmark of a modern society. The advanced technology which to some extent liberates the Russian people from the animal imprisonment of nature cannot liberate them from the menagerie instituted by an orthodox Communist party. The Russian people face the absolute power of the Communist apparatus with the same fatalistic submissiveness and superstitious dread with which primitive humanity faces the inexorable and inscrutable powers of nature.

One of the startling discoveries of our time is that revolutions are not revolutionary. We have been slow to realize that revolutions lead not to a wholly new future but back to a distant past. The most revolutionary changes during the last several decades have occurred in nonrevolutionary countries. Think of what has happened in the United States: since the Second World War we have been transported into a new age. Nineteen fifty seems far off and semi-mythical. Incredible psychological transformations have taken place in other nonrevolutionary countries. The warlike Japanese and Germans have become the world's foremost traders, and the Jews the foremost warriors. Hereditary enemies like France and Germany have become close collaborators; former imperial powers are learning to function as dynamic small countries. Tendencies toward affiliation and federation are concurrent with tendencies toward loosening of long-established unions. The nonrevolutionary world is a seething alembic in which nations are transmuted and new entities synthesized.

The revolutionary countries seem stuck in the mud. When Communist Czechoslovakia tried to shake off its torpor in 1968, it became self-evident that it had to join the nonrevolutionary world. There is fear of change in all revolutionary countries.

3

The spirit of an age is the product not of achievements and happenings but of the type of humanity that makes things happen.

It is vital to remember that, in the West, the passage from the management of men to the administration of things coincided with the transfer of power from traditional elites to the middle class. The ageless spirit of most of history is due to the fact that, from the beginning of history until well into the first half of the nineteenth century, events were shaped and dominated by elites of kings, nobles, soldiers, priests, and intellectuals. The coming to power of the middle class in the middle of the nineteenth century mattered more than the coming of the machine. Had the machine age been inaugurated by aristocrats or intellectuals, the last hundred years would have had a different temper and spirit.

To an elite, power means power over men. It cannot savor power by dominating nature, by moving mountains and telling rivers whither to flow. Even when, as in Soviet Russia, an elite sets in motion vast projects to tame and master nature, it uses these projects as a means for mastering and regimenting men. No elite would countenance, let alone promote, a state of affairs in which things happen of themselves, without command and obedience.

The middle class is the least elitist ruling class we know. Not only is it wide open to all comers, but it aspires to a state of affairs in which things happen of themselves and regulate themselves. Unlike any other ruling class, the middle class has found it convenient to operate on the assumption that if you leave people alone they will perform tolerably well; and under no other ruling class have common people shown such willingness to exert themselves to the utmost. It is this fabulously productive, more or less self-regulating chaos of a society that has given the modern age its singular spirit and set it off from all preceding centuries. Regimentation and minute regulation are as ancient as civilization. Small wonder that elitists of every stripe—aristocrats, Marxists, Fascists, priests, power-hungry intellectuals—have viewed middle-class society and the modern age as abominations.

4

Just now, middle-class society is in deep trouble. Several paradoxes of the human condition have combined to turn its successes into critical failures. Affluence is showing itself to be a greater threat to social stability than poverty. The accelerating rate of change, though the change is mostly for the better, is upsetting and weakening traditions, customs, habits, routines—all the arrangements which make everyday life self-starting and self-regulating. At a time when miracles are becoming commonplace, the commonplaces of everyday life can no longer be taken for granted. Finally, the education explosion is enormously increasing the number of people who want to live meaningful, relevant, and important lives but lack the ability to attain relevance and significance by individual achievements.

To cope with these difficulties the middle class must learn how to contain anarchy, how to regulate and manipulate everyday life, and, above all, how to concoct a faith, a philosophy, and a style of life to suit the needs of a noncreative horde hungering for meaningful, weighty lives. In short, in order to win, the middle class must lose itself. It must shape itself in the image of the elitists who hope and work for its destruction.

There is much talk now of the death of an age and the birth of a new one. My hunch is that, whether the middle class resolves the present crisis or is pushed aside by a new class, the age that is waiting for us around the corner will be not new but ancient. It will be an age preoccupied with the mastery of men—static and ageless despite its advanced technology.

Thus the indications are that the spirit of an age is not only a new phenomenon in history but a short-lived one-time thing. The trajectory into which the Occident was catapulted over a hundred years ago is turning out to be a loop that curves back to where it started. And when we get back to the ancient rutted highway of history we shall find that the revolutionary countries have arrived there before us, making good their boast that they are the wave of the future.

2   BROTHERHOOD

IT IS EASIER to love humanity as a whole than to love one's neighbor. There may even be a certain antagonism between love of
humanity and love of neighbor; a low capacity for getting along
with those near us often goes hand in hand with a high receptivity
to the idea of the brotherhood of men. About a hundred years ago
a Russian landowner by the name of Mikhail Petrashevski recorded a remarkable conclusion: "Finding nothing worthy of my attachment either among women or among men, I have vowed myself to the service of mankind." He became a follower of Fourier
and installed a phalanstery on his estate. The end of the experiment was sad, but what one might perhaps have expected: the
peasants—Petrashevski's neighbors—burned the phalanstery.

Some of the worst tyrannies of our day genuinely are "vowed"
to the service of mankind yet can function only by pitting neighbor against neighbor. The all-seeing eye of a totalitarian regime is
usually the watchful eye of the next-door neighbor. In a Communist state, love of neighbor may be classed as counterrevolution-
ary. Mao Tse-tung counted it a sin of the liberals that they would
not report the misdeeds of "acquaintances, relatives, schoolmates,
friends, loved ones." To promote solidarity among neighbors is as
good a way as any to block the diffusion of totalitarianism in a
society.

The capacity for getting along with our neighbor depends to a

From *The Ordeal of Change.*

large extent on the capacity for getting along with ourselves. The self-respecting individual will try to be as tolerant of his neighbor's shortcomings as he is of his own. Self-righteousness is a manifestation of self-contempt. When we are conscious of our worthlessness, we naturally expect others to be finer and better than we are. We demand more of them than we do of ourselves, as if we wished to be disappointed in them. Rudeness luxuriates in the absence of self-respect.

Now it is the tragedy of our time that the enormous shrinkage in distance, both geographical and social, that has made neighbors of all nations, races, and classes coincides with an enormous increase in the difficulties encountered by the individual in maintaining his self-respect. In the Communist part of the world, government policies are designed not only to eliminate actual and potential opponents but to turn the population into a plastic mass that can be molded at will. A Communist regime cannot tolerate self-respecting individuals who will not transgress certain bounds in dealing with their fellowmen. Such individuals, even when few in number, render a population uncontrollable. "Every despotism," wrote the nineteenth-century philosopher Henri Amiel, "has a specially keen and hostile instinct for whatever keeps up human dignity and independence."

This hostility is particularly pronounced in a despotism that is doctrinaire. Because of its professed faith in the irresistibility of the doctrine that supposedly shapes its course, such a despotism cannot be satisfied with mere obedience. It wants to obtain by coercion the type of consent that is usually obtained only by the most effective persuasion and this requires a population made up of individuals totally devoid of self-respect.

Nor is it at present easy for the individual to maintain his self-respect in the non-Communist part of the world. In the underdeveloped countries the poignant awareness of backwardness keeps even the exceptional individual from attaining "the unbought grace of life" that is the true expression of an unconscious and an unquestioned sense of worth. Similarly, individual self-respect cannot thrive in an atmosphere charged with racial or religious discrimination. Both the oppressors and the oppressed are blemished. The oppressed are corroded by an inner agreement with the prevailing prejudice against them, while the oppressors are infected with the fear they induce in others. Finally, even in advanced and egalitarian societies, millions of people are robbed of their sense of worth by unemployment and by the obsolescence of skills as the result of revolutionary advances in technology.

Thus it seems that under the conditions current in the world the nearer people get to each other, and the more alike they become, the dimmer grows their awareness of the oneness of mankind. The human image is clear to us when it is a silhouette against a distant horizon. When we come close so that we can look into a fellowman's eyes, we find there mirrored an image of ourselves, and we do not like what we see.

The unattainability of self-respect has other grave consequences. In man's life the lack of an essential component usually leads to the adoption of a substitute. The substitute is usually embraced with vehemence and extremism, for we have to convince ourselves that what we took as second choice is the best there ever was. Thus blind faith is to a considerable extent a substitute for the lost faith in ourselves, insatiable desire a substitute for hope, accumulation a substitute for growth, fervent hustling a substitute for purposeful action, and pride a substitute for unattainable self-respect. The pride that at present pervades the world is the claim that one is a member of a chosen group—be it a nation, race, church, or party. No other attitude has so impaired the oneness of the human species and contributed so much to the savage strife of our time.

Goodwill and peace have their roots in the conditions of the individual's existence. But the terrible fact seems to be that with our present standards of usefulness and worth there is no certainty that economic and social betterment can cure the individual's private ills. The new industrial revolution holds the promise of an unprecedented abundance for all, and there is a chance that in the free world the masses, though largely unemployed, will still get their share of the good things of life. But unless there is a radical change in our conception of what is useful, worthwhile, and efficient, it is hard to see how an economic millennium could possibly create optimal conditions for general tolerance and benevolence.

Under our scheme of values, affluence and leisure may well intensify tendencies toward national and racial exclusiveness. In an indolent population living off the fat of the land, the vital need for an unquestioned sense of worth and usefulness is bound to find expression in an intensified pursuit of explosive substitutes.

At bottom, a country's efficiency must be measured by the degree to which it realizes its human potentialities. Industry, agriculture, and the exploitation of natural resources cannot be deemed efficient if they do not serve as a means for the realization of the intellectual, artistic, and manipulative capacities inherent in a population.

Now that the new industrial revolution is on the way to solving the problem of means, and we can catch our breath, it behooves us to remember that man's only legitimate end in life is to finish God's work—to bring to full growth the capacities and talents implanted in us. A population dedicated to this end will not necessarily overflow with the milk of human kindness, but it will not try to prove its worth by proclaiming the superiority and exclusiveness of its nation, race, or doctrine.

3 SHAME

THE ANCIENT HEBREWS were alone in envisioning a troubled paradise. The Garden of Eden was not an abode of bliss but a place tense with suspicion and anxiety. For no sooner did God, in a moment of divine recklessness, create man in his own image than he was filled with misgivings. There was no telling what a creature thus made would do next. So God placed Adam and Eve in the Garden of Eden, where he could watch them.

It is plain that Adam and Eve were ill at ease under constant observation and in their isolation from other living things. They welcomed the snake's visit, confided in him, and listened to his advice. The expulsion from Eden was not the terrible fall it has been made out to be. It was actually a liberation from the stifling confines of a celestial zoo.

What concerns me is the puzzling fact that when Adam and Eve followed the snake's advice, disobeyed God's commandment, and ate from "the tree of the knowledge of good and evil," they felt not guilty but ashamed—ashamed of their nakedness. What connection could there be between the knowledge of good and evil and the impulse to cover the genitals with fig leaves?

It is conceivable that, to begin with, good and evil were not individual but social concepts. That was good which preserved the group, and that evil which threatened its survival. Now, there is one dangerous threat that no society can escape: the recurrent

---

A slightly different version of this essay appeared in *In Our Time*.

threat of disruption by juveniles as a young generation passes from boyhood to manhood. Since sexual drives are at the core of the destructive impulses characteristic of the juvenile phase, sex is seen as a threat, hence an evil. The primeval association of sex with shame is like the taboos of incest and endogamy, part of an apparatus devised to defend a society against rape by the juveniles of the tribe. Through the millennia, societies have acted as if their safety depended upon the preservation of female chastity.

Sex, of course, is not the sole threat to the group. Cowardice, weakness, bad manners are as dangerous, and they, too, are associated with shame.

Shame, far more than guilt, involves an awareness by the individual of being watched and judged by the group. It is to be expected, therefore, that the more compact the group, the more pronounced the sense of shame. The member of a compact group carries the group within him and never feels alone.

Some anthropologists distinguish between the "shame culture" of primitive groups and the "guilt culture" of advanced societies. Actually, what comes here in question is not social primitiveness but social compactness. It is true that the most perfect examples of social compactness are found in primitive societies. But a technically advanced country like Japan, in which the individual is totally integrated with the group, has as strong a sense of shame as any primitive tribe.

By the same token, one would expect the sense of shame to be blurred where socialization of the young becomes ineffectual and social cohesion is weakened. In this country in the 1960s the inability of adults to socialize their young made it possible for juveniles to follow their bents, act on their impulses, and materialize their fantasies. The result was a youth culture flauntingly shameless.

Even more disconcerting is the fact that the loss of shame is not confined to juveniles. The adult majority is not ashamed of its cowardice, workers are not ashamed of negligence, manufacturers of marketing shoddy products, nor the rich of dodging taxes. We have become a shameless society.

Our intellectual mentors strive to infect us with a sense of guilt—about Vietnam, the Negro, the poor, pollution—and frown on shame as reactionary and repressive. But whether or not a sense of guilt will make us a better people, the loss of shame threatens our survival as a civilized society. For most of the acts we are ashamed of are not punishable by law, and civilized living depends upon the observance of unenforceable rules.

One also has the feeling that shame is more uniquely human than guilt. There is more fear in guilt than in shame, and animals know fear. We blanch with guilt as we do with fear, but we blush with shame. Did not Aristotle define man as "the beast with red cheeks"?

Shame is a social manifestation, and the more compact a society the more intense the sense of shame. Yet no society is so shameless as monolithic Soviet Russia. In Russia everybody lies, everybody betrays, everybody confesses—no one feels shame. It is legitimate to wonder whether Soviet Russia with all its totalitarian compactness constitutes a genuine society. Mihailo Mihailov maintains "there is no society at all in communist countries."

Hesiod foresaw the day when Aidos (the goddess of shame) and Nemesis (the goddess who avenges offenses against shame) would forsake mankind "and bitter sorrow will be left for mortal man, and there will be no help against evil."

4 MONEY

Most of us spend much of our time satisfying other people's needs. To a visitor from another planet it would seem that human beings, like bees, are engaged in selfless toil. It would take him some time to discover that this self-sacrificing behavior is induced by a magic drug called money.

Whoever originated the cliché that money is the root of all evil knew hardly anything about the nature of evil and very little about human beings. The monstrous evils of the twentieth century have shown us that the greediest money grubbers are gentle doves compared with money-hating wolves like Lenin, Stalin, and Hitler, who in less than three decades killed or maimed nearly a hundred million men, women, and children and brought untold suffering to a large portion of mankind.

The middle class was relatively harmless as a ruling class because money could cure all that ailed it. But the passage from the nineteenth to the twentieth century saw a shift from a preoccupation with money to a preoccupation with power, and centuries ago Sir Francis Bacon saw such a shift as "the origin of all evil."

It is part of the sickness of our time that money has lost its magic power. What ails societies at present is not that everybody wants as much money as possible but that everybody wants to do as little as possible. We used to wonder how in the nineteenth century it was possible for so few to have so much at the expense

---

From *In Our Time*.

of the many. Now the wonder is that so many get so much at the expense of the few. A showdown between the few who work and the many who don't will make a strange sort of revolution.

What will life be like in a society without money? Men will try to assert and prove themselves by all sorts of means and under all sorts of conditions. The question is what means for the demonstration of individual worth are likely to develop in a nonacquisitive society. Vying in creativeness is not a likely substitute for vying in acquisitiveness—not only because creativity is accessible to the relatively few but because creative work is without automatic recognition and is not easily measured. Rather, the nonacquisitive society is likely to develop into a combination of army and school. People will prove themselves by winning degrees, medals, and rank. There will be as much, if not more, self-seeking, envy, and malice as in a moneyed society.

A society without money will be largely preoccupied with managing people. There will be little social automatism. Sowing, harvesting, mining, manufacturing, and so on will become burning national problems. Instead of the harmless drug of money there will be the black magic of brainwashing and soul-raping. Eventually the medicine men will be replaced by slave drivers.

5   A NEW RULING CLASS

I WAS PAST MIDDLE AGE when the "Free Speech" movement exploded on the Berkeley campus in 1964. Like most older people I was outraged by the sight of history made by juvenile delinquents. Yet, from the beginning, part of me was straining for a detached view. I became interested in the role the young had played in history, and it did not take much research to show me that we can hardly know how things happened in the past unless we keep in mind that much of the time it was juveniles who made them happen.

The discovery did not turn me into a champion of the young. Watching the happenings of the 1960s I shuddered at the thought of a world run by self-important, self-indulgent, self-righteous, violent, and clownish punks. Nevertheless, I find myself now and then believing that history made by the young may help us solve some otherwise insoluble problems.

Until the middle of the nineteenth century the young were prominent in politics and acted effectively as creators of business enterprises, advocates of new philosophical doctrines, and leaders of armies. The middle-aged came to the fore with the Industrial Revolution. The experience and capital necessary to make a successful capitalist in an industrial age required a long period of apprenticeship. One might say that from the middle of the nineteenth century the world has been run by and for the middle-aged. This era seems now to be nearing its end.

From *In Our Time*.

The golden century of the middle-aged was a century of colossal achievements but also of unprecedented global exploitation and global wars. In no other era have the young been sacrificed so recklessly by their elders. And the middle-aged were bunglers as history makers. Does anyone believe that the course of history would have been any more destructive had the young of the warring nations come together in 1919 and written a peace treaty instead of leaving peacemaking to the middle-aged and the old?

The most fateful fact at this moment is that over half the population of the planet is under twenty-five—an age group that clamors for action and power. In the past, the predominance of the young coincided with a short life span: the young had opportunities for action because the older people were eliminated by death. Today, longevity combined with the driving creativity of the young produces an explosive situation. But we need not adopt Stalin's practice of killing the old to make room for the young. Instead, we could have an upper age limit for holding public office. We could retire people at forty.

In an age of ceaseless change, people over forty are no longer flexible enough to take things in their stride. Feeling the strain, they may not mind stepping back. They can stand the separation from action and power much better than the young, bursting with energy and driven by the need to prove themselves. And, should compulsory retirement breed frustration and bitterness, it stands to reason that people over forty would have neither the energy nor the recklessness to tear the world apart.

Retirement at forty would have to be linked with an earlier start for adulthood—say, at thirteen. But after doing the everyday world's work for twenty-seven years one would gain entrance into another world of creative leisure. For it is likely that retirement at forty would result in something like a cultural renaissance. People over forty are more attuned to learning and more patient in application than the young. The need to compensate themselves in the realm of thought and imagination for what they have had to give up in the world of action ought to generate a potent creative ferment. One would also expect a flowering of scholarship when the over-forty go back to the universities to mesh what they have learned in the book of the world with what they can find in the world of books.

6   NEW SCHOOLS

Sᴏᴍᴇ ᴛɪᴍᴇ ᴀɢᴏ, while writing an essay on the young, I was surprised by the discovery that the young in this country do not constitute a higher percentage of the population now than they did in
the past. The percentage of the young has remained remarkably
constant through many decades. What has changed is the percentage of teenagers.

We used to count as teenagers those between the ages of thirteen and nineteen. Now the teenage group includes those between
the ages of ten and thirty. Television is giving ten-year-olds the
style of life of juveniles, while the post-sputnik education explosion has been keeping students in their late twenties on the campuses in a state of prolonged adolescence. There are no children
any more. Our public schools are packed with mini-men hungering for the prerogatives and probably the responsibilities of adults.

The poet W. H. Auden said that what America needs are pu-
berty rites and a council of elders—which are probably beyond
our reach. What this country needs and can have is child labor.
The mini-men, bored by meaningless book learning, are hungry
for action, hungry to acquire all kinds of skills. There will be no
peace in the schools and no effective learning until the curriculum
is reformed to meet the needs of the new type of students.

There is evidence that a student in his early twenties, when he
is eager to learn, can master in less than a year all the book learn-

---

From *In Our Time*.

ing that teachers try to force into unwilling, bored minds through grammar and high school. There is also evidence that forced book learning in public schools, rather than preparing students for a fuller mastery of subjects later in college, often makes them unfit for it. When the great British physicist Sir Joseph Thomson was asked why England produced great scientists, he answered, "Because we hardly teach science at all in schools. Over here the minds that come to physics arrive in the laboratory with a freshness untarnished by routine." Reading and writing are a different matter; if these are not thoroughly mastered early in life we will continue to have what we have now: college students who can neither read nor write.

I propose, then, that half the school day be given to book learning—reading and writing, elementary mathematics, a familiarization with the geography of the planet, and a bird's-eye view of history—and the other half to the mastery of skills. Retired carpenters, masons, plumbers, electricians, mechanics, gardeners, architects, city planners, and their like could teach the young how to build houses and roads, how to landscape and garden, how to operate all sorts of machines. Retired bankers, manufacturers, merchants, and politicians could familiarize the young with finance and management.

In small towns where there is only one school it would be easy to set aside a hundred acres or so on which generations of students could build a model neighborhood, plant gardens, and raise crops. In large cities the work would have to be done on the outskirts or on land made available by slum clearance. By the time they graduated from high school, the young would be equipped not only to earn a living but to run the world.

7   A RETURN TO THE PAST?

ALTHOUGH IT SEEMS REASONABLE to expect a post-Christian world to revert in some degree to pre-Christian paganism, hardly anyone is hospitable to the idea that post-industrial society might revert in some degree to pre-industrial days. What kinship could there be between an automated affluent society and a hand-run society immersed in scarcity? Yet even a cursory reading of the social history of the early decades of the nineteenth century reveals startling similarities with our time. The London and Paris of those days had the same insoluble problems that at present confront our big cities. There were slums, overcrowding, and violent crime in the streets. The well-to-do middle class became obsessed with the new dangers and the explosive social situation. The nightly muggings, beatings, and holdups were the chief topic of conversation. The poor were seen not simply as people without money but as a race of savages and barbarians. There was also a chorus of complaints from employers about the indolence and negligence of workers. There was a stubborn resistance among workers to dull, repetitive factory work. Coleridge observed in 1833 that, in Manchester and Birmingham, "the most skillful artisans are constantly in the habit of working but a few days a week and idling the rest." Absenteeism was high, especially on Mondays, and the high turnover of labor crippled production.

In nineteenth-century England the reconciliation of the work-

---

From *In Our Time*.

ing population with factory routine occurred in the late 1840s, in the wake of the railroad boom. Railroad-building stimulated a whole range of new metal industries which, unlike the textile mills, employed only men and paid high wages. Around 1850 the illusion was born that there was a comfortable, secure, middle-class existence ahead for the steady worker. The illusion lasted until the Great Depression of the 1930s, when the conviction spread among unemployed workers on the dole that hard, steady work does not get one anywhere.

It is remarkable that whereas books on the coming of the Industrial Revolution usually have a clear recognition that the willingness to work, as much as anything else, gave modern civilization its unique character and marked it off from all its predecessors, there is rarely a reference to the changed attitude toward work in books on post-industrial society. They mention the educational attainments of the new generation of workers, the shift from blue-collar to white-collar work, the role of the unions, but not a word about an impending human-energy crisis. So axiomatic is the assumption that history is made by elites that it simply does not enter the forecaster's mind that a revulsion from work is likely to give the post-industrial society a backward pre-industrial aspect.

8   A JOB TO DO

You ASK YOURSELF: what are the essential attributes a country must have if it is to remain vigorous? The answer is simple: so long as a country has courage and a passion for excellence, it can face the future confidently no matter how fearsome its difficulties. Courage is not only a serviceable substitute for hope but also, as we shall see, a chief factor in the maintenance of personal security. As to the passion for excellence, it may sound highfalutin but it actually concerns common, everyday affairs. I have spent fifty years doing backbreaking work in the fields, in lumber camps, and on the waterfront. Many of the people I lived and worked with had courage and, whether they knew it or not, a passion for excellence.

The word "job" used to have a magical connotation in this country. It was something you had to do the best way you knew how. A job might be unpleasant, dangerous, or trivial, but it still had to be done, and it had a claim on your skill and ingenuity. Even the simplest job had its mysteries; and once you fathomed them, time flew.

As one would expect, the formula "There is a job to do" cropped up in situations that had nothing to do with work. The American's performance on the battlefield, for instance, had a matter-of-fact, job-doing quality. He did not fight for a motherland, a fatherland, or some ideal. There was a job to do and he

---

From *In Our Time*.

did it. Field Marshal Rommel was astonished by the prosaic, practical manner in which Americans mastered modern warfare.

The manner in which the word "job" lost its magical potency illustrates the irony of history. I remember how scornful I felt when I first read Marx's description of the worker's attitude toward work in a capitalist society. The worker, he said, feels physically and morally debased by his work. He is like an exile in his place of work and feels at home only when away from his job. Marx never did a day's work in his life and never took the trouble to find out how a worker really feels when on the job. He naturally assumed that workers were a lesser breed of intellectuals. Yet one hundred years after Marx, by an ironic twist of history, a toylike sputnik launched in Marxist Russia set off a chain of events which eventually made Marx's false diagnosis come true in capitalist America.

On October 4, 1957, we woke up to discover that the clodhopping, backward Russians were ahead of us. We reacted hysterically. Catching up was a new and frightening experience. We poured billions of dollars into universities to produce scientists and technicians wholesale. There were soon seven million university students, and this mass of semester intellectuals set the tone for the young in every walk of life.

By now, American workers have indeed become a lesser breed of intellectuals, and their attitude toward work fits Marx's description. They feel demeaned and dehumanized by the work they have to do, and see a job as a trap. Workingmen who have never read a book talk glibly about frustration, alienation, and relevance. Like intellectuals, they expect a job not only to give them the wherewithal of a living but to fill their lives with meaning.

The fact that the word "job" has lost its magic is affecting America's performance and style in every field. Will we now need the tribal magic of charismatic leaders and medicine men to get things done in peacetime and in war?

9   A MEANINGFUL LIFE

ONE OF THE LESSONS of our times has been that abundance, freedom, equality, and justice are not the most vital ingredients of a satisfactory individual existence. We begin to realize that from now on a society will be able to stay on an even keel only when it makes it possible for a majority of its people to live meaningful lives.

Now there is no doubt that in a modern society there is not enough meaningful work to make it possible for most people to derive the meaning in their lives from the work they do to earn a living. For it is a peculiarity of a modern society that the existence of millions depends on being paid for doing what seems like nothing when done. The demand that the work we do for a living should be worth doing, though not "a human impertinence," as Santayana thinks, is unrealizable.

There is a widely held assumption that the way to inject meaning into an individual existence is by participation in communal affairs. Good citizenship, it is true, involves a concern for the welfare of one's community, one's country, and probably of humanity in general. But to make such a concern the main content of an individual life is, in normal times, unnatural and unhealthy. With the majority of people, participation in communal affairs cannot be more than a condiment.

In a healthy society the craving for acting with others becomes

From In Our Time.

an aid to the realization and cultivation of the individual. One joins others in a relatively small circle to learn a skill, master a subject, or exercise a talent. It is the acquisition of skills in particular, irrespective of their utility, that is potent in making life meaningful. Since man has no inborn skills, the survival of the species has depended on the ability to acquire and perfect skills. Hence the mastery of skills is a uniquely human activity and yields deep satisfaction.

I am also convinced that the mastery of skills can be therapeutic. Skill-healing should be particularly effective in the reconstruction and human renewal of the chronically poor, the unemployable, and people who cannot cope with life. The acquisition of a skill generates confidence, and, since people enjoy doing what they are good at, it may have an energizing effect.

Were I the mayor of San Francisco, I would have a square or a street lined with small shops where subsidized experts would practice and display every imaginable skill. I would comb the globe for little-known or half-forgotten skills in order to revive them. And I would have children apprenticed to the experts. It is most fitting that in an automated world the human hand, a most unique organ, should come back into its own and again perform wonders. It may well be the hand that will save us.

THERE WAS A TIME when I doubted whether tragedy was at all possible in America, and whether a person born and bred in this country could produce a genuinely tragic novel, play, or film. Our equality is such that a comedown in the world cannot have the tragic import it has in other countries. In no other society are there so many topics on which people from every walk of life can talk with equal expertise. Moreover, the language of skid row or prison is not substantially different from the language one hears in a bankers' club or even in the White House. Thus a banker who lands on skid row or in prison finds life familiar enough not to feel wholly cast out. No matter how low one has fallen, one can still argue, beef, and laugh in the old manner.

However, the fact that a personal comedown cannot be as tragic here as in other countries became irrelevant when tragedy did come to America in the 1960s. In that terrible decade, the sober report of a day's events became the chronicle of individual and communal tragedies: the wasting of young lives by rebellion, drugs, and drift; the despair of parents; the humbling of the deans and presidents of universities; the savage beatings of old men and women by murderous punks; the wreckage of two presidencies; the agony of a drawn-out, no-win war.

Though the war is now over, the campuses quiet, and the presidency back on the rails, the tragic sense is still with us. We can-

---

From *In Our Time.*

not defend our old against juvenile savagery in the big cities, and we cannot safeguard our young. The erosion of traditional authority goes on and it is difficult to see how it can be stopped, let alone reversed. This is particularly true of the family. We are at the mercy of our children. They hold the threat of self-destruction over our heads, and we are afraid to discipline them. It is doubtful whether a society can be buoyant and hopeful as long as there are pitfalls and snares to decimate the young, and parents can do little to protect and direct their children.

Thus it looks as though the tragic sense will become a permanent part of our inner landscape. It will darken our spirit, but it may also deepen and mature our view of life. It may make us

> Face the world as a wise man should,
> And train for ill and not for good.

It may also expand our capacity for compassion.

VI

DIARIES

1 WORKING AND THINKING

ON THE WATERFRONT:

JUNE 1958–MAY 1959

While rummaging recently through a pile of old notebooks, I came upon a diary I had kept during 1958–1959. I had completely forgotten about it. Nineteen fifty-eight and fifty-nine were difficult years. I was trying to write a book on intellectuals, the "men of words." Since it was not going to be a scholarly history, it soon became clear that my theories and insights would not come to more than forty pages of manuscript—enough for a chapter but not a book. Obviously, the intellectual would have to be part of a larger subject. I began to suspect that all my thinking life I had had only one train of thought, that everything I had written stemmed from a central preoccupation, and that I might go through life and never discover what it was.

I had to sort things out, talk to somebody. So on June 1, 1958, I began a diary. Toward the end of March 1959, I realized that my central subject was *change*.

The diary eventually filled seven notebooks. The entry on the last pages of the seventh notebook was for May 21, 1959. I cannot remember what decided me not to go on with the diary. I did not start another notebook. . . .

June 1, 1958, 5 A.M.

I am getting self-righteous. This usually happens after a long stretch of work. I remember Tolstoy saying somewhere that work makes not only ants but men, too, cruel.

10 P.M. Went to the union meeting. Again the contrast between the shallowness of the discussion of the abstract and the
originality in tackling the practical. There were weariness and
boredom in the first half of the meeting, which dealt with the
Sobell[1] case. In the second half the subject was the hiring hall and
how to deal with chiselers on the scrap-iron jobs. The solutions
offered were original and wonderfully simple. The simplicity
gave an impression of subtlety.

It would be fascinating to see whether the longshoremen's
originality in solving practical problems could be canalized into
theorizing, into play with ideas. We know of a canalization in the
opposite direction. The feats of practical organization of the
Rockefellers, Morgans, and even the Carnegies were the feats of
potential philosophers plunged into an atmosphere of action.

I am aware of how much I have to watch myself. The pitfalls
are all around me: not only self-righteousness but also a deprecation of others. The others are not the people I work and live with
but intellectuals in general. There is a danger I might come to
think of most of them as sterile, pretentious, and futile. And it is
strange that this attitude should become pronounced at a time
when my creative flow is at its thinnest.

June 2

I am cheered when I realize that things vital for my welfare or prospects have completely escaped my mind. Preoccupation with the self has always seemed to me unhealthy.

June 4

Nine hours on the German ship *Dortheim* at Pier 26.

On the way to the job it occurred to me that the homogenizing
effect of communism is partly due to its inducement of passionate
rudeness. People of all nationalities become somewhat alike when
swept away by a fit of rudeness.

---

[1] Morton Sobell was convicted as a spy in 1951, in connection with the Rosenberg
case. Radical factions in the West Coast longshoremen's union were agitating for his
release.

On the job I had for a partner the voluble "Cigar" Barlow. He is a fairly effective speaker at union meetings, somewhat of a rabble-rouser, but his conversation is pretentious and empty. He had gone to see and hear Billy Graham but could not tell me why he was so impressed.

June 5

Finished the German ship at Pier 26. Six hours. I have the impression that many Scandinavian longshoremen are anti-British. They speak of the British the way the anti-Semites speak of the Jews. According to Axel (the Swede I talked with today), the British own every mine, mill, and factory in Sweden, Norway, and Denmark. How come then that Britain seems to be hard up? Answer: it's only the poor in Britain who are hard up.

It is perhaps true that ignorance tends to be extremist. Our opinions about things we do not know are not likely to be balanced and moderate.

My mind went back to the possibility of canalizing practical intelligence into intellectual channels. One of the peculiarities of the Occident has been the ability to distill spiritual impulses from practical pursuits. The Italian Renaissance was born in the marketplace, in the workshops of artisans. Pure science emerged from the pursuits of architects, navigators, and craftsmen. The Greeks extracted geometry from surveying, and their philosophy probably received its first impetus from the invention of coinage about 700 B.C. It was but a step from seeing coins as the common denominator of all values to the speculation that the manifold appearance of things is due to different states and arrangements of a fundamental substance.

June 6

Four hours on the *Lurline* at Pier 35. In the afternoon I took Lili and the boy to the circus.[2] The child seemed hardly interested in the stunts and spectacles. My impression is that he can

---

[2] The boy is my godson, Eric, son of Selden Osborne and Lili Fabilli Osborne.

get excited only about something that has a direct relationship to him. In the zoo and in the park there is a personal confrontation between the animals and himself. His lack of enthusiasm for the circus reminded me that he shows no interest in animated toys such as pecking birds and other mechanical animals. He becomes passionately attached to the sculpture of a bird or an animal, no matter how crude, and he spends hours tinkering with wheels and gears.

June 8

A long day, loading rice on the *Hawaiian Pilot* in Encinal. There have been intermittent downpours. Had it not been for the pleasantness of my partner it would have been a miserable day. Between loads I watched sparrows feeding on patches of scattered rice on the dock. How timid they are! Are there blobs of life without fear? They come down from the edge of the roof like a cloud and spread out like a carpet. They seem to keep away from spots where the rice is thick, as if fearing a snare.

June 10

Didn't do a thing! Took Lili and the child to lunch and then to the Indian exhibition at the Palace of the Legion of Honor.

I was roused by an article in the latest *Nation*. It was written by a fellow named Halevy who is obviously an American writer living in Mexico. He has recently paid a visit to the U.S., and his article deals with Disneyland and Las Vegas. My impression is as follows: the man is some sort of a radical and is extremely money-conscious. He is contemptuous of people who throw away their money. Chances are he made some money in real estate and went to Mexico, where living is cheap, to write. His contempt for America is standard. In one sentence he says we worship the almighty buck, and in the next he grinds his teeth at the levity and stupidity with which we throw away our money. He resolves the paradox by saying that our wasting is a way of punishing our idols.

The article tells little about this country but a lot about the writer. I am struck by the money-consciousness of many radicals and their skill in business. The radicals on the waterfront have left-wing principles and right-wing bank accounts.

June 11

Eight hours on the sorting pile at Pier 29. As hard a day as I have had in a long time. This company has finally figured out how to keep people going without a pause. No sooner is one row of loads started than another row is all lined up waiting for you. I ran up a sweat all day long, partly because of the heat but mostly because of the rushing.

The *Manchester Guardian Weekly* is suggesting that De Gaulle, if not a fool, is a weak sister. Some letter writer sees De Gaulle as a Hindenburg who unknowingly prepares the ground for a Hitler. My feeling is that whatever authoritarian regime may arise in France, it will be tempered by rationality and good sense.

June 13

Seven hours on the Norwegian ship *Hoegh Silverstream*. Rubber wrapped in burlap or paper. Partner one of the laziest men on the waterfront, yet he worked well and was pleasant. He is, however, a total pathological liar, hence conversation with him is meaningless. For a moment it seemed to me that only conversation about ideas can be honest. Most other talk is nine tenths make-believe.

At noon I heard a Sicilian proverb: "The tongue has no bones, but it can break bones."

In the afternoon a young clerk came over to talk with me. He is a graduate of the University of San Francisco, fairly intelligent, pious, and superficial. I talked a lot and it did me good. Yesterday I spent twenty-four hours without talking to anyone, so I needed talking.

June 14

Pier 26. British ship. Discharging meat and apples from New Zealand. The apples, Rome Beauties, are as fine as any I have seen.

The British crew on this ship makes an excellent impression. Compared with average-run Americans, these British sailors have a freshness about them and an individual distinctness. They have not spent their lives running, and they have not been run over by life. One wonders whether America will continue to exist when we stop running. There is a streak of extremism in us: we either run or do not move at all. To stop running might edge most of us toward inertness and stagnation.

June 15

Danish ship at Pier 31. More meat from New Zealand.

I have been feeling quite well the last couple of days—light of heart and alert.

Charles Diehl's book on Byzantium is sometimes stimulating. Here and there Byzantium reminded me of today's America. For example, Diehl quotes a sixth-century writer about the popular preoccupation with chariot races in the Hippodrome, which roused men to inordinate heights of passion: "Should the green charioteer take the lead, some are in despair; should the blue overtake him, half the city is in mourning. People with no personal interest in the matter utter frantic imprecations; those who have suffered nothing feel grievously wounded." He adds, "The most serious men declared that without theatre and Hippodrome life would have been virtually joyless." The emperor himself took sides in the contest as passionately as anyone.

I have always wondered whether it is vital for a society that all its members should have some common subjects in which they are equally interested and in which they all have some expertise. In Byzantium the common subjects were theology and chariot races. In this country they are machines and sports.

On the way home, in the bus, it struck me that Eric is the only human being I have grown onto—that the relation between us is that of a graft. Many elements went into the making of this graft, not the least of which is that he is my namesake. The fact is also important that he is still to me, after 2½ years, a new human being—a newly arrived visitor on this planet. Now and then I feel like asking him how he likes this country.

June 16

In this morning's *Chronicle*, Tito is quoted as saying of the Chinese Communists that in attacking Yugoslavia they are using "such insulting language that even Marx and Lenin, if they could hear it, would turn over in their graves." Unintentionally, Tito is here pointing at Marx and Lenin as paragons of rudeness. Good manners are inconceivable without a degree of objectivity and the give-and-take of compromise. He who clings with all his might to an absolute truth fears compromise more than the devil. He throttles the soft amenities which would dovetail him with others and blur his uncompromising stance. Thus it happens that when a faith loses its potency, rudeness often serves as a substitute.

June 22

Nine and three-quarter hours on the *Hawaiian Wholesaler* in Encinal. Steady grind but the loads moved slowly. A good bunch. I felt better at 6 P.M. than I did in the morning.

I spoke with a tall Montenegrin whom I call Negus. He is Communist in his sympathies, bitter about this country, chock-full of grievances, but we get along. I asked him how many years ago Stephen Dushan lived. He answered correctly: about six hundred years ago. I felt I could discuss with this barely literate Montenegrin some of the things I have learned from Dichl's *Byzantium*. I pointed out that the Bible was translated into Serbian, Bulgarian, and Russian before it was translated into German, French, and English. How come? Because in the West the Catholic Church was an independent power, an imperial power, and it did not want to see the formation of national churches, which might be promoted by a translation of the Bible into common speech. On the other hand, the Byzantine church, being under the thumb of the emperor, was interested solely in the Christianization of the warlike barbarians, and this could be effected more readily by the formation of national churches.

Eventually, national churches came into being also in the West, and nations crystallized around these churches. This is a significant point: the compact churchly organization of Christianity promoted nation formation, while Islam, being without a churchly organization, could not supply a nucleus for national crystallization. This suggests that compact Communist parties, rather than promote internationalism, may in the long run foster nationalist separatism.

He was listening attentively and shaking his head, but I had no way of telling whether he got the hang of what I said. Of one thing I am sure: he will always remember, and brag about it, that the Bible was translated into Serbian long before it was translated into English—that Serbian literature is more ancient than English literature.

June 23

The kink in my back is gone. Yesterday's work did it. The world looks clean and fresh after last night's rain. I have a long list of chores to do, and I am just getting ready to clean my room. Before starting I read the last few pages of *Byzantium*. I cannot tell as yet what I got out of the book, but it corrected my view of the Byzantine Empire as a stagnant body. It needed vigor to last a thousand years.

5 P.M. Spent a hectic day getting things done. Now I am caught up. After a meal of lettuce salad and pea soup I sat down to drink a glass of tea and read. I happened to read the latest issue of the *Nation*. Suddenly I threw it away as a distasteful thing (whining, self-righteous, carping, petulant) and turned to a new travel book by Lord Kinross. This is a continuation of his book on the interior of Asia Minor.

7 P.M. The second Kinross book, so far as I read, is inferior to the first. Since I am in the mood to make it easy for myself, I switched to another book—a delightful one. It is a book of letters written by an American woman who lived in Jerusalem in 1953–54. It is a warm, sensitive, honest book. My first reaction is: what delightful people Americans are. I ought perhaps to say fine people. And saying this, I reflect that I certainly am not an American. Under similar circumstances I would have been neither delightful nor fine. Here she is among total strangers, and she does not carp or criticize or betray the least trace of bad temper. The American's capacity for fraternization is a noble feature, a true foretaste of the brotherhood of man. The book is *Letters from Jerusalem* by Mary Clawson. I shall probably sit up all night reading it.

July 1

Nine hours on the *Flying Enterprise* at Pier 34. A busy day but not unpleasant. The work though steady was not rushed.

Both morning and evening are now cold and wet, but the middle of the day has a warm brilliance. The bay as seen through the huge open door in the back of the dock seemed a fairyland. I don't think a landscape can come into a room through a window. It can come in only through a door.

The fact that I accomplish little when I take time off disqualifies me as a writer. I do have an original idea now and then. If I hang on with all my might, I eventually put together a few thousand words. It may take a year. I lack a flow of words. The most crucial words are never at my service. I have to search and recruit them anew every time.

July 2

Followed the *Flying Enterprise* to Oakland. An easy day in warm weather. A discussion with several Slavonians on the relative merits of America and the old country. What it comes to is that this is not a country for the old. After twenty some years in America, these Slavonians are still homesick for their native village. They are excellent workers—skilled and conscientious. They look healthy and young for their age. But the American tempo grates on them. They talk of the ease and the slowness back home, and how men over fifty no longer work but sit around talking and sipping coffee, letting their children take care of things, and remain hale till they are eighty or more. Actually, none of these Slavonians would be happy if he went home. A few tried and rushed back to America. I mentioned the fact. One of them said, "It may be so, but it will be our greed that will drag us here."

Early this morning on my way to work I felt a burning pain in the arms. It seemed to me for a moment that had I been without this pain I would have been wholly happy. In a moment like this I realize how lucky we are when nothing at all—good or bad—happens to us.

July 3
Worked the same ship the same place. A cold wet gale is just now blowing outside, and the world is lost in thick fog.

More talk with the Slavonians. As I said, they are extremely competent people. I found that most of them built their own houses, have small vegetable gardens, and each has a well-appointed workshop in the basement. I cannot see how people of their kind back in the old country need a totalitarian government to tell them what to do. Even the most perfect central planning could not achieve anything approaching what these people manage to do on their own.

Returning to the talk about the old country, I remarked that there is nothing to prevent them from getting together and re-creating somewhere in California a replica of the village they came from. They are all of them well off, and it should not be impossible to obtain the required financing from a bank or even from a government agency. One of them said, "It can't be done. The air here is not clear. Even in the mountains there is gas and smoke. In the old country the air is sweet."

July 6
Nine hours on the Chilean ship *Almagro* in Encinal. Quite a number of people on the Chilean ship look like intellectuals. I don't think they are passengers. In several Latin-American countries the intellectuals go not only into teaching and the civil service but also into the army. This is probably one reason why army officers are meddling in government. It could be that lack of employment prompted some intellectuals to become sailors on merchant ships.

I am reading *An American in India* by Saunders Redding. The author is an American Negro sent by the State Department to India. It is a perplexing and depressing book. When facing the most preposterous questions and defamatory insinuations, he remains speechless. He tells us that he identifies himself with America, yet here is a man of words without words. I suspect that for an American audience this is probably the most anti-Indian book they could read.

July 7

Same ship, same place. Six hours. In the morning as I walked down the several blocks from the bus stop to the docks, I was impressed by the gardens in front of the houses. The houses, of average size, are fairly old yet in excellent shape. The people living here are mostly workingmen. The sight of the gardens and houses turned my mind to the question of maintenance. It is the capacity for maintenance which is the best test for the vigor and stamina of a society. Any society can be galvanized for a while to build something, but the will and the skill to keep things in good repair day in, day out, are fairly rare. I wonder how true it is that after the Second World War the countries with the best maintenance were the first to recover. I am thinking of Holland, Belgium, and Germany. I don't know how it is in Japan. The Incas had an intense awareness of maintenance. They assigned whole villages and tribes to keep roads, bridges, and buildings in good repair. I read somewhere that in ancient Rome a man was disqualified as a candidate for office because his garden showed neglect.

Saunders Redding's book is worth reading for its detailed recording of the talk of the Indian intellectuals both young and old. He reproduces minutely their arguments, rudeness, sarcasm, and self-righteousness. Since he seldom essayed a rebuttal, his recording comes out sharp and forceful.

July 9

I had several good hours with Lili and the boy. He is growing up fast and is becoming reasonable. He ate a frozen boysenberry tart which he greatly enjoyed. For the first time I saw him attack food methodically—eating first the loose berries on the plate and, after cleaning them up, tackling the tart. I savor being with him the way I savor food and drink. Tonight I feel as if nothing can go wrong. Everything we do is adequate, everything we say meaningful, everything we see memorable.

July 10

There is something in the air. You come to expect America to fail, whether it be in the launching of a satellite, the exhibition at the Brussels Fair, the intervention in the Near East, the revival of the slumping economy. We are not in the van, and we are not going anywhere in a hurry. To those in the van much is forgiven; their blemishes and shortcomings are temporary, since they are growing and rushing into the future. But to those who are not going anywhere, the present (made up of vulgarity, senseless haste, juvenility, dishonesty) is all there is. You are suddenly aware that the country is in dire need of an exceptional leader. The need is an unhealthy symptom.

July 12

Pier 38. One o'clock start. The five-hour shift (1–6) passed without the least strain.

Reading Ivan Bunin's little book *Memories and Portraits* reinforced my conviction that life with writers, artists, and intellectuals in general is most likely to be irritating and unpleasant. Wherever these people come together the air will be charged with envy and malice. It could be that the air thus charged stimulates the creative flow. Yet what a strained and miserable life it would be!

July 15, 5 A.M.

It is wonderfully good that I don't have to go to work. A four-day stretch of work gives a special flavor to a free morning. Come to think of it, no particular place or particular day has ever had a special flavor for me. No homesickness for a place, and no looking forward to a holiday.

Yesterday five thousand American marines landed near Beirut. No one knows how the Russians will react. The idea occurred to me that the present confused goings-on in the Near East made good sense to members of Jehovah's Witnesses. According to them, all that is happening in the world at present is a prelude to the battle of Armageddon, which will take place on the plain of

Jezreel. The return of the Jews to Israel has for its chief purpose the readying of the battlefield. The kibbutzim which now dot the plain of Jezreel are clearing and leveling the ground and draining the swamps. Movements of troops, whether in the frozen expanse of Russia or in the heart of America, are preliminary stages in the unfolding of the drama. Yesterday's landing of five thousand marines is a meaningful development. I wonder how many hypotheses which make sense in nuclear physics are more valid than the meaningful hypothesis of Jehovah's Witnesses.

July 20

I have just returned from a union meeting. The discussion about the newly instituted eight-hour shift was as intelligent and absorbing as any I have heard. Several of the speakers, though plain longshoremen, would not have been out of place as delegates to the United Nations or as representatives at difficult negotiations of whatever nature. Details of organization fascinate the average American, and dealing with them brings out his subtle originality. Could this organizational intelligence be effective in science or philosophical speculations?

August 4

Five hours on the *Mikagesan Maru* at Pier 23. I did some composing during the short shift. The reason for today's composing was partly that we had hardly anything to do, since it was all heavy lifts, and partly that I had nothing to read.

It is important that I should note the difficulty and pain I experience in writing. It is incredible how vague is my memory of past difficulties. It is only now, when I am beginning to go through it again, that there is a revival of faded memories. Since the publishing of a couple of books I have been cast in the role of a writer and, without being aware of the utter absurdity of it, I have come to expect words to flow out of my fingertips. The truth is that I have to hammer out each sentence and must hang on to an idea for ages if aught worthwhile is to be written.

Last evening I sat down at the table to write and could make no headway at all. The irritation was such that I had to dress and get out of my room. I drifted to a cheap movie and saw an old Western (*The Far Horizon*). It was eleven before I went to bed, and I was up at four thirty.

August 15

Nine hours on the Dutch ship *Batjan*. As easy a day as one could wish and no sort of unpleasantness. Still the depression this evening is as black as yesterday. I must face the fact that the chief reason for the depression is that I cannot write.

August 16

Still on the *Batjan* at Pier 23. Today I somehow managed to make some progress on "Intellectuals as Schoolmasters." In Jewish history between the return from the Babylonian captivity and the destruction of the second temple, the schoolmasters prevailed against kings, nobles, and priests. The result was a school possessing a nation rather than a nation possessing a school. In China, too, during the period of the contending states, the schoolmen were on the march. Confucius, Mo Ti, and their disciples felt themselves qualified as rulers. The schoolmaster Mo Ti organized his disciples into an army of experts in all departments of government. In Greece, schoolmaster Plato maintained that cities would never have rest until schoolmasters became kings. All through the ages schoolmasters seem to have had the delusion that they could order society as readily as they could a classroom. But it is probably the twentieth century that will be seen in retrospect as the golden age of the schoolmaster.

In all contemporary mass movements, schoolmasters played a vital and often leading role. I am willing to bet that more than half the leaders in Africa are ex-schoolmasters. In the Nazi movement, grammar-school teachers played a prominent and fateful role. Now and then I am inclined to think that the passion to teach, which is far more powerful and primitive than the passion to learn, is a factor in the rise of mass movements. For what do we see in the Communist world? Half the globe has been turned into a vast schoolroom with a thousand million pupils at the mercy of a band of maniacal schoolmasters.

August 17

Still at Pier 23. Nine hours. Fishing fever has seized many of the people working on this ship. The striped bass are running, and they have been catching real big ones. The result was that half of the time we were short-handed on a big pile of drums. The strain and the irritation combined to make it an unpleasant day. Of course, I didn't write a line.

August 27

Eight hours on the Norwegian ship *Evanger* at Pier 41. Steady grind all day long, and I had neither the time nor the inclination to write a line.

In the morning on the bus, I heard a man argue that the "No Smoking" signs are put up by the fire insurance companies. Pretty soon they'll have "No Smoking" signs inside the house, even in the bedroom. In other countries people smoke wherever they please, but here the insurance companies are running things.

I haven't had a good look at the bay all day. The feeling of being rushed drains the capacity for savoring things.

In the morning I read an article by Max Nomad on "Masters Old and New." Writing in 1937, he clearly discerns the intelligentsia as the coming elite in both capitalist and noncapitalist countries. But the article is without a hint of the intellectual's role in history, and the significance of his dramatic comeback in the twentieth century.

September 1

I just read the introduction to *Men of Words.* It is not bad. I also copied Sections 8 to 11. I have so far forty pages of manuscript. The thing is crude and fragmented, but it is a beginning.

September 3

Eight hours on the *Arizona Maru* at Pier 24. An easy day, and I am off tomorrow. My head worked in spasms. The beginning of Part 2 must tackle the problem of the optimal milieu for literature. I shall trace the chain of events which led to the appearance of written literature in Egypt, Sumer, Palestine, Greece, and China. But the main thing is to outline the conditions optimal for literary creativeness.

After all, the chief value of history is not that it helps us understand the present or decipher the future but that it furnishes us clues concerning the manner in which man is affected by his natural and social environment. We cannot experiment with humanity, but history is a record of how man reacted under a variety of conditions.

September 29

What is the optimal milieu for creativeness in literature, art, music, etc.? It is a milieu which rewards excellence. Cosimo the Elder reverenced talent the way the pious reverence saints. When Arab civilization was at its height, the Ommiad caliphs gave poets and scholars precedence over officials, and some of them were made governors of provinces. To Louis XIV a good sentence was a major achievement.

In an optimal milieu there is considerable leisure. Where people are engrossed in some feverish pursuit so that they neither are bored nor dream dreams nor nurse grievances, creativeness will be anemic.

Finally, an optimal milieu is one in which the creative are in close intercourse with each other—hating, loving, envying, admiring; where faces flush, hearts flutter, and minds swell with the passion to rival and emulate.

October 1

Eight hours on the *Wonorato* at Pier 23. My partner was the old Slavonian with the big nose and squinting eyes. He has a chip on his shoulder, but his aggressiveness is actually defensive. We got to talking about the achievements of the different nationalities. He said, "You heard about the Slavonian inventor Nikola Tesla? He was greater than Edison, but he remained poor because he was a foreigner. When Edison was trying to make an electric bulb he asked Tesla whether it could be done. Tesla answered in Slavonian: '*mazda*,' which means 'maybe.' This is why they have the word 'mazda' on the electric bulbs."

He also told me of a Slavonian longshoreman who went to the old country and just returned. Among the stories he tells is the following one: he was standing on the sidewalk in some town watching a gang of pipefitters at work. They guessed he was an American and one of them asked, "What would they pay us an hour for this kind of work in America?" He answered, "They would not give you five cents."

October 3

It is funny that on my days off I don't feel like keeping the diary.

Today I worked eight hours sorting cargo at Pier 29. It was a steady grind, but we had a good bunch.

Yesterday I received a letter from an editor of the *Saturday Evening Post* offering me $2,500 for an article on fanaticism. I shall not answer until I have an article to send him. It won't do to rehash the old stuff.

This morning I happened to think of the possibility that a virulent outburst of fanaticism may precede the death of a faith. Southern fanaticism on the issue of slavery was at its height when slavery became untenable, and the same is true of the present segregationist fervor. The fanaticism of the Crusades preceded the coming of the Renaissance, and the religious fervor of the Thirty Years' War was followed by the skepticism of the seventeenth and eighteenth centuries. It is also true that the rabid chauvinism of the second quarter of the twentieth century has been followed by a considerable cooling of the nationalist spirit in the West. The question is how fast do burning problems burn themselves out?

October 6

Cleaned the room, took care of the laundry, went down to the hall to sign up and pay dues. The rest of the time I just fiddled around. In the evening I went to see a movie.

Lili brought over the boy for a few minutes. He has become demonstratively affectionate. At three years he has an astounding range of understanding and feeling. His capacity for utmost remembrance and utmost forgetting is a puzzle. He forgets his grievances and hurts in a jiffy. He cannot be inflated durably, nor can he be humbled and crushed. Yet he has a phenomenal memory for sights and sounds. He knows most of the letters of the alphabet, the names of a hundred animals, can easily identify any number of melodies, and knows quite a number of nursery rhymes by heart. He learns rapidly. But, as I said, he forgets in a flash many things, even those which caused him pain enough to make him cry.

October 8

Eight hours on a Japanese ship at Ninth Avenue loading onions. The heat and sweat have left me limp. I can't even read, let alone write. There is no use changing course ten days before the vacation. It is conceivable that thoughts are dammed up within me, and once the flow of words starts all will be well. I have had the feeling for months that steady work has settled a thick carpet of dust over my mind—a dust bowl.

October 13

This has been the sixth straight day of work, and I probably feel more chipper and limber now than when I started last Wednesday. Chances are if I went on working day after day I might notice cycles of tiredness, a curve of fatigue. I might get over my tiredness even as I work. How my mind would fare is hard to say. Long periods of rest have not had a stimulating effect. Unless I have my teeth into a subject, and a body of manuscript to rethink and rewrite, there is no guarantee that leisure will be productive. I am even afraid to try it and find out. Have I a subject right now? I know that the intellectual is not it. Nor is it fanaticism. Chances are that the intellectual, the true believer, mass movements, etc., are facets of a larger problem. None of these topics can stir and excite me just now.

October 18

Eight hours at Pier 29 on a Luckenbach ship. I am replacing a regular dockman in Rekula's gang. Most of the gang are Finns, and when I am with them they stuff me full of Finnish words. Today I learned to count up to ten and a dozen words or so concerning the weather, ships, and the work.

It occurred to me during the day that in my present state of weariness I ought not to make any plans. My mind is not in good shape. After catching my breath and spending some time with myself I may be able to gauge things and decide what to do. Tomorrow is my last day of work. Perhaps for the first time in my life I am looking forward to a vacation.

I seem to be afraid to make an outline of what I am going to say to the editors and journalists from Southeast Asia next Thursday. I ought to speak about the American worker—his readiness to work, his skill, his ability to get things done with a minimum of supervision, and his attitude toward the pencil pushers.

October 20

Thinking in my case is like sluicing poor placer dirt. You must trap every flake of gold if you are to get anything. The final lump is not a nugget but a "button" made up of innumerable flakes each so slight that it floats.

October 21, 8 A.M.

This is the second day of my vacation, and already I feel as if I had spent a whole month doing nothing. I have forgotten how to rest and not give a damn. Went to sleep last night at three. A book written by a group of German generals kept me up. When I finally went to bed I slept fitfully.

October 23

Today I have to meet the journalists from Southeast Asia, and it preys on my mind. It seems to me that I shall be carefree when it is over.

6:30 P.M. It was a hell of a meeting. These people came to us to look and learn, but as men of words they were contemptuous of our practicalness and our addiction to acts rather than words. Since America was shaped by the masses, it seems to them that we have no civilization at all. I responded with an attack on the sort of civilization they cherish—a civilization shaped and dominated by scribes—and warned them to beware of American influence. For Americanization affects mainly the masses, stiffens their backbone, and infects them with a passion to act on their own, get their full share of the good things of life, and dispense with the tutelage of scribes and clerks. I remembered Saunders Redding, the American Negro in India, and the sort of baiting he had to endure without hitting back. I struck out in all directions. Bill Stucky of the American Press Institute said it was the first time anyone had talked back to them. They had needled and baited everyone from Dulles down. Americans don't know how to be rude to foreigners. I am glad I let them have it.

October 24

Spent hours in the Mechanics Library. When I returned, my room seemed cheerful and I said "Hello" to the four walls. I am going to boil up some pea soup with Vienna sausages, drink hot tea, and read a book by Van der Post on the Kalahari Desert and the Bushmen.

Many topics have gone stale on me, while others remain fresh. I know that the field of self-awareness is about played out. The origin of the modern Occident has become a somewhat dim subject, perhaps from neglect. The intellectual is still in the center, though I am aware of a deep reluctance to go on with it. The uniqueness of man and the nature of change are subjects I would love to tackle.

During the whole day I have not spoken half a dozen sentences, yet I feel as if I have been engaged in an interminable dialogue. The optimal milieu for me is to be surrounded by people and not be part of them.

October 26

I woke up with the idea that it was Monday. It cheered me somewhat to realize that it was not yet. I spent several hours downtown eating breakfast and strolling about.

I wonder how much of the feeling of well-being that I have had now and then during the past two days comes from the book I am reading—Van der Post's *The Lost World of the Kalahari*. Nothing this man ever writes could be without the excitement of life. And even as he brings to life the landscape, the plants, the animals, and the human beings he also manages to put the quality of himself in every word. His prose though unlabored is genuine poetry. You begin to realize that the chief function of poetry is to use words as charms to evoke life and colors and smells—a sense of joy, of awe, of compassion, and so on.

Yet all the time you know that it is the man and not his words that count. Wherever he puts his foot the earth becomes portentous. It is as if his presence has diverted the elements and forces from their routine pursuits. The whole world is addressing him, and concerning itself with his tastes and intentions.

October 28

One can achieve more in a few fruitful minutes than in months of effort. The same problem which confronts the cultural historian also baffles the individual facing himself. What is it that releases our energies, kindles our mind, illumines our soul, and gives wingèd words to dim stirrings inside us? Creativeness has both a social and an individual aspect. Flowering and decline are cycles which occur both in the history of a society and in the life span of the individual.

I derive a subtle pleasure from the conviction that the world does not owe me anything. I need little to be contented: two good meals, tobacco, books that hold my interest, and a little writing every day. This to me is a full life.

October 29

I have not worked out in detail the differences between Islam and Christianity. Whereas Christianity, both in the West and in the East, promoted national crystallization, Islam had on the whole a denationalizing effect. Only in Persia, with its awareness of a superior culture and its memories of past glories, did national consciousness persist after conversion to Islam. Both Islam and the Roman Empire were denationalizing agents. Both incorporated the elites everywhere into the conquering ruling class. After two centuries of Islam, the bureaucracy and the military were wholly in the keeping of non-Arabs. The bureaucracy, known as "the people of the pen," was largely responsible for the flowering of Islamic culture. The converted masses, too, found pride and fulfillment in Islam. Renan's theory that it was the denationalization caused by the Roman Empire which brought about an increased interest in social problems and a receptivity to new religious movements does not hold true of Islam. Islam seemed to fulfill every need and had a tranquilizing effect. The end result was stagnation.

Compared with Christianity, Islam is almost without inner contradictions—between church and state, profession and performance, the spirit and the flesh. We somehow assume that inner contradictions, if severe enough, may bring about the breakdown of a society or a system. Actually, vigor and creative flow have their source in internal strains and tensions.

October 30, 6:30 A.M.

You accept certain unlovely things about yourself and manage to live with them. The atonement for such an acceptance is that you make allowances for others—that you cleanse yourself of the sin of self-righteousness.

November 1

I notice wild fluctuations of confidence. Ten minutes after I have finished writing something passably good I wonder how I managed to do it.

A stranger spoke to me on Powell Street. He knew my name and wanted to talk. We went into Compton's and talked for a while over a cup of coffee. He was a typical lesser intellectual: interested in ideas, but without an inkling of what an original idea is. What role do ideas play in his life? They perhaps give him the feeling that he is walking in higher regions, that he is above the noise, stench, and pain of the present. I am quite certain that had I chosen my illustrations from petty everyday life rather than from history and world politics he would have felt it as a desecration. Ideas and words are to him a badge of distinction.

Fair play with others is primarily the practice of not blaming them for anything that is wrong with us. We tend to rub our guilty conscience against others the way we wipe dirty fingers on a rag. This is as evil a misuse of others as the practice of exploitation.

November 7
What would life be without coincidences? Actually, all prayers and hopes are a reaching out for coincidences. Most of the time, too, it is the timely occurrence of chance which gives us the feeling that we are really going somewhere. For all I know, a life is great because it is a crossroad of coincidences.

Where sheer survival is concerned, accidents are less decisive in the case of man than in the case of animals. Much of the time, society shields a person against death by accident. But in the shaping of a life, chance and the ability to respond to chance are everything.

The idea that man is a stranger on this planet always excites me. To feel wholly at home in the world is to partake of the nature of an animal. I play with the fancy that some contagion from outer space was perhaps the seed of man. The present fascination with outer space and the eternal preoccupation with stars, heaven, and God are a sort of homing impulse which draws us back to where we came from.

November 11

Went down to the hall but wasn't dispatched. I called Lili and she, the boy, and I spent a pleasant morning in the park. We walked from 8th Avenue to the ocean, and then uphill to Cliff House, where we had an enormous breakfast. The boy began by being unusually affectionate. But as he wearied of the long walk he became moody.

I have begun to read Van der Post's *Dark Eye in Africa*. I do not as yet know what the book is about. The introduction is a tissue of existentialist double-talk. But as I leafed through the text it seemed I might find here something about the prehistory and history of Africa.

6:30 P.M. No. There is hardly any history. It is a discussion of African unrest in mystical terms. Van der Post objects to our "causalistic concept of life, our linear idea of a chain of cause and effect." He thinks that such an approach "to the mercurial soul and nature of man is dangerously limited." Yet to me there is a singular beauty in the lucid exposition of a linear chain of cause and effect. It can encompass intuitive insights and vague intimations and need not be "dangerously limited."

November 13

Eight hours on the *Samadinda* at Pier 19. Loading lumber, mostly with a good bunch. The bay, seen from the dock, had surprising colors: leaf green of a most delicate shade along the bay bridge, and a band of pale purple on the Oakland side. The wires of the bridge have been painted with red lead, but they look pure pink. Toward evening you could see the rain coming down, as a gray smear, across the bay.

Just now it is raining outside. I have eaten a light supper of crackers, avocado, tuna, and a can of beer. I shall take a hot shower and then sit down to read *Flamingo Feather*, a novel by Van der Post. This is the first novel I have touched in years.

November 16

Eight and three-quarter hours on the *Hawaiian Merchant*. It was steady going all day. The pineapple discharged was of many marks, and the loads came out badly mixed. Luckily, I had Joe Monitz for a partner. We get along fine, and we both did our utmost. Time passed rapidly. I had no time to read or scribble. Nor did I have time to talk with anyone.

Finished *Flamingo Feather*—long-winded and unconvincing.

November 17

I took out from the library a book of essays by Georges Bernanos (*Last Essays*). At last a genuine Frenchman. His directness and lucidity come as a surprise in these days of existentialist double-talk. One is no longer used to writing that says exactly what it means. Rivarol said that anything that's not lucid is not French. Most contemporary French writers are writing like Germans.

Finished Section 12. Very short. I know what Section 13 has to be.

9 P.M. Finished Section 13. A peculiar dejection settled on me this afternoon. It may have something to do with my upset stomach. I am easily irritated. Going down Market Street in the afternoon I was fuming at the clumsy deception practiced by even the most reputable stores. It is an old trick which twenty years ago was confined to shady shopkeepers on skid row. Now it is practiced by all. The infuriating thing is that the trick works. An article marked $1.99 sticks in the mind as costing one dollar and a few cents. It is not in me to view things with alarm, yet this spread of deception affects me as if I were witnessing the spread of corruption and decay.

November 22

Eight hours on the *Hawaiian Packer* in Encinal. At noontime in the lunchroom the canteen man came over to talk with me. He asked whether I was interested in psychos. I said no, since normal people are more interesting and stimulating than the abnormal. Then he plunged into a weird discussion of the goings-on in the world since the beginning of time. There is something outside the world, he said, some sort of agency which at intervals infects our earth with a feverish agitation. Even the molecules of a piece of wood are affected by it. When such an agitating influence is on, history explodes. This is the reason why history is made in spurts.

It was only after half an hour of talk that I realized that his original question was whether I was interested in *cycles*, not psychos.

The gang I worked with today was all Negro. My partner was an excellent worker—conscientious and extremely willing. All day long people from other gangs came visiting, and I overheard some of the talk. One elderly fellow eulogized chiropractors, and particularly the one who was treating him. "Anyone says chiropractors are no good will get his ass whipped." His chiropractor had been treating him for arthritis, tonsilitis, and ulcers. "I never felt so good in forty years. He charges $250, and I am paying $25 a week. It's worth every penny."

November 23

I can't sit down to write. I can sit down to rewrite. I usually sit down to read or to copy, and then at intervals insert a sentence or so in the manuscript.

This morning I went down to the hall and wasn't dispatched. Only a few dockmen were called. I returned to my room, reworked Section 14, then took a shower and went to see *The Seventh Seal*. Though the movie has no story, I found it wholly absorbing. The re-creation of the Middle Ages was fascinating and the acting excellent. Actually, when a moving picture deals with a remote era, the mere breathing of life into any common episode of that time is enough. A story might perhaps diminish the authenticity, since all stories are contemporary. The reactions and responses of individuals are timeless.

November 24

Didn't feel like going to work. I spent most of the day shopping. A huge tiger for Eric, and a wooden tray for Lili. It cost about $25.

At noon I noticed the headlines about a terrific slump in the prices of stocks. I felt quite cheered. There is no doubt malice in this attitude, but my gloating had also a legitimate reason. Rising stock prices have often meant a rise in prices generally. A devaluation of wages and savings is a more general and grievous calamity than the busting of thousands of gamblers.

I wrote very little during the day. Section 15 will deal with scribes as sages and prophets, and Section 16 with scribes as schoolmasters. It will need vigorous writing to show that the scribe began to shape history when he lost power. Creativeness and moral fervor are phenomena of a stretched soul, and the stretching of the soul is brought about not by the possession of power but by the insecurity of individual autonomy—by detaching the scribe from either church or state apparatus.

It goes without saying that the scribe does not relish his insecurity. He strives with all his might, whether he knows it or not, to create an order of things in which the scribes' usefulness is unequivocal—which is to say, an order run and dominated by scribes.

November 25, 11:30 A.M.

Bought *Doctor Zhivago* at the Bonanza bookstore. The girl at the store seemed glad to see me. She gave me the only copy on hand, which she was apparently reading. The book is a Christmas present for Selden.

The stock market is still falling. No one seems panicked. It is a peculiarity of our time that crises simmer but do not come to boil.

November 26

Eight hours on the Norwegian ship *I Gadi* at Pier 9. I felt in good shape. Though tired toward the end, I was not irritable.

All through the day I was worked up by an article in the latest issue of the *Nation*. A would-be maker of history by the name of Birnbaum vents his irritation with the mass of people in the Western democracies. What riles him is that the common people "consume," seem to enjoy their private lives, and show no interest in "general political programs." Here is a mediocre mind throwing its weight around.

9 P.M. I am more tired than I had imagined. I am reading *Doctor Zhivago*—181 pages so far. Interesting but not soul-stirring.

November 27, 6:30 P.M.

Finished *Doctor Zhivago*. The book reads easily, never drags, and holds one's interest. But it is only in the last hundred pages that one's heart becomes involved. It is not in a class with Dostoevski and Tolstoy. Still, no other book gave me so poignant a picture of the criminal magnitude of the Russian Revolution. But Russia has recovered. The aftermath of the revolution has not been like the aftermath of the great calamities of the past, such as the Mongol invasion. One can decry nationalism and damn it as a monstrous perversion. Yet it gives immortality to the societies of the present. It is national pride that raised Germany from the ashes, and it was a chief factor in Russia's recovery from revolution and war.

November 29

I have been reading a book on the Aztecs, *Burning Water* by Séjourné Laurette.

One gains the impression that the rise of cities and civilization was the result of a fusion of a sedentary, highly skilled population, and an invading population of warrior hunters who knew little of crafts. The substance of civilization was furnished by the conquered; the organization, particularly the evolvement of cities, was largely the work of the conquerors. It is conceivable that the priesthood was of the conquered population, and the fusion between conquered and conquerors was consummated by an alliance between the priestly and the warrior hierarchies.

In Egypt, the skills and crafts came from the delta and the organization from the south, from upper Egypt. In Mesopotamia the situation was similar: the native dwellers of the lowlands, on the Persian Gulf, had the skills, and the Sumerians brought the organization. In Greece, the crafts came from the Pelasgians and the organization from the invading Achaeans and later the Dorians. In Mexico the fusion was between the native Toltecs (a word which in Nahuatl means "master craftsmen") and the invading Aztec warriors.

November 30

Doctor Zhivago fills one with compassion for the Russian people. Has there ever been a happy period, a golden age, in Russian history? The presence of an obedient, long-suffering vast population can be a deadly peril to mankind.

My impression is that in the Western democracies just now people are weary of history. They view the future as a leech sucking the lifeblood of the present. Even the leaders are weary of history-making. In Eastern Europe, too, people are hungry for the joys of the present and see their leaders' preoccupation with history as a worship of Moloch.

December 2

It is fantastic how much of a feeling of well-being I can derive from performing duties. Today I took care of the laundry; mailed figs, dates, and money to Sara; paid dues and signed up in the hall; drew a hundred dollars from the bank for Lili. By the time I got through I was so much at peace with myself that I went and bought half a dozen roses for the room.

Recently I came across several instances where the term Americanization was used in connection with workingmen. When a workingman becomes Americanized you no longer can spot him on the street as a workingman. He beings to look and act like everyone else, and only by looking at his hands can you tell he is a workingman. In business, Americanization means a cut in red tape and probably also in supervisory personnel. There is also a blurring of the division between different kinds of business. The workingman benefits more from Americanization than any other segment of the population. The one who suffers most is, of course, the intellectual. Not only is the American attitude disdainful of the intellectual, but by curtailing supervision it robs him of many opportunities for positions of prestige and power.

December 4

Eight hours on the German ship *Henriette Wilhelmine Schulte* at Pier 31. It was a very easy and pleasant day. We discharged sixty cars. Time went by fine.

Yesterday I found a telegram from the *New York Times Magazine* asking for an article (two thousand words) on the brotherhood of man. My feeling is that I could not write more than five hundred words, and it would be on how much easier it is to love humanity as a whole than to love one's neighbor.

Most of the day I felt in a particularly playful mood, and at one with the people around me. Have I missed much by spending my life with barely literate people? I need intellectual isolation to work out my ideas. I get my stimulation from both the world of books and the book of the world. I cannot see how living with educated, articulate people, skilled in argument, would have helped me develop my ideas.

December 5

Six hours on the *Dowa Maru* at Pier 23. We started 10 A.M. and finished 5 P.M. There was little to do—about eighty tons for two gangs.

During the day I tried to follow a train of thought started by the telegram from the *New York Times*. Are we likely to love our fellowmen most if we consider them our brothers? Actually, it is not a question of love but of tolerance—of putting up with people and managing to be pleasant and benevolent. It seems to me that the attitude most fruitful of benevolence is the viewing of ourselves and others as strangers on this planet—as tourists (fellow travelers) on a journey. Tourists are usually brotherly with each other. In the latest *Reporter* there is an interview with Boris Pasternak in which he says that we are "guests of existence."

December 6

Eight and half hours on a Grace Line ship at Pier 37. We discharged canned tuna from Peru. A busy but not a hard day. I did not touch a pencil the whole time.

I could stop working for the rest of the year, but I am afraid to do it. My plan is to work one more week, until the 15th, and then take it easy. I have on hand the following sums:

Cash	$103
Check	59
Check coming	100
Check for next week	100
	$362

If I lay off on the 15th I won't have any new money coming until the middle of January. This means that the money must last me for five weeks. This makes out to $72 a week. Actually it will come to less since I have to pay rent, dues, etc. So it comes to $60 a week, which is not enough. I'll be spending money like water around Christmas. I must keep on working until December 21, take off ten days, and go back to work January 2. This will give me $100 more.

December 7

I am reading Trotsky's *Diary in Exile*. A perpetual juvenile. He values seriousness and dedication above all virtues. An engineer, he says, can build a machine reluctantly, but you cannot write a poem reluctantly. It does not occur to him that you can invent a machine or write a fine poem playfully.

He is convinced that people cannot be decent unless they have a great idea which raises them "above personal misery, above weakness, above all kinds of perfidy and baseness." To a Trotsky, the mass of people who do the world's work without fuss and feathers are morally debased.

I wonder how many share my loathing for self-appointed soul engineers who see it as their sacred duty to operate on mankind with an ax.

December 8

Eight hours on the Dutch ship *Lombock* at Pier 19. A pleasant day, and since I am to be off two days I felt lighthearted.

During the day I had two afterthoughts which I like. The first is connected with the relation between the playful and the utilitarian. I have harped on the primacy of the playful: that most utilitarian devices had their ancestry in playful practices; that the clay figurine preceded the clay pot, and that the bow was a musical instrument before it became a weapon. Actually the relation is circular—the utilitarian may give rise to the playful. Playful pictures preceded utilitarian picture writing, but hieroglyphic writing often served an ornamental purpose. The same is true of the relation between ornaments and clothes: Ornaments preceded utilitarian clothes, but clothes often became ornamental.

The second afterthought concerns the relation between originality and borrowing. Our originality shows itself most strikingly not in what we wholly originate but in what we do with that which we borrow from others. If this be true, it is obvious that second-rate writers or artists may stimulate our originality more than first-rate ones, since we borrow more readily from the former.

December 10

A whore must have moved into the room underneath me. First night she did a gold-rush business which kept me awake until past midnight. Tonight, the moment I hear somebody knocking on her door I open the window and call out into the dark, "She don't live here any more!"

Living among people yet being alone is the most favorable condition for the creative flow. It is a condition found in a city but not in a village or a small town. Routine, lack of excitement, plus a modicum of boredom and disgust are other ingredients of the creative situation. Most of the time the creative impulse is a mild reaction against a mild continuous irritation. Just so the oyster reacts with a pearl against the continuous irritation of a grain of sand lodged in its flesh.

Is commonness compatible with uncommon achievements? Does the creative person need a sense of uniqueness, a clearly marked separation from the common mass, in order to realize and exercise his talents? I snort any time I come across the statement that "All artists want fame, glory, immortality." My feeling is that once cultural achievements were considered as worthwhile and useful, and were as munificently rewarded as achievements in business, technology, and politics, a mass civilization would be as culturally creative as an aristocratic civilization.

December 11

Eight hours on the *Santa Anita* at Pier 37. It was an easy, pleasant day and my mind was working. I can now see my way to write the article on brotherhood for the *New York Times*. I might push it through before the new year.

I am reading the memoirs of Tolstoy's sister-in-law. In 1869, on a trip away from Yasnaya Polyana, Tolstoy was suddenly seized by an overwhelming fear of death. What he feared most, she says, was to die on the road or in a strange house. He wanted to return as quickly as possible to his wife and children. The whole thing does not sound true. Is it really easier to die among relatives and loved ones? We die alone. Compare this with Montaigne's feeling when away from home: "I think I should rather die on horseback than in a bed; out of my own house and far from my own people. Let us live and be merry among our friends, but let us go and die among strangers. A man may find those, for his money, who will shift his pillow and rub his feet, and will trouble him no more than he would have them."

December 13

Four hours on the *Santa Anita*. Finished the job. In the afternoon I spent several hours with Lili and the boy shopping. The boy is a delight. Any day now he will be talking fluently.

The quality of a social order may be gauged by several criteria: by how effectively it realizes its human resources; by how well it maintains its social plant; and, above all, by the quality of its people—how self-respecting, benevolent, self-reliant, energetic, etc.

The elimination of the profit motive in Communist countries has not made people less greedy and selfish. The increased dependence of the many on the will and whim of the few has not made people more gentle, forbearing, and carefree. From all that I read it seems that the attitude of every man for himself is more pronounced in a Communist than in a capitalist society. The compact unity imposed from above has weakened the impulse toward mutual help and voluntary cooperation. Moreover, where failure may have fatal consequences, vying will not proceed in an atmosphere of good fellowship.

And yet, on the whole, there is less loneliness in a Communist than in a capitalist society. People do not feel abandoned and forgotten in a regimented society. This perhaps keeps people from cutting loose from the Communist fatherland. The afterthought is that there is no loneliness in prison.

December 22

I cannot tell with certitude whether Little Eric imitates me or I him. It would be difficult to exaggerate the degree to which we are influenced by those we influence.

My attachment to the boy is as much a constant as there has ever been in my life. Yet at his birth there was no reason to assume that I could become attached to anyone. For I had been wholly alone for thirty-five years.

December 27

I have finished the article on the brotherhood of man for the *New York Times Magazine*. I don't know whether it is good. The train of thought is cohesive and original. I have copied it, and it should be typed and mailed next week.

What the finishing of the article demonstrates is that by hanging on I can make things grow—that this is the secret of composing. I need time and leisure to hang on.

January 3

So long as we were ahead of everybody, America's banalities, vulgarities, and inanities could be accepted as perhaps an unavoidable by-product. Since Sputnik, our shortcomings and blemishes have become conspicuous and portentous. The need to catch up with Russia will have profound effects on our temper, and probably also on the social landscape. There is more talk now than ever before about the need for a national purpose. Our preoccupation with business, a high living standard, sport, etc., suddenly seems childish.

I am reading *Eastern Exposure* by Marvin L. Kalb, who spent the year 1956 in Moscow. The most absorbing part of the book is the record of conversations with educated Russians. The hunger for material things is greater among Russians than among us. The most important things in Russia are "money and connections." To hear them talk you would think that the young generation in Russia would barter its soul for a private, individual existence. Yet it is doubtful whether they could endure such an existence once they had it. They are not inured to the burden of free choice.

January 8

Six hours on the Dutch ship *Sarangan* at Pier 19. Loading lumber. Last night I hardly slept because of the ruckus underneath. I have to rent a room to sleep in until I find a new apartment. The upset stomach and the inability to sleep have frayed my nerves. Perhaps it is all to the good: I shall be forced to get out of this cursed place.

Worse perhaps than the noise is the expectation of noise: the straining of the ears even when there is absolute quiet—so much so that I mistake the rumblings of my stomach for an approaching disturbance.

January 10

The rented room in a hotel on Seventh Street was a bust. It was like moving from the frying pan into the fire. The earth-shaking noise of trucks and buses and the rattle of cars kept me awake.

Yesterday we worked eleven hours to finish the *Sarangan*. By the time I went to bed it was eleven o'clock. The noise downstairs woke me at twelve thirty, and I was probably awake for half an hour. This means I had about five hours' sleep last night.

Today I worked eight hours on the *Tar Heel Mariner* at Pier 41. I return there tomorrow.

January 12

Six and a half hours on the *Tar Heel Mariner*. An easy day. I had a heated argument with several longshoremen about the trustworthiness of what Mikoyan and Khrushchev say. It is a waste of time to try to analyze a Russian statement. No one will remember a week from now what Khrushchev said—not even he himself.

January 15

Five hours on a Dutch ship at Pier 23. My head was not busy with anything in particular, yet I felt as if I was mulling over something of utmost importance.

January 16

Eight hours on the *Hakonesan Maru* at Pier 40. Hard work: nails, pipe fittings, and porcelain.

January 17

Four hours. Finished *Hakonesan Maru*. I returned to my room at noon, cleaned up, and went to bed. Lili and the boy woke me up at four o'clock.

It is good that I live alone, for I have a tendency to allow my inner discontent to color my attitude toward the people around me. I also seem to feel that a strong attachment to others narrows and stifles. Yet if I am not to sour and shrivel as I grow old, I must see my attachment to Lili and the boy as a blessing.

January 18

Four hours on the *Wonorato* at Pier 19. I volunteered for the job. Working five days, since Thursday, I barely made $70 take-home pay.

I have been reading Herbert J. Muller's *The Loom of History*. The book gives a feeling of the passionate life which once animated the now desolate western coast of Asia Minor, and the striving for beauty, grandeur, knowledge, and power which stretched souls there for centuries. What concerns me is the fact that the trader—an essentially trivial human type—played a major role in the birth and growth of Ionian civilization. This civilization was the product of a fusion between the native population and fugitive immigrants from the Greek archipelago—the debris of communities shattered by the Dorian invasion. The significant point is that about the same time the coast of Syria and Palestine was also seized by immigrants—the Phoenicians and the Philistines—yet only in Ionia was there a cultural explosion.

January 20

Yesterday I spent nine hours with Sir Andrew Cohen and his wife and the Iranian Consul, Rahenema, and his wife. Somebody in New York arranged the meeting. I talked too much and made an ass of myself. Spinoza was right when he said that every time we open our mouths it is because of our vanity. It did not occur to me to listen and learn. Sir Andrew was governor of Uganda, and later British representative at the United Nations. Rahenema is the son of a Persian grandee and spent much of his life in Paris. I ought to have asked questions about Africa, about Britain, about Persia. These two highly intelligent people had much to teach me. Instead, I talked ceaselessly.

Strangely, I felt elated when I returned to my room after nine hours of talking. It is only now that I see the ghastliness of the performance.

January 22

Today I went down to the new hall, near Fisherman's Wharf, but was not dispatched. How disturbing the change in routine due to the removal of the hall! Of course, in a few weeks the new routine will be firmly established and seem eternal.

My head is still buzzing with speculations about the role of the trader in history. My impression is that we know less about the origins of the trader than about the origins of other human types. The first traders were probably strangers—fugitives, exiles, and the like. Even in modern times, trade in many parts of the world is the monopoly of strangers: Parsees in India, Chinese in Southeast Asia, Indians in East Africa, Syrians and Greeks in West Africa. For all we know, the trader is more ancient than the warrior. He certainly antedates the cultivator and the herdsman. The Ionian traders came to trade by way of piracy. The Phoenician traders practiced piracy whenever they could. The Philistines constituted a warrior aristocracy and were not known as traders.

January 24

Did not get dispatched, and hurried back to my room before the rain got started. Now, at 9 A.M., I am at my table watching a gentle rain washing the world outside my window.

It strikes me as significant that the conditions which produced the first trader also produced the first individual. The emergence of the individual does not come as a result of social maturing, but usually in the wake of catastrophe. The first individual was an exile, a fugitive, an outcast, a straggler—someone cut off from the clan, tribe, or village. The incursion of strangers into a country will have one effect if the strangers come as individuals, and another if they come as a compact tribe or organized band. My hunch is that the Greek fugitives came to the Ionian coast as individuals, while the Phoenicians and the Philistines settled on the eastern coast of the Mediterranean as organized groups and not as a conglomerate of stragglers and fugitives.

What makes an explanation of the creative situation so difficult and uncertain is the role of example, of which in most cases we know nothing. The presence of a small group or even a single individual capable of setting the tone and of shaping attitudes may decide the nature of the resulting social, cultural, or economic pattern. I don't say that they who play such a shaping role have to be possessed of exceptional capacities and talent. They must have the knack of influencing others.

January 29
>Eight hours on the German ship *Thorstein* at Pier 26.

Something struck me today. Precisely at the moment when the world seems to leap into an unknown future, there is an enormous eruption of the past. Not only do archaeologists uncover just now cities of unimagined antiquity (Jericho), but in the political field, too, the past is rising from the grave. In Eastern Europe we have a revival of the German-Slav conflict of A.D. 900–1200. In Palestine the dormant past of the Old Testament has come to life, and the stirrings of the Arab world echo the happenings of A.D. 600–1300.

January 30
>Eight hours on the *Thorstein*. Finished the job.

In my room I found a check for $300 from the *New York Times* for the article on brotherhood. I was not satisfied with the article when I mailed it; indeed, I didn't think they would take it. Reading it now I can see its merits. Still, the fact that it is better than I had thought it to be may affect my judgment in the future. It may stifle stirrings of justified misgivings.

January 31
>Eight hours on the *Hawaiian Refiner* in Encinal. This is going to be a big money week. I am going back to the ship tomorrow, and if I get a full day I shall have a take-home paycheck of $125 next Friday.

February 2, 6 A.M.
>Yesterday I worked 7½ hours on the *Hawaiian Refiner*. I went straight from the job to the Osbornes. Little Eric has chicken pox. He is covered with red blisters, but his vitality is not diminished in the least. Lili has had to keep him in the house since

Friday, and as a result he is restless and full of mischief. I had a fine time until ten o'clock.

What strikes me again and again is the number of excellent people, people of gentle character and inner gracefulness, one meets on the waterfront. I spent some time on the last job with Ernie and Mac, two elderly fellows I have known slightly. I found myself thinking what fine persons the two are—generous, competent, and intelligent. I have watched them tackle jobs not only intelligently but with striking originality. And all the time they work as if at play.

February 6

Eight hours on the Chilean ship *Almargo*. A very easy day and quite pleasant. As I have noticed before, the men at this Chilean ship are more like intellectuals than sailors. Assembled together they give the impression of a university group. Our chief clerk told me that the second mate speaks English with an Oxford accent and that all ratings have shelves of books in their cabins. Obviously the intellectuals in Chile are hard pressed for jobs befitting their status. The inadequate employment of intellectuals is a potent revolutionary factor.

I am beginning to think that the activation of the masses—their readiness to work and strive—is a function of individual freedom. When the masses are left more or less to themselves, they turn to work as the most accessible means of providing their worth and usefulness. On the other hand, the ideal condition for the creativeness of the intellectual is apparently an aristocratic social order which appreciates his work and accords him rank and dignity. The intellectual does not want to be left alone, and this is perhaps the reason why he cannot leave others alone.

February 11

Seven hours on a Luckenbach ship at Pier 29. I worked with the bulkhead swampers on the breakup pile. It was steady going all day, yet the feeling at the end was one of pleasure. The pleasantness was due largely to the presence of Jack, the head-up man—a highly competent and soft-spoken person. We did an enormous amount of work but did not feel driven or frustrated. It made me realize again how a single individual can count in the development of a pattern of life. Yet we are told that it is circumstances and not men that make history.

9:30 P.M. What is it that can grip my interest, concentrate my attention, and get my thoughts flowing? Judicious praise? Not quite. Verification of my theories and hunches? More so. Actually, the most durable and effective source of stimulation is a hefty body of manuscript wanting to grow.

I live in a society full of blemishes and deformities. But it is a society that gives every man elbow room to do the things near to his heart. In no other country is it so possible for a man of determination to go ahead, with whatever it is that he sets his heart on, without compromising his integrity. Of course, those who set their heart on acclaim and fortune must cater to other people's demands. But for those who want to be left alone to realize their capacities and talents, this is an ideal country. It is incredible how easy it is in this country to cut oneself off from what one disapproves—from all vulgarity, mendacity, conformity, subservience, speciousness, and other corrupting influences and infections.

February 12, 7:45 P.M.

I am reading Irving Babbitt's *The Masters of Modern French Criticism*. The essay on Renan confirmed my impression that no Anglo-Saxon can truly appreciate him. They cannot take him seriously. I wonder whether an esssay on Renan written in the 1950s could be as patronizing. The Bolshevik and the Nazi revolutions have shown how profound and unerring were Renan's insights into the mind of the fanatic. The Babbitts, Santayanas, Arnolds, etc., were without forebodings of the future. Renan's grasp of the fanatical mentality, and the dovetailing of his interest in the past and the present, made him a good prophet. Like Dostoevski, Renan becomes more timely with the passage of time. Yet who reads Renan nowadays? No one could convince an American that Renan's five volumes of the history of the people of Israel, written in the 1880s, are a greater aid to an understanding of the present than any number of volumes by outstanding political scientists, sociologists, psychiatrists, or any other experts. Renan's expertise was in the human condition, which is eternal.

February 13

Five hours on the Norwegian ship *Tancred* at Pier 26. A drunken Slavonian made life miserable for everybody. My irritation was intense, while the other members of the gang took the day-long nuisance in their stride. By quitting time I felt weary and dejected.

8 P.M. I am still reading Babbitt's book. A mediocre man, but I pick up a few things. I found a remarkable quotation from Brunetière: "The great error of the 19th century, in morality as well as in science and art, has been to mingle and confound man and nature without pausing to consider that in art as in science and morality he is a man only in so far as he distinguishes himself from nature, and makes himself an exception to it." He paraphrases him also as saying that man becomes good not by obeying but by resisting nature. I cannot think at this moment of a single book or even an essay that makes the opposition between man and nature the cornerstone of a train of thought. My hunch is that in human affairs all true opposites reflect in some degree the archetypical opposition between man and nature. God and man are on one side, the devil and nature on the other. From this point of view the mechanical and the natural are not true opposites, since both are opposed to that which is uniquely human. Moreover, nature is wholly mechanical and automated. To build something in the image of nature is to build a machine.

February 14

Nine hours on the *Turnadot*. One of the hardest days I have had in a long time. Seventeen hundred sacks of copra came out in 3½ hours. The rest of the day we spent sorting cargo. My partner was George Saraback, a Russian Armenian with an unexcelled technique for labor faking. The sacks felt twice their weight, and the sorting was done in spite of the partner. Still, I felt good when the day was over. In 4½ days I managed to make almost $105 take-home pay.

9:15 P.M. Still reading Babbitt. I am repelled by his smugness. He has a position, connections, and "truths" which he will not offend by letting himself go. He lives in the midst of a herd of holy cows.

10:30 P.M. You can remember a feeling only when you have put it in words, or when it is connected in your mind with some sentence, no matter what. We remember readily what we see, hear, smell, or touch. But we cannot remember what we felt when we were humiliated or praised, when we hoped or despaired.

February 16

Four hours on a Norwegian ship at Pier 26. A beautiful job. We discharged fifteen cars and sixty-six drums of cyanide. No strain and no discord.

Another suggestive sentence from Babbitt's book (p. 181): "Science and Romanticism have cooperated during the last century in the dehumanization of man." What have science and romanticism in common? Obviously, a return to nature. Both science and romanticism are based on the equation *human nature = nature.*

February 21

Seven hours on a Japanese ship at Pier 23. I have been lucky this week with my fellow workers. Not a cross word or an unpleasant incident. It nourishes and enhances my benevolence toward people.

The waterfront is the only place where I have felt at home. All my life, wherever I went, I felt an outsider. Here I have a strong feeling of belonging. One of the reasons is of course that I have tarried here long enough to take root. Yet it seems to me that I have felt at home here from the first month.

February 27

Four and a half hours on the Norwegian ship *Besseggen.* Back in my room at noon.

My brevity as a writer is partly the result of a reluctance or inability to write. Delight in the act of writing breeds expansiveness. One shudders at the thought of the innumerable thick volumes which come into existence as the result of the sheer habit of writing. How many people with nothing to say keep writing so many pages a day in order that their body, particularly in old age, should perform its functions?

March 4

Five and a half hours on the *Matsonia* at Pier 35. Kolin's gang. Little to do, and a cheerful bunch.

As I was reading about Khrushchev's juvenile shenanigans this morning, it struck me that there has been a process of juvenilization going on all over the world for decades. Almost all the leaders of the new or renovated countries have an element of juvenility or even juvenile delinquency in their make-up: Khrushchev, Castro, Sukarno, Nkrumah, Nasser, Sékou Touré—you name them. Arthur Koestler maintains that revolutionaries are perpetual juveniles—that there is something in them that keeps them from growing up. Now it is possible to see some family likeness between the adolescent who steps out of the warmth of the family into a cold world, and knows not how to come to terms with it, and the revolutionary who cannot come to terms with the status quo. Then you look around you, and you realize that the American go-getter who has no quarrel with the status quo is as much a juvenile as any revolutionary. Finally there is the juvenile character of most artists and writers. What quality can these diverse human types have in common? The answer that suggests itself is that all of them have a vivid awareness of the possibility of a new beginning; of a sudden, drastic, miraculous change. To a mature person, drastic change is not only something unpleasant, he denies its reality. He sees drastic change as a falling down on the face: when we get up we are back where we started plus bruises and dishevelment. The change that endures is that of growth—a change that proceeds quietly, and by degrees hardly to be perceived. To the juvenile mentality, continuity and gradualness are synonymous with stagnation, while drastic change is a mark of dynamism, vigor, and freedom. To be fully alive is to feel that everything is possible.

March 5

It is good to be vividly aware that what seems impossible at one moment may seem easy at another. This drastic change in mood is perhaps a symptom of a weakened mechanism. But so long as the awareness is there, the unhealthy fluctuation in confidence is endurable. I doubt whether anyone has worked out the rules which govern the flow of creative energy. What I know is that once I have waded into a subject and piled up a hefty body of manuscript, the thing wants to grow of its own accord.

March 7

Seven hours discharging frozen fish at Pier 17. During the day I put together a few more paragraphs on freedom. If you judge a society by its books, paintings, music, science, etc., you are not likely to get excited about freedom. A regimented society run by a literate ruling class that rewards excellence and reverences talent might be an ideal milieu for cultural creativeness. Only the masses are energized by freedom. It is of interest that freedom is apparently vital for the readiness to work but not for the readiness to fight and die. De Tocqueville's magnificent sentence about freedom, that "it infuses throughout the body social an activity, a force, and an energy which never exist without it and bring forth wonders," refers mainly to the performance of common folk. And yet it should be possible to create great works of the spirit in a totally free and equal society where he who writes books need not feel infinitely superior to he who sweeps the streets or prints and binds the books. The trouble is that some people do not want to be left alone; they feel oppressed when they are left alone.

March 8

Eight hours on the *Dona Alicia* at Pier 9. A very pleasant day. My partner was a Negro by the name of Flat Top. He is easy to work with. It seems to me that much of the day we talked about the problems of large families. Flat Top has five children, while the Negro winch driver Jimmy has seven. Both Flat Top and Jimmy are hard drinkers, although Flat Top is just now on the wagon.

Not a thought all day, and not a sentence.

March 11

Five and a half hours on the *Lurline*. I felt sleepy and tired. Through the haze of weariness, I felt welling up within me a murderous rage against Khrushchev and the Russians. What do words mean to them? With us it holds true that even a lie tells some truth about the person who tells it. With the Russians it is not so: they lie on principle. It is significant that the dehumanization caused by communism should be linked with the murder of words. It is perhaps a general rule that where human uniqueness is impaired, words are emptied of meaning.

March 12

Eight hours on the *Oceania Maru* at Pier 41. Frenchie for a partner—an incurable drunk but of a pleasant disposition. He can't watch the game. Had an unpleasant beef with the steward of the gang. The man talks and acts like a schoolmaster. I resented every word he said. He is going to put me "on the carpet." It will be an interesting experience.

For some reason my mind reverted to the problem of the readiness to work. I am itching to write a chapter on the subject. To me it is a miracle that 200 million people who are largely the descendants of rejects and dropouts from Europe should have created in this country the most important material power on the planet. I do not think that our engineers, scientists, and technologists are markedly superior to their kind elsewhere or that our natural resources are vaster or more accessible than those anywhere else. The unprecedented thing in America is what has happened to the masses. Never since the beginning of time have the masses had a chance to show what they could do on their own. It needed the discovery of a new world to give them the chance. It is the performance of the common people that made America what it is—the only new thing in the universe. I remember what Charlie Sorensen (*My Forty Years with Ford*) wrote about his visit to Leningrad in the 1920s. He found that in the higher field of engineering, like turbine building, the Russians were doing a pretty good job, but anything that had to be done by common people was in an awful mess. This was forty years ago, and it is still so today. Chances are it will be so forty years from now. Sorensen's conclusion was that we need not worry about Russia catching up with us so long as the common people are kept under the thumb of commissars. When you think of the marvels of food production achieved by Russian peasants on tiny plots of ground, and of the unmatched ingenuity displayed by Russian black marketeers, you realize what a release of boundless energy would take place if the Russian people were told to come and get it the way this country told the millions of immigrants from Europe.

Soviet Russia knows how to foster the exceptional skills requisite for the manufacture of complex machinery and instruments, even the harnessing of the atom and the launching of Sputniks. But it seems helpless in anything which requires an automatic readiness on the part of the masses to work day in, day out.

To a somewhat lesser degree this holds true even of Britain. There, too, the scientists and top technicians perform uncommonly well, while the mass of people see no reason to bestir themselves.

March 13

Eight hours on the Dutch ship *Friesland* at Pier 23. Hard work all day—asbestos from East Africa. We have to come back tomorrow to finish the ship.

Despite the hard work I do not feel too tired. Though not elated, I feel a certain lightness of heart, and I take delight in the neatness of my room. I had Emilio for a partner. He is an excellent worker, but he keeps up all day long a peculiar line of propaganda—propaganda for himself. It is not bragging, but he naturally assumes that every good thing that happens is due to his presence on the job. He is very good-natured and goes out of his way to be helpful to others. His English is fantastically garbled. But when I try my Spanish on him he makes fun of the slightest mistake. I like him a lot.

I have on my table a bunch of grape hyacinths in a green vase.

I have had it since Monday, and it still looks fresh and beautiful. All evening I have been conscious of the beauty of this combination of green and blue. Had I the ability I would have painted it again and again.

March 14

Seven and a half hours on the *Friesland*. Finished the job. About the hardest two days I have put in, in a long while. On the bus returning from work I had a sudden attack of compassion— for the young and the old, the successful and the failures. It seemed to me that in the whole world there was not one soul without its share of misery. I cannot connect the attack with anything that happened to me.

I am reading a small book by Klaus Mehnert on *Stalin versus Marx*. It is exciting reading despite my lack of interest in ideological subtleties. I cannot hate the dead—not even Stalin and Hitler. Yet my heart often rages with murderous fury against the living malefactors. My hunch is that the twentieth century will be a continuous hell to the end—one crisis after another—until all passions have burned themselves out.

March 16, 6 A.M.

Yesterday I worked on the Norwegian ship *Tudor* at Pier 26. Sacks again—this time copra. In the evening I went straight from the job to the Osbornes'. I had a fine time drinking, eating, and talking. We were all of us in a benevolent mood. On returning to my room I took a shower and fell immediately asleep. Just now I am at my table feeling rested.

There is not going to be a book on the intellectual. This is certain. Every article I have written during this decade seems to fit into a pattern. My subject is change: why it is so difficult in the Communist countries and in the new nations. The intellectual is trying to direct and master the process of change. If I manage to write a few more articles—on the readiness to work, freedom, the connection between technical modernization and social primitivization—I will have a book. Its title should be *Explosive Change*.[3]

---

[3] Published in 1963 under the title *The Ordeal of Change*.

A comprehensive theory of change should be applicable not only to the change from backwardness to modernity but also the change from boyhood to manhood, from poverty to affluence, from subjection to equality, and even to the menopause.

March 17

At noon I took Eric from the nursery school and traveled to the Hitchrack restaurant on the beach. I am beginning to realize that I cannot be impulsive with the boy. I must be deliberate and learn to impress him. I tried to be reserved, not show too much affection, and he behaved excellently.

8:45 P.M. The readiness to work is still tugging at my mind. Pride undoubtedly plays a considerable role. It is a mark of modern man's desperate need for pride that he finds the weight of sin much lighter than the weight of weakness. It is disconcerting that despite its monstrous transgressions under Hitler, Germany seems yet to be the one European country with an unimpaired pride. Defeat in the Second World War has not blurred the awareness in most German minds that no nation by itself—however vast in territory, population, and resources—is Germany's match; that it needed the mobilization of the whole world to bring Germany to its knees. Thus the Germans alone among the Europeans are not oppressed by a vitiating sense of impotence, and it is their unimpaired pride that accounts for their astounding capacity for recovery.

March 18

Eight hours on the *Banggai* at Pier 19. I am having a run of bad luck. Everything I touch is hard work. Last week I had two days of asbestos, one day of copra, and one day tough sorting on the Japanese ship. Today I found myself working in the only hatch that had tapioca. I did not have anything to read, so I made myself write.

Right now we ought to know all we can about the chemistry of pride. Pride—in a nation, a race, a religion, a party, or a leader—is a substitute for individual self-respect. In other words, pride is a vital necessity when we are in the antechamber of self-respect, and it matters not whether we are in the antechamber on the way in or on the way out. The present fierce craving for pride is indicative of the enormous difficulty experienced by people (particularly educated people) in maintaining their self-respect.

March 19

Eight hours on the *Banggai*. An easy day.

I am too familiar with my ideas to savor their originality. The article on brotherhood for the *New York Times* was a mosaic of ideas I have lived with for a long time. I had great misgivings about the piece. The fact that the article made some impression on all sorts of people has revived my awareness of it. If, then, intercourse with other people can be stimulating, it will be partly because it makes it possible for me to savor again the originality of my ideas. But for this you need people who will know an original idea when they see it.

March 20, 6:30 P.M.

Five and a half hours to finish the *Banggai*. On returning to my room I was seized by a fit of drowsiness which I could not resist. Now rested and bathed I am at my table itching to sort out the train of thought that has been trying to emerge for the past several days.

If, as seems to be true, my chief preoccupation is with change, then practically everything I have written should be connected with this theme. Mass movements, the true believer, the intellectual, the masses, freedom, America, the Occident, the antagonism between man and nature should all be facets and phases of the phenomenon of change. All the movements which have convulsed the Occident for 150 years, all the human types that came to dominate the scene, all the views and doctrines and theories that found acceptance should be in one way or another connected with the inducement of human plasticity indispensable for survival in ceaselessly changing societies. I can see the dovetailing of nationalism, industrialization, militarism, revolution, the scientific view of man and his soul, the romantic return to nature, the proliferation of cartels and unions—I can see the dovetailing of all these into a vast unconscious effort to induce unbounded human plasticity. The originators of these movements, organizations, processes, methods, doctrines, views, and tendencies were often pulling in opposite directions; each had his own motives and aims, yet they all tended toward a common goal.

Put in a few simple words, the idea has a strange impact: change has been the cause of revolution, of world wars, of Lenin and Hitler, of Marx, Nietzsche, Wagner, and Freud.

March 23

No country is a good country for its juveniles. Like newly arrived immigrants, the juveniles will adjust themselves to the status quo when they are given unlimited opportunities for successful action—for proving their manhood. There is a fascinating circular process involved. The strain of drastic change cracks the uppermost mature layers of the mind and lays bare the less mature layers. Drastic change juvenilizes or even infantilizes. The infant is plastic. But the crucial point is that the juvenile will adjust himself to the new only when he is given abundant opportunities to prove his manhood. The explosions and convulsions which attend change are a sort of juvenile delinquency. Another way of putting it is that every drastic change recapitulates to some extent the change from boyhood to manhood.

March 26

Was there ever a utopia which visualized a society free of planning, regulation, and supervision? Utopias are usually visualized by potential planners, organizers, directors, leaders. The envisioned new society is the ideal milieu for bureaucrats.

My feeling is that the age of utopia writing is over. We have lost our innocence and naïveté. We know something that most of the historians, sociologists, and dreamers of the nineteenth century did not know. We know the end of the story.

March 28

Eight hours on the *Waitenata*. Finished the job.

I have been mulling over the opposites of freedom and power.

If it be true that the human uniqueness of an aspiration or an achievement should be gauged by how much it accentuates the distinction between human affairs and nonhuman nature, then the aspiration toward freedom is the most human of all human manifestations. Freedom means freedom from forces and circumstances which would turn man into a thing, which would impose on man the passivity and predictability of matter. By this test, absolute power is the manifestation most inimical to human uniqueness. Absolute power wants to turn people into malleable clay.

The significant point is that people unfit for freedom—who cannot do much with it—are hungry for power. The desire for freedom is an attribute of a "have" type of self. It says: leave me alone and I shall grow, learn, and realize my capacities. The desire for power is basically an attribute of a "have-not" type of self. If Hitler had had the talents and the temperament of a genuine artist, if Stalin had had the capacity to become a first-rate theoretician, if Napoleon had had the makings of a great poet or philosopher—they would hardly have developed the all-consuming lust for absolute power.

Freedom gives us a chance to realize our human and individual uniqueness. Absolute power can also bestow uniqueness: to have absolute power is to have the power to reduce all the people around us to puppets, robots, toys, or animals and be the only man in sight. Absolute power achieves uniqueness by dehumanizing others.

To sum up: those who lack the capacity to achieve much in an atmosphere of freedom will clamor for power.

March 31

A beautiful day. In the morning I had an unusual feeling of well-being. I don't know what caused it. After breakfast I went around shopping for flowers, but I didn't find anything to satisfy me. In my room I copied out several sections (mainly on freedom) and read Alexander Campbell's *The Heart of India*. Can a country so poor afford freedom? And are not the strains and tensions of freedom too much for a new country not oversupplied with technical, social, and political skills? To me it is axiomatic that a nation has to be affluent enough before it can afford freedom, and vigorous enough to stand up under the ceaseless tug of willful parties and free individuals. Above all, to stay free, a society needs skills so that its apparatus of everyday life functions smoothly.

April 1

Eight hours on the German ship *Birkenau* at Pier 28. An easy job, but I strained my back. Last night the union meeting went on until 11 P.M. I didn't fall asleep until past midnight, and I was up at 4:30 A.M. The result is that I am not feeling well. In addition to the pain in the back I seem to have a touch of the flu.

7:30 P.M. The problem of change is getting mixed up in my mind with the problem of man and nature. The human plasticity required by drastic change involves some dehumanization. In a sense, to become plastic, man must become matter—malleable clay. Thus drastic change, even when it is a leap forward, results in primitivization, in a return to nature. And since absolute power tends to turn people into matter, you can see how the absolute despot fits into the picture of change.

One thing is certain: absolute power turns its possessor not into a God but an anti-God. For God turned clay into men, while the absolute despot turns men into clay.

April 2

Alexander Campbell's book gives me the smell and taste of India. Asia is not only a graveyard but also a dust bin. Everything is crumbling and in a state of decay. Yet the Taj Mahal is kept in good repair. He quotes Nehru (p. 59). "It is folly to talk about culture, or even to talk about God, while human beings starve and rot and die." He could have added freedom.

I have always had the feeling that American aid to backward countries should concern itself almost solely with food: teach the mass of people how to raise crops efficiently, give them the technical and social skills which would enable them to get bread, human dignity, and strength by their own efforts. The common people are our allies. If the intellectuals want steel mills, skyscrapers, and other twentieth-century toys, let them go to the Russians. America should be synonymous with bread.

April 5

I am beginning to believe that human uniqueness can unfold and endure only in an environment of stability and continuity. The incessant, drastic changes in all departments of life characteristic of modern society are hostile to human nature. It was probably inevitable that when change was beginning to gain momentum in the second half of the nineteenth century there was also set in motion a process of dehumanization.

What puzzles me is the passionate, blind effort by scientists, psychologists, historians, economists, businessmen, industrialists, revolutionaries, and military men to hack away at man's uniqueness—to demonstrate that there is no basic difference between man and the rest of creation. It is a blind, concerted effort to downgrade man, and it goes hand in hand with an unprecedented increase of man's power over nature. Fantastic!

April 6

I am getting used to leisure. It is now five days since I worked last, I have not written much, yet I feel I am making some progress. I am free of restlessness and fear.

I have never taken time off to write. Yet the fact remains that the crucial advances in writing *The True Believer* occurred during the strikes in 1946 and 1948—three months each. The strained back may give me a couple of weeks of leisure.

10 P.M. I am fascinated by the enormous dovetailing among the participants in the historic process. Take for instance the lustful dovetailing between the manipulators and the manipulated. The absolute despot lusts to dehumanize—to turn people into things—while the weak, weary of the strain of human uniqueness, long to drop the burden of free choice. All the metaphysical double-talk about the *Zeitgeist*, world spirit, historic necessity, super-individual tendencies, and the like cluster around. I would love to spend the rest of my life playing with this puzzle.

There is such a thing as fashion in thinking. There was something in the air that Darwin and Marx and others picked up when they elaborated their theories. The integration of man with non-human nature which preoccupied scientists, philosophers, and writers in the nineteenth century—the romantics and the realists, the idealists and the cynics—had perhaps a common origin, and I have to find it. To say that the onset of the Industrial Revolution created a demand for a new type of man, malleable and mechanized, does not explain anything. Darwin and Freud had nothing to do with the Industrial Revolution, and the romantics were violently against it. The industrialists wanted money, the politicians power, the scientists searched for regularities. Each one of the actors wanted something different, yet they all labored at the same task.

April 9

Six and a half hours on the *Lurline*. A very easy day.

I am rereading Jaspers's *Origin and Goal of History*. He is blind to trivial motives and causes. Something momentous, he is sure, started the axial period. To suggest that unemployed scribes set the whole thing in motion would be to blaspheme. The more or less sudden breakdown of the bureaucratic apparatus in many countries in the early part of the first millennium B.C. brought into being the unattached scribe—a scribe without status and identity. Amos, Hesiod, Confucius, Zoroaster were probably unemployed scribes. Jaspers also fails to recognize that the inception of the axial period marks also the birth of written literature in Palestine, Greece, Persia, and China.

April 11

Not dispatched. A letter from Norman Jacobson. He is going to give a series of seminars on mass democracy and the creative individual. From his outline it is obvious that he will deal mainly with creativeness in science. He wants me to give one of the seminars: I should describe the manner in which I first stumbled into thinking and writing. It will choke me to repeat the oft-told tale. However, I am interested in the creative potentialities of common people, and in the creative process in general, and should have enough ideas to play with for an hour or so.

Lili and the boy came about four o'clock. He is wonderfully alert, and his mind works much faster than his capacity for speech. He wants to ask all sorts of questions but has not enough words.

April 12

Ten hours on the *Golden Gate* at Pier 37. It was a long but not unpleasant day. My back seems to have straightened out.

How I rage against Khrushchev in my reveries. It is almost as it was in the 1930s when I raged against Hitler. Does my heart need an enemy to vent its fury on? And I can't separate Russia from Khrushchev. Russia: founded on a cesspool of bondage and gore. Whatever is built on this foundation is soon impregnated with an ancient stench and made leprous with the ancient rot. Westernization means here cleaning up—a hopeless task. Culture: an interaction between the exhalations from the dark depths and elements introduced from the Occident. There is a crackling and hissing and a giving off of varicolored flashes and of fabulous odors and perfumes.

Martin Luther found that the rage against his enemies helped him to pray well. I ought to drain my rage against Khrushchev into thinking and writing.

April 14

I do not want to feel that I know best. I hope that other people—many of them—know better. For the counsel of my heart is often savage. And what do I really know about this country? I am without instinctive tolerance. The fact that I have not been to grammar school disqualifies me as a prompter of genuinely democratic behavior. When others counsel patience, forbearance, and kindness, I ought to keep my mouth shut.

April 15

Eight hours on the *Keito Maru*. A surprisingly easy day, yet in the evening I felt dejected. It is so easy to be dissatisfied with myself. The least transgression weighs on me. To preserve my sense of well-being I must lean backward in my dealings with others. A sensitive conscience is probably a symptom of old age. I must be scrupulously decent not in order to feel noble but to feel well.

April 17

Eight hours on the *C. E. Dant*. Finished the job. Had a new partner, a Negro, very conscientious and nice to be with.

Something I read in the *Manchester Guardian Weekly* started me thinking about the attitude of the masses toward the intellectuals. There is no doubt that to most Portuguese and Italian longshoremen a schoolmaster is an important person, almost as much a dignitary as the priest. But through most of history the common people resented the educated as exploiters and oppressors. Rabbi Akiba, who started life as a roustabout, recalled how he used to cry out, "Give me one of the learned and I shall bite him like a jackass." During the peasant uprisings, the clerks were given short shrift by the mobs. When in the fourteenth century the mob burned the charters and manuscripts of the University of Cambridge, an old hag tossed the ashes into the wind crying, "Away with the learning of the clerks, away with it."

April 20

Back to Pier 19 to finish the ship we started Saturday. It is a Norwegian ship—the *Hoegh Silverstream*. An easy day, but the stretch of six days' work is beginning to tell. I am very tired.

I have to remind myself that I have not the temperament of a scholar. I am not going to pile up carefully documented facts. If I can't swing out with theories, hunches, and guesses I am lost.

April 21

The fact that I have read a lot and that I think and write has never generated in me the conviction that I could teach and guide others. Even in a union meeting of unlearned longshoremen it has never occurred to me that I could tell them what to do. This reluctance to teach and guide is the result not of a lack of confidence in myself but rather of a confidence in the competence of the run-of-the-mill American.

The important point is that the lack of the conviction that I have the ability and the right to teach others marks me as a non-intellectual. For the intellectual is above all a teacher and considers it his God-given right to tell the ignorant majority what to do. To ignore this teacher complex is to ignore the intellectual's central characteristic and miss the key to his aspirations and grievances. I am sure that the passion to teach has been a crucial factor in the rise of the revolutionary movements of our time. In most cases when a revolutionary takes over a country, he turns it into a vast schoolroom with a population of cowed, captive pupils cringing at his feet. When he speaks the whole country listens.

April 24, 5 A.M.

Karl Jaspers's grandiloquence moves me: "At the termination of history in the existing sense we are witnessing the radical metamorphosis of humanity itself." Or "Our age is of the most incisive significance. It requires the whole history of mankind to furnish us with standards by which to measure the meaning of what is happening at the present time." Does not mean much, yet for a moment you feel as if he had given you a glimpse of the awesome spectacle that is unfolding in the whole of the world at this moment. There is a stirring of depths and a jostling of nations all over the earth.

And yet what a shabby, crummy, vain, and posturing lot are the men who engineer and preside over this spectacle.

The meaning of technology, he says, "is freedom in relation to nature. Its purpose is to liberate man from animal imprisonment in nature, with its wants, its menace, and its bondage."

April 27, 9 P.M.

I am reading *The Privilege Was Mine* by Zinaida Shakovskoi. She comes from a Russian aristocratic family (a princess), was brought up in France, and married a Frenchman. She visited Moscow in 1957. Her writing is delightful—lucid, precise, intelligent. To be civilized is perhaps to rise above passion; to be able to observe and report without giving way to anger or enthusiasm, and let the reader react as he will. Her book crystallized in my mind something I have known for a long time. The change in Russia has been not mainly ideological, political, or economic, but biological. Stalin liquidated the most-civilized segment of the Russian population and made of Russia a nation of lower muzhiks. Most of the city-bred Russians were killed off, imprisoned, or exiled. She searched the faces in the streets of Moscow. "It was hopeless trying to find one single face which clearly belonged to a born city dweller." How was the pattern of life of these newcomers formed? It has the appearance of an old-fashioned bourgeois world harking back to the period of 1900.

You get the impression that the suspicion and the rudeness which manifest themselves in Russia's foreign dealings are a reflection of the suspicion and rudeness which permeate the lives of the people high and low. Whom does Khrushchev trust? In Russia "even the most commonplace activities assume a sinister air of secrecy." What she holds against the Soviet government is not that it has not been able to provide the citizens of such a rich country with a good life but "the fear which rules men's lives in Russia today." The fear, she thinks, is more degrading than hunger and cold and is a sign of something rotten within the regime.

Now, Soviet Russia is undoubtedly a going concern with an air of permanence. It does not operate smoothly and efficiently, but it manages to feed, clothe, house, and educate its millions. She was aware of an "all-pervading atmosphere of latent discontent" and of "a clear division between government and people, as if the latter were making a point of dissociating themselves from the former." But my feeling is that if a drastic change takes place in Russia it will come from above. Despite their education, the Russians are still as submissive as Lenin knew them, "so patient, so accustomed to privation."

May 3

Can the human species ever adjust itself to endless, drastic change? Are there instances of living organisms enduring and thriving in an environment without stability and continuity?

I compared the stretched soul to the stretched string of a musical instrument when I said that only a stretched soul makes music. Nietzsche likened the stretched soul to a tensely strained bow with which one can aim at the furthest goals.

May 6

Eight hours on the *Samadinda* at Pier 19. An easy and very pleasant day. Head does not work.

May 7

Eight hours on the *Samadinda*. Finished the job.

10 P.M. On the way home I picked up a book in a secondhand bookstore. The title caught my eye: *The Vanished Pomp of Yesterday* by Lord Frederic Hamilton. Quite often of late there has welled up in me a craving to live in a stable, stagnant, and even decaying society where values and ways have remained unchanged for generations and no one is going anywhere. Actually the book is about life in the diplomatic world of the last decades of the nineteenth century. It is a chatty book, but on page 135 I found something that startled me: the record of a conversation between the author and a young muzhik in a village in northern Russia. What startled me were the similarities between the opinions of a Russian muzhik eighty years ago and present-day Communist propaganda. The muzhik thought there was no electric light outside Russia, since Jablochkov, a Russian, had invented that. Were there roads outside Russia? Could people read and write? Certainly there were no towns as large as Petrograd. Clearly, Communist propaganda has not been cooked up in the Kremlin but echoes attitudes and beliefs indigenous to a nation made up of peasants. It is probably true that in thinking of Russia one ought not to confuse the victims with their executioners. But it is also true that the two have an awful lot in common.

May 11

I just discovered that the last few entries in this diary were dated March instead of May. I apparently forgot the month.

Yesterday I was dispatched to Pier 41, but the ship did not come in. They gave us four hours, sent us home, and ordered us back for today. This morning I found the beautiful French ship *Maryland* tied at the pier. We had an easy, delightful day.

The article on man and nature which I am writing for the *Saturday Evening Post* is coming along fine. Almost every idea in the train of thought has been worked out long ago. What I have to do is dovetail them more or less smoothly. There are a few gaps to be filled. One is the idea that man's creativeness originates in the characteristics which distinguish man from other forms of life. In other words, human creativeness is basically unlike any creative process that may be found in the rest of creation. I also must have a pithy section on the role of magic (words) in human affairs. The title of the article will be "The Unnaturalness of Human Nature." I ought to have it finished and typed before the end of this month.

The fact that I can put together a good article by fitting ideas into a mosaic bothers me a little. It would have done me a world of good to be able to pour forth a stream of writing, to have new ideas gush from my mind onto paper. My sort of writing lacks the quality of catharsis. Yet only writing—any sort of writing—can justify my existence.

May 12

When exploring the differences between civilizations, their attitude toward nature must be given a prominent place. This attitude affects not only religion and the mechanics of everyday life but the position of the individual and the pattern of freedom and power. The same environment made a nomad of the American Indian and a pioneer of the European immigrant, and in the makeup of the pioneer the Old Testament was a pronounced ingredient.

May 20

I twisted the wrist of my right hand six days ago while heaving sacks of nails. Today is the first day's work after a week of oppressive leisure. The bruised hand is almost well.

Today I worked 6½ hours on the *Harunassan Maru* at Pier 26. An easy and pleasant job, and my head is beginning to work.

There is something like a Moses pattern in every instance of drastic change. Moses wanted to turn a tribe of enslaved Hebrews into free men. You would think that all he had to do was gather the slaves and tell them that they were free. But Moses knew better. He knew that the transformation of slaves into free men was more difficult and painful than the transformation of free men into slaves. The change from slavery to freedom requires many other drastic changes. To begin with, a leap from one country to another—a migration. Hence the Exodus. More vital was the endowment of the ex-slave with a new identity and a sense of rebirth. The whole Pentateuch deals with the staging of the drama of rebirth. No playwright and no impresario has ever staged such a grandiose drama. The setting had a live volcano as a backdrop, and the cast included the mighty Jehovah himself.

What was the denouement? Moses discovered that no migration, no drama, no spectacle, no myth, and no miracles could turn slaves into free men. It cannot be done. So he led the slaves back into the desert and waited forty years, until the slave generation died and a new generation, desert born and bred, was ready to enter the promised land.

All revolutionary leaders, though they fervently preach change, know that people cannot change. Unlike Moses, they have neither a handy desert nor the patience to wait forty years. Hence the purges and the terror to get rid of the grown-up generation.

It is of interest that even in the objective world of science, man's mind is not more malleable than in the habit-bound world of everyday life. Max Planck maintained that a new scientific truth does not triumph by convincing its opponents, but because its opponents eventually die and a new generation grows up that is familiar with it. Here, too, you need forty years in the desert.

May 21

Eight hours on the Pope & Talbot *Voyager* at Pier 38. An easy and pleasant day. Indeed, I was in something like a festive mood all day long. It was partly due to the fact that I had on new working clothes. No one has fully investigated the effect of clothes on man's moods and behavior. Nietzsche said somewhere that a woman who feels well-dressed would not catch a cold even if she were half naked. Emerson quotes a lady saying that when she is perfectly dressed she has a feeling of inner tranquillity which religion is powerless to bestow. I have never been well-dressed, never had on things of perfect fit and excellent material.

The union has taken in five hundred new longshoremen. They have been sifted out of several thousand applicants and make an excellent impression. It was pleasant to see fresh faces, mostly young, on the dock.

2 BEFORE THE SABBATH:

NOVEMBER 1974–JUNE 1975

November 26, 1974, 10:00 P.M.

The other day I finished the first draft of a slim collection of short essays. I suddenly had the feeling that I had been scraping the bottom of the barrel, and that the slim volume might mark my end as a thinker. I doubted whether I would ever get involved in a new, seminal train of thought. It was legitimate to assume that at the age of seventy-two my mind was played out.

I did not panic. As a retired workingman I now have the right to do what I have denied myself since 1940—read novels; thousands of them. There are only a few years left anyhow. But first I have to get a clear picture of the manner in which age affects my mind. The reasoning capacity is unimpaired. I can still tell sense from nonsense, and my judgment of books I am reading and of my own writing is sound. It is true that I have noticed a tendency toward wishful thinking, a lessened interest in what is happening in the world, and a marked weakening of memory. But I sense that the crucial difference lies elsewhere, in the loss of alertness.

I remembered something I wrote in *Reflections on the Human Condition:* "That which is unique and worthwhile in us makes itself felt only in flashes. If we do not know how to catch and savor the flashes, we are without growth and exhilaration." Would it be possible to reanimate and cultivate the alertness to the first, faint stirrings of thought? What would happen if I forced myself over a period of several months to sluice my mind the way I sluiced dirt in my gold-hunting days, using a diary as a sluicebox to trap whatever flakes of insight might turn up?

This, then, is why I am starting this diary today. I intend to keep it for at least six months, and I have promised my weary mind a blissful Sabbath when the task is done.

November 28, 7:30 A.M.

A letter from Eric[1] yesterday. The hard work of planting trees on the cold mountains justifies his existence, hardens his body, and seems to stimulate his mind. Here is a striking example of the double function of work in our society: to do what needs to be done, and to give the worker a sense of usefulness. In the case of a young workingman, hard work gives a sense of manliness, and the earned money an exhilarating feeling of independence.

9:30 P.M. One of the surprising privileges of intellectuals is that they are free to be scandalously asinine without harming their reputations. The intellectuals who idolized Stalin while he was purging millions and stifling the least stirring of freedom have not been discredited. They are still holding forth on every topic under the sun and listened to with deference. Sartre returned in 1939 from Germany, where he studied philosophy, and told the world that there was little to choose between Hitler's Germany and France. Yet Sartre went on to become an intellectual pope revered by the educated in every land. The metaphysical grammarian Noam Chomsky, who went to Hanoi to worship there at the altar of human rights and democracy, was not discredited and silenced when the humanitarian Communists staged their nightmare in South Vietnam and Cambodia. Is there a greater freedom than the right to be wrong?

November 29, 7:00 A.M.

I cannot see myself living in a socialist society. My passion is to be left alone and only a capitalist society does so. Capitalism

---

[1] Eric Osborne. He and his brother Steven, who were children when I wrote *Working and Thinking on the Waterfront*, are young men now. When this was written, Steven and his wife, Beatrice, were living in San Francisco, not far from the home of Steven's and Eric's mother, Lili Osborne. Eric was working in Oregon.

is ideally equipped for mastering things but awkward in mastering men. It hugs the assumption that people will perform tolerably well when left to themselves.

The curious thing is that the reluctance or inability to manage men makes capitalist society uniquely modern. Managing men is a primitive thing. It partakes of magic and is the domain of medicine men and tribal chieftains. Socialist and Communist societies are a throwback to the primitive in their passion for managing men.

Idealists never weary of decrying capitalism for its trivial motivation. Yet a discrepancy between trivial motives and weighty consequences is an essential trait of human uniqueness and is particularly pronounced in the creative individual. Not only in the marketplace and on the battlefield but also in the world of thought and imagination, men who set their hearts on toys often accomplish great things. The idealists prize seriousness and weightiness. Let them go to the animal kingdom! Animals are deadly serious.

November 30, 6:00 A.M.
What will the flood of money do to the Arabs? A flood of gold hastened the decline of Spain and Portugal while the inflow of riches during the first half of the nineteenth century propelled Britain to economic and political supremacy.

It is a striking fact that up to now no Islamic country has achieved anything remotely comparable to the rapid modernization of Japan, Taiwan, South Korea, Singapore, Hong Kong, and India. Egypt began to modernize itself early in the nineteenth century, fifty years before Japan, yet Egypt is still a backward country. It is probably safe to predict that the expensive industrial hardware piled up in Iran and Saudi Arabia will end up as piles of junk.

Islam creates a way of life incompatible with the modern temper. It does not generate tensions which goad the individual to ceaseless effort. No other religion gives its adherents such unshakable pride: just being a Muslim makes the individual superior and he is not under the pressing need to prove his worth anew each day. Thus to a Muslim the plunge into the hectic atmosphere of a modern industrial society must seem like an expulsion from Eden.

5:30 P.M. I have a hunch that the Arabs will use their oil billions not to modernize their countries but to redress the balance between the Christian West and the Islamic East. They are financing the pressure against the non-Muslim enclaves of Lebanon, Israel, and Ethiopia. Idi Amin is a Muslim kept in power by Arab money in largely Christian Uganda. Muslims are also gaining the upper hand in the republic of Chad and in Nigeria. The Islamization of Africa is a dream to fire Arab hearts.

December 2, 8:00 A.M.

It is almost eight years since I retired from the waterfront, but in my dreams I still load and unload ships. I sometimes wake up in the morning aching all over from a night's hard work. One might maintain that a pension is pay for the work we keep on doing in our dreams after we retire.

I am inclined to think that at present it is the inefficient societies that are likely to be more stable. By inefficient I mean societies that employ as many workers as possible to do a job. Such societies have a wide distribution of a sense of usefulness, which is more vital to the maintenance of social stability than the distribution of wealth or power.

December 3, 4:00 P.M.

A world that did not lift a finger when Hitler was wiping out six million Jewish men, women, and children is now saying that the Jewish state of Israel will not survive if it does not come to terms with the Arabs. My feeling is that no one in this universe has the right and the competence to tell Israel what it has to do in order to survive. On the contrary, it is Israel that can tell us what to do. It can tell us that we shall not survive if we do not cultivate and celebrate courage, if we coddle traitors and deserters, bargain with terrorists, court enemies, and scorn friends.

December 4, 7:00 A.M.

The Chinese Far East (which includes Japan, Korea, Vietnam, and Mongolia) is at present the last refuge of the work ethic.

In the rest of the world labor faking is the rule. It matters not whether a country is feudal, capitalist, socialist, Communist, backward or advanced, rich or poor, its people will do as little as possible. Here is a description of the situation in Russia: "At any time, in any office, 80 percent of the staff is in the corridors or the bathrooms. No one works." Something similar is taking place in capitalist societies. The fateful event of our time is not the advancement of backward countries but the leveling down of advanced countries.

I am curious about Pechorin, a Russian intellectual of the mid-nineteenth century who wrote a poem on "How sweet it is to hate one's native land and eagerly await its annihilation." Pechorin became a Catholic and ended his days as a monk in a monastery. In a letter to Alexander Herzen he predicted that "the material civilization will lead to a tyranny from which there will be no shelter." He thought that a greedy bourgeoisie would sell its soul for material rewards. Actually, the logic of events has been more subtle. Our materialist civilization is edging toward tyranny because the elimination of scarcity also eliminates the hidden hand of circumstances that kept the wheels turning. The coming of abundance has weakened social automatism and discipline. Societies now need forceful authority in order to function tolerably well.

December 5, 6:30 A.M.

We should have been on the lookout for the snake to pop up when we were given a taste of paradisiacal affluence. And, remembering that the snake was "more subtle [hence more learned] than any beast in the field," we might have guessed that he would come out of the universities.

It is now the fashion to contrast authority with human rights. But we are learning that the moment authority becomes ineffectual most of our rights are nullified by the many-headed tyranny of anarchy.

December 6, 7:00 A.M.

The proponents of change claim that they aim to make

society more responsive to what people want. Actually, what people want most is stability and continuity rather than change.

December 7, 5:00 A.M.

A revulsion from work is a fundamental component of human nature. It is natural to feel work to be a curse. A social order that grants only minimal necessities but asks for little effort will be more stable than a system that offers superfluities but demands ceaseless striving. One reason Communist governments seem so stable is that they no longer insist on hard work. Islam too is markedly stable because it functions tolerably well in an atmosphere of indolence.

In the period between the two World Wars Czechoslovakia was one of the most progressive and prosperous countries in Europe. It had an industrious, skilled population that kept the economic and social plant in good repair. In 1948 the Communists took over, and twenty years later, when the lid came off during the Dubcek interlude, the world could see the changes that had taken place under Communist rule. The chief change was the loss of the work ethic. The Czechoslovaks took to labor faking with gusto. Hard work was looked upon as a violation of the fraternal code. It was also startling to discover how easily the workers had adjusted themselves to a lower standard of living. It seemed doubtful whether an offer of higher wages could wean them from their meager brand of *la dolce vita*.

In Britain workers are immune to the blandishments of a higher living standard, and this attitude is spreading to other democracies, particularly among the young. I suspect that the present chatter about quality of life is an attempt to mask the fact that to the new generation the good life is a life of little effort.

December 8, 7:00 A.M.

How strange the nineteenth century! It was a century in which ceaseless, drastic change went hand in hand with a strong sense of continuity—even of immutability. There was a widespread assumption that prevailing patterns would persist indefinitely. Even the people who dreamed wild dreams and foresaw apocalyptic denouements lived regular, stable lives.

Nowhere and at no time have people of all sorts become rich so quickly as in Britain during the first half of the nineteenth century. Rapid industrialization not only opened fabulous opportunities for enrichment to the middle classes, but the landowning aristocrats had more than their share of the explosion of prosperity. It was this unprecedented outburst of moneymaking that gave Britain's ruling class its confidence during a time of drastic change.

December 9, 8:00 A.M.

When Americans do not act the way I think they ought to, my reaction depends on whether I feel one of them or see myself as an outsider. When I feel one of them I tend to accuse them of cowardice, gullibility, mindless conformity, and the like. But as an outsider I wonder whether the reason Americans do not act the way I expect them to is that they "know" more. I am aware that I lack their social instincts and skills. Their forbearance and patience derive from their deep-seated belief that, given time, situations work themselves out.

December 12, 3:00 P.M.

Kemal Atatürk knew that Islam is incompatible with modernization. He deliberately tried to uproot Islam by laicizing everyday life and banishing Arab influences. He persecuted Islam with a personal passion.

Has he succeeded? Today, almost forty years after Atatürk's death, Islam is gaining ground in Turkey. It is apparently easier to de-Christianize than to de-Islamize. Islam's rapid and total de-Christianization of the Middle East and North Africa contrasts with the ineffectuality of Christian proselytizing in Islamic lands. Islam caters to basic human needs and is without inner contradictions and tensions. It legitimizes an easygoing, even indolent life. I doubt whether any Islamic country can be durably modernized.

December 13, 10:20 A.M.

I say to myself: Lenin and Stalin between them liquidated at least sixty million Russians in order to build factories and dams.

America welcomed thirty million immigrants to help build factories and dams.

Capitalism is fueled by the individual's appetites, ambitions, fears, hopes, and illusions. Communism forces people to hate what they love and love what they hate. Imagine a country of land-hungry peasants forced to renounce ownership of land. Imagine a system that frowns on friendship, free association, and individual enterprise. It is no wonder that after sixty years the Russian Communist party must still coerce, suspect, and minutely regulate the Russian people.

Can anyone visualize the time when the unemployed of a Western Europe made stagnant by a shortage of energy and raw materials would storm the borders of Russia, where there is no unemployment, the way thousands of unemployed Mexicans are risking their lives to steal into capitalist America? Should the unlikely happen and Communist Russia become truly prosperous, it will still have to guard its borders to prevent Russians from running away.

We underestimate the passion of common people for freedom. We see every day common people doing their utmost to escape from nonfree to free countries.

December 14, 9:15 A.M.

The day before he died, Renoir painted anemones with a brush strapped to his crippled fingers. When he finished, he said: "I am beginning to learn how to paint anemones."

On his deathbed Michelangelo said to Cardinal Salivati: "I regret that I die just as I am beginning to learn the alphabet of my profession."

I cannot see a writer saying toward the end of his life that he is just beginning to learn how to write. A writer never knows he can write the way a painter knows he can paint or a sculptor knows he can sculpt or even a composer knows he can compose. Not long before his death Adam Smith observed that after all his practice in writing he composed as slowly and with as much difficulty as he had at first. V. S. Pritchett sees it as "one of the disgusts of the writer's life that he finds himself having to learn from the beginning again every time he puts pen to paper."

December 15, 10:00 A.M.

Through most of history laborers must have lived soul-emptying lives. The Greeks did not believe a laborer could think, let alone contemplate beauty. Yet men have sung as they worked from the beginning of time, and work has its ancestry in play.

According to the Bible God placed Adam in the Garden of Eden "to dress it and keep it." It was pleasant, playful work. With the expulsion from Eden man came face to face with hard, monotonous, endless work.

Disraeli was certain there is no greater misfortune than to have a heart that will not grow old. Actually, when we have someone we dearly love and who loves us a young heart is no misfortune. Sensuality reconciles us with humanity. The misanthropy of the old comes from the fading of the magic glow of desire.

December 16, 8:00 A.M.

The historian Herbert Butterfield asks for "a more scientific analysis of the reasons why the twentieth century became an age of conflict." Could a scientific analysis explain why the Occident blundered into the First World War? There was nothing inevitable about the coming of the war and the terrible mess of its aftermath. Nor were Lenin's and Hitler's revolutions inevitable. How many people knew in 1914 that they were in the last year of a dying age?

The great casualty of the First World War was hope. The belief in the perfectibility of man and the certainty of progress which began with the French Encyclopedists died with the war.

December 17, 8:20 A.M.

Both the Hapsburg and the Ottoman empires dominated the Balkans for centuries. Yet in the Balkans today there is little left of the Austrian presence, while a number of towns in Macedonia and Serbia have Turkish mosques and retain the Turkish language. Could it be that the more foreign an influence, the more enduring its mark? The Turkish influence in the Balkans was the more foreign. Would the same hold true of British influence in India? The Turks intermarried more with their subjects than did the Austrians. But perhaps the persistence of Turkish influence is another instance of the persistence of Islam (December 12). Spain still shows strong traces of Islam seven centuries after its de-Islamization, whereas few signs of Christianity are left in Islamized North Africa.

10:45 P.M. I went over by taxicab to meet Eric's train in Oakland and spent the whole day at Lili's house.

It seems preposterous that I who landed on Skid Row at the age of eighteen, and spent twenty years on the bum, one step ahead of hunger, should worry about Eric going out into a cold world at the age of nineteen. It is an instance of the truth that we tend to see those we love as brittle and vulnerable.

Eric is the only human being I have known from the word go. I shall always think of him as a child—perpetually vulnerable and inexperienced. I shall always tremble for his fate and fear the worst. Paradoxically, though I have watched Eric closely from the day he was born, I understand him less than I do others.

December 18, 7:15 A.M.

I am reading the autobiography of Norman Bentwich, an English Jew. It has puzzled me that English Jewry has not produced until recently outstanding scientists, writers, and artists. When you compare this with the accomplishments of Jews in Germany, France, Austria, Italy, and America you feel that you are up against a seminal problem. Even Russia has produced two Jewish Nobel Prize winners—Pasternak and Landau.

England has been an ideal milieu for outsiders. Scotsmen, Irishmen, Australians, New Zealanders, Canadians, Americans, and nationals from several European countries have been prominent in many fields. Jews excelled in business, manufacturing, and to some extent in public life. England is perhaps the only Western country where Jews have not played a central role in the development of nuclear physics. Are there any famous Jewish names associated with Oxford and Cambridge? I can think only of Wittgenstein (an Austrian Jew), Sir Isaiah Berlin, and Max Beloff. My hunch is that Jews did not feel at ease in Oxford and Cambridge, where social intercourse is as vital as the process of learning.

Is there a difference in style between English and Jewish nuclear physics? Einstein's scientific thinking had a metaphysical undertone. He wanted to rethink God's thoughts. He felt that "behind all discernible concatenations there remains something subtle, intangible and inexplicable. Veneration for this force beyond anything we can comprehend is my religion." To Rutherford, the mysterious rays emitted from a substance were "the debris of decaying atoms."

December 20, 7:45 A.M.

We had a fine time last night. Eric, barefoot in the kitchen, experimented with a mixture of calf's brains, figs, and nuts. The mess did not taste good but we had plenty of baked chicken. I was high on Wild Turkey.

I wonder how I would react if someone demonstrated to me beyond the least doubt that I am mean, deceitful, selfish, and ruthless. The answer is: so long as there is a person I love and who loves me, and so long as I have some ability to think and write, I would go on uncrushed, accepting the fact that I am without the capacity to see myself as I am. I doubt whether I am capable of mortifying remorse. I might even quote St. Paul: "No one does good; not even one."

December 21, 6:30 A.M.

It comes as a surprise to find that Clausewitz saw a kinship between traders and warriors. In the essay on the trader in my new book I dwell on the interchange of roles between warriors and traders in the aftermath of the Second World War, when German and Japanese warriors became the world's foremost traders, and the Jews foremost warriors. I thought it was a new idea, but here is Clausewitz, a Prussian Junker, maintaining that the talents which make for success in business are similar to the talents of a successful military commander.

December 23, 7:30 A.M.

Communism was invented by highbrows while capitalism was initiated by lowbrows. A capitalist society can be run by anybody whereas it needs exceptional leaders to make a Communist society work. If the vigor of an organization is measured by the ability to function well without an outstanding leader then, clearly, a Communist society is less vigorous—less well made—than a capitalist society.

Churchill saw Communist Russia ruled by a band of "bloody-minded professors." And, indeed, the contrast between a Communist and a capitalist government is the contrast between a government by schoolmasters and a government by schoolboys. Churchill himself was one of the fabulous schoolboys who ruled Britain during the nineteenth century and up to the First World War. Apparently, lowbrows and schoolboys are better social builders than highbrows and schoolmasters.

Communism can reconstruct the chronically poor and launch backward countries on a road to modernization. Capitalism is ideal for enterprising, self-starting people but cannot do much for people who cannot help themselves. Clearly, where communism succeeds it makes the helpless fit for capitalism.

December 24, 7:45 A.M.

William McNeill's *The Shape of European History* has so far been a disappointment. The first two chapters, dealing with theory, are pale and unimpressive. Some vague ideas about the nature of change. Not one sentence sticks in the mind. McNeill will be better when describing events and conveying information.

Despite its remarkable achievements in the Late Paleolithic (cave paintings) and Megalithic eras, Europe became a backward subcontinent during the Neolithic. Europe did not domesticate a single animal or plant, did not invent any sort of script, did not invent anything comparable to the wheel, sail, or plow. Greece and Rome, though geographically part of Europe, were Mediterranean in spirit. Even their attitude toward Christianity was Mediterranean. Christianity did not create in Greece and Rome the tension of the soul which manifested itself in Europe when warrior tribes were made to adopt a religion of meekness and love.

McNeill asks: "What literature excels Homer, Aeschylus, Sophocles, Euripides?" I wonder whether these Greek masterpieces can engage the hearts and minds of people the way the literature of the Old Testament does.

My most vivid memories are of the middle twenty years of my life, 1920–1940. I was then on the bum and most of the time one step ahead of hunger. Those years seem to me eventful although life on the bum was actually endlessly repetitive. My stretched mind was exaggerating and fitting together slight happenings into fabulous, hilarious tales. And I was talking all the time, telling people about all that happened to me. They listened and roared with laughter. Sometimes when I came to a lumber camp or a work barrack, people would ask me to tell them about my adventures. So in retrospect those twenty years are a procession of stories in which truth and fiction are so interwoven that I cannot tell them apart. I might almost say that I remember most minutely and distinctly things that did not happen to me.

December 27, 7:10 A.M.
One could write a beautiful essay or even a small book on "The Flow of Influence."

The fact that the influence of the Occident is world-wide inclines us to assume that the flow of influence follows a hydraulic model; that it flows from the high points of the human landscape to the low. We take it for granted that the learned influence the ignorant, the advanced influence the backward, adults influence the young, and so on. It seems natural that the Occident being more learned, advanced, rich, and so on should influence the rest of the world.

Actually, the flow of influence has followed a hydraulic model only for a short interval—after the coming of the Industrial Revolution. Up to A.D. 1800 the flow of influence was from the East to the West although the Occident had been pulling ahead since 1400. Through most of history it was the weak who influenced the strong. Not only did conquerors learn most readily from the conquered, but small countries most often shaped history. Israel, Greece, and the small states of Italy gave the Occident its religion and the essential elements of its civilization. There is also the crucial fact that civilizations become most influential when they begin to decline. McNeill speaks of the cultural primacy which comes with economic decline as an "ecological succession": "The spread of classical Greek culture throughout the Mediterranean came after the economic power of Athens had broken down. Latin thought and letters penetrated the Western provinces of the Roman empire when Italy's economy was already in trouble." He adds that the influence of Muslim Spain and Byzantium became stronger "after military and economic disaster had struck the heartlands of both civilizations." It is also true that Italy's influence at the time of the Renaissance was at its height when Italian economic hegemony was in decline due to the self-assertion of native entrepreneurs in England, France, Germany, Spain, and also in the Ottoman Empire.

Thus it is reasonable to assume that a decline of the Occident will not mean a diminution of its influence. On the contrary, the Occident's loss of military and economic supremacy will enhance its attractiveness as a model. Countries are most at ease when they imitate a defeated or dead model.

December 28, 6:45 A.M.

There is one more example of the link between material decline and increased cultural influence: the city of Vienna exerted its widest influence when it was the capital of a decaying Hapsburg empire.

In the past there were potential great leaders waiting in the wings. This was true of Hitler, Churchill, de Gaulle, Adenauer, Ben Gurion, and others. Right now the wings are empty. Does the quality of the population have something to do with the absence of leaders? Hardly so. It is true that when there are leaders waiting in the wings their entrance onto the stage and their effectiveness depend on the character and attitudes of the people. Lenin knew his revolution was possible because of the inordinate submissiveness of the Russian people. Churchill had to wait for Dunkirk to prepare the British people for their finest hour. Hitler was possible only in Germany. De Gaulle did not get far because of the nature of the French.

I like to compare what Lenin said about the Russians with what de Gaulle said about the French. Lenin: "How can you compare the masses of Western Europe with our people—so patient, so accustomed to privation?" De Gaulle: "What can you do with a country that has 315 different kinds of cheese?"

December 30, 7:50 A.M.

Back to the flow of influence: No foreign influence spread so rapidly and found such wholehearted acceptance as Romanization. Gaul was Romanized in less than fifty years. The Roman way of life was embraced with ardor both in the East and in the West. It must have been breathtaking to see Roman cities spring out of the soil with their forums, colonnades, theatres, and baths. Rome had a state-forming influence. Its success in influencing primitive people was due to its social effectiveness. Someone compared the two Celtic nations France and Ireland: France formed the first European state and Ireland the last, and the difference is due to the fact that Ireland had no Roman experience.

Greek influence was altogether different. The Greeks made an impact only on people with long-established civilizations. They had little effect on the Scythians, Illyrians, and Thracians. The Greeks at Marseilles had little influence on Celtic Gaul. Greek influence was largely esthetic and intellectual and was no factor in crystallizing and bolstering authority.

December 31, 8:00 A.M.

The nineteenth century despite its unprecedented changes was a century of law and order. In Britain, where the changes were most spectacular, the lower orders who early in the century had turned the cities into savage jungles became meek and law-abiding. In this country during the absorption of thirty million immigrants, the cities were relatively peaceful and safe.

The First World War was a watershed of effective authority in the Occident. Was it the terrible slaughter and waste of the war that shook authority? Hardly so. It was the loss of hope. Hope unites people and induces patience. Hope was probably one of the most striking characteristics of Western humanity prior to the First World War. It was the loss of hope rather than its mere absence that drained authority of its effectiveness.

January 1, 1975, 9:00 P.M.

I have spent a fortune this Christmas yet I do not feel impoverished. We shall celebrate every Christmas as if it were my last. The sky is the limit.

We spent the afternoon with Lili's family in Cupertino. The Fabilli women delight in singing together the songs they used to sing as children. The ninety-year-old mother joined in. It occurred to me that singing together could be a means of cultivating esprit de corps, of creating family ties among strangers. So would occasional common meals and opportunities for good conversation.

January 2, 9:10 A.M.

Through most of his existence man's survival depended on his ability to cope with nature. If the mind evolved as an aid in human survival it was primarily as an instrument for the mastery of nature. The mind is still at its best when tinkering with the mathematics that rule nature. It is awkward and often misleading when confronted with the task of comprehending and mastering man. Hence in a time like ours when man has become the main threat to human survival, intellectual faculties alone cannot solve our problems. Imagination, intuitive insights, and the lessons of experience are more critical than logic.

Revolutionaries are as a rule logicians, and when the dreams shaped by their logic come true they turn into nightmares. The harm done by self-appointed experts in human affairs is usually a product of a priori logic. Progressive experts in child-rearing assume logically that to raise independent adults children must be made self-reliant as early as possible. Events have proved, however, that children left to get in and out of trouble on their own feel abandoned. Where parents fail to exercise authority the peer group takes over, and members of a peer group are most conformist and least confident. Many young parents after the end of the Second World War, particularly the better educated and more affluent, were receptive to avant-garde ideas and followed the advice of know-all child-rearing experts who frowned on authority and exalted spontaneity. The 1960s saw the result: an adolescent counterculture of drift, drugs, and appallingly conformist nonconformity.

In a society dominated by the human factor, events have a logic of their own more subtle and profound than a priori logic. Perhaps the reason that economists and sociologists are at present consistently wrong in their predictions is that they are logicians.

January 4, 6:30 P.M.

Most social thinkers of the nineteenth century were afraid that the entrance of the masses onto the stage of history would make democratic government impossible. Even the most liberal among the thinkers were obsessed with this fear. Bagehot, so insightful in other matters, thought that once the masses were given political power only education and prosperity could preserve social stability.

Bagehot's faith in the stabilizing effect of affluence and education must seem naïve to us who have seen how, during the 1960s, abundance and a multitude of semester intellectuals produced by the post-Sputnik education explosion brought this country to the brink of chaos.

It is puzzling that Disraeli should have known more about the nature of the masses than his liberal contemporaries. He sensed the conservatism and patriotism of common folk. It is perhaps true that a genuine conservative is more attuned to the eternal verities of human nature and of society. He is aware that the logic of events may draw from man's actions consequences which a priori logic cannot foresee. Disraeli's forebodings about England's future and his ideas on what keeps a nation vigorous and great have a poignant relevance at present. Must one be conservative or even reactionary if one wants to be thought up-to-date tomorrow?

January 5, 6:50 A.M.

    I am both moved and irritated by Randolph Hearst's effort to justify himself in the eyes of his daughter Patty, despite her unspeakable behavior. He is not the kind of parent who can renounce his child. It reminds me of David and Absalom.

    The nineteenth century was rich in new beginnings while the twentieth is a century of endings and harvests. Both the achievements and the crimes of the twentieth century are a harvest of what the nineteenth century sowed.

    Guglielmo Ferrero, when describing the fabulous stability of the nineteenth century, says that "it could dream of anarchy, worship revolution, and amuse itself by destroying and reworking the world with its thought, while enjoying the most solid and perfect order that had ever been established on earth." The dreamers, schemers, and thinkers were planting the seed of the apocalyptic events of the twentieth century.

    As hard as breaking an ingrained habit is the discarding of a reform that is no longer relevant. Our time cries out for child labor—there are no children any more—but no one dares propose it.

January 6, 10:00 A.M.

    The task of a united Germany should have been to enlarge Europe: to push Russia beyond the Urals, back into Asia. It was a fateful flaw of German statesmanship not to work for a whole-hearted reconciliation with France and Britain at any price so as to be able to canalize all German energies eastward. It was also a flaw of French and British statesmanship not to encourage a German *Drang nach Osten.*

    During the second quarter of the nineteenth century, de Tocqueville, Jules Michelet and František Palacký knew that the role of a united Germany and of the Hapsburg empire was to serve as a buffer against Russia. But with the outburst of chauvinism after 1848 Europe's energies went into internal rivalries which culminated in the catastrophic civil war we know as the two World Wars.

One wonders whether a civilized, truly European Hitler might have rallied Europe in a grand undertaking to free western Russia of Stalinist slavery and tap the fabulous resources of the Eurasian land mass. Chances are that an envious France would have defeated such an attempt. Still, it was a crowning absurdity of the absurd twentieth century that Germany, instead of pushing the Russian slave empire back into Asia, set in motion the chain of events which brought the Russians to the bank of the Elbe.

January 10, 7:30 A.M.

The great cloth merchants of Florence and the great shipowners of Venice passionately loved their cities. They were greedy for gold but they also strived to make their cities beautiful and famous. They saw it as their natural task to govern their cities and employed great artists and poets to commemorate their rule with immortal works. They saw it as their duty to spot and nurture talent and reward greatness.

In the Netherlands, too, the great cloth merchants and shipowners built a society in which wealth and power justified themselves by patronizing learning and the arts.

In America up to now the wealthy and powerful have shied away from personal involvement in the cultural life of their country. The foundations which bear their names are administered by intellectuals often not in sympathy with the ideals and goals of their capitalist benefactors. Yet the need for justifying the wealth and power of great corporations in the eyes of the people has never been greater. Why not hark back to Florence, Venice, Antwerp, and Amsterdam? The great corporations could devote wealth and energies to cleaning up, improving, and adorning our cities. Each large corporation might adopt a city and vie with other corporations to see whose city shines brightest. In the center of each financial district there should be a large plaza in which periodically poets, singers, storytellers and artists of every sort would compete for rich prizes. The corporations should see it as their duty to spot and encourage talent, and celebrate greatness. There should be social intimacy between the powerful and the creative.

January 11, 6:30 A.M.

The crisis of our time stems from the fact that social institutions have become as vulnerable as individuals. The attributes which made institutions less subject to the vicissitudes of chance and circumstances have lost much of their effectiveness. Traditions and axioms no longer find unquestioned acceptance.

I wonder whether the fences and taboos which used to surround institutions, and the savage sanctions against anyone who laid hands on them, originated in an awareness of their vulnerability. We have seen how a scratch on an institution easily develops into a cancer.

January 12, 1:00 P.M.

There is a leveling process going on at present all over the globe. There are now rich backward countries dictating to poor advanced countries. The revulsion from work is bringing capitalist economies down to the Communist level. Freedom no longer energizes people and no longer creates plenty. One wonders whether, once the leveling process has run its course, freedom will still matter. Will people continue to run from nonfree to free countries?

It is uncanny how when trying to make sense of what happened to America in the 1960s we find the nearest analogies in Weimar Germany, pre-revolutionary Russia, and Britain in the early decades of the Industrial Revolution. America is becoming not so much like other countries as like other countries' pasts.

In a preceding entry on the flow of influence (Dec. 27) I should have pointed out that influence flows from the high points of the human landscape to the low (that it follows a hydraulic model) only in the rare cases when one segment of mankind executes a leap that changes the quality of history. The domestication of plants and animals in the Fertile Crescent was such a leap, and so were the founding of the earliest cities in Sumer and the coming of the Industrial Revolution in the Occident.

January 13, 9:30 A.M.

I am reading a book on Hegel by Professor Walter Kaufman. After a hundred and fifty-four pages I still have not an inkling of what Hegel was after. The time he lived in (1770–1831) was as eventful and unsettled as our own. No one knew what the next morning would bring. Yet here were a number of German professors, living practically on the battlefield (Jena), who were totally absorbed in producing thousands of pages of abstruse philosophy, convinced that they alone had a hold on the ultimate truth. They were drunk with words.

Hegel wrote his *Phenomenology of the Mind* in an incredibly short time—in the time it would take to transcribe the manuscript. He finished the book during the battle of Jena. Starting for the publisher in the morning he was surprised to see the streets of Jena full of French soldiers. Here is what Professor Kaufman has to say about the book. "The whole style of the *Phenomenology* is such that students and scholars are almost bound to ask themselves: What is the man talking about? Whom does he have in mind? Indeed—and this is crucial—the obscurity and whole manner are such that these questions are almost bound to replace the question whether what Hegel says is right."

It never ceases to amaze me that for over a century brilliant people derived a sense of chosenness from their ability to understand Hegel's *Phenomenology*.

I said that the time Hegel lived in was like our own. Actually there was a vital difference. The people who lived through the French Revolution and its Napoleonic aftermath were full of hopes and illusions. They felt they were at the birth of a new world far superior to anything that had been in the past. We have the feeling that we are living in an absurd century with a dark age waiting for us at the end.

January 14, 6:30 A.M.

Americans have often been accused by Europeans of confusing quality with quantity. Yet this has been the sin of European philosophers, particularly the Germans. The main idea is to produce a thick book.

Ballet dancers are the only creative people who accept retirement as natural. It occurs to me that if thinking is a ballet of ideas, the thinking mind too should accept the fact that age makes dancing difficult.

To God eternity is as a day while to a one-day fly a day is an eternity. Our time is getting near to that of a one-day fly. A year now is as a century. We measure eras not in centuries nor even in decades. Every five years or so we have a new era. We have two or three turning points in a decade.

January 15, 6:40 A.M.

The fact that there is no such thing as happiness does not mean that there is no unhappiness.

January 17, 10:20 A.M.

The generation that plunged into the First World War was up to its neck in axioms. It took civilization, progress, monetary stability, freedom, order, rationality for granted. There were, it is true, intellectuals who lusted to tear down all that existed and create a perfect world. But they too had a belief in the lastingness of things. They did not expect their words to become flesh. The war saw the wholesale slaughter of axioms.

Actually, the slaughter of axioms was as much the work of the Russian Revolution as of the war. Indeed, the revolution marked a sharper break with the past than did the war. Despite the frightful bloodshed, the First World War remained within a civilized framework. The treatment of prisoners and of civilians followed international agreements. To Lenin, all civilized usages were bourgeois tricks. He made a mockery of honor, truth, freedom, and democracy.

Had there been no Lenin, there would have been no Hitler.

January 19, 2:30 P.M.

America has never ceased to be an experiment. In every generation America has still to prove that a society founded on values cherished by common people can endure, and that it is possible to fuse hordes of heterogeneous immigrants into one nation indivisible.

The attitude toward theory: Late in the eighteenth century there were many who thought theory more potent than action, that in the words of Hegel: "Once the realm of notion is revolutionized, actuality does not hold out." Heine predicted that the words piled up by German philosophers would eventually bring about a revolution compared with which all other revolutions would seem a storm in a teacup.

The men of action who initiated the Industrial Revolution made light of theory. They discovered how things worked by trial and error, and had faith in feel and know-how. However, the atomic bomb and Sputnik have made theory supreme. The practical lowbrows who made fun of theory as a species of wind now see it as a mighty explosive that may blow up the universe. Has this awe of theory undermined capitalist confidence?

January 21, 6:40 A.M.

Of late I have been losing my way in my dreams. Suddenly I do not know where I am. Dreaming with me is not an escape from an untenable existence. Sometimes when I lie down to sleep, I am overcome by weariness at the thought of what's ahead of me.

I have always felt that the people I love could easily renounce me. How often have I felt that the connection had been cut and that I was a stranger, alone in the world. Yet how often too has my heart glowed with the knowledge that I am unconditionally and unalterably loved and cherished.

The best education will not immunize a person against corruption by power. The best education does not automatically make people compassionate. We know this more clearly than any preceding generation. Our time has seen the best-educated society, situated in the heart of the most civilized part of the world, give birth to the most murderously vengeful government in history.

Forty years ago the philosopher Alfred North Whitehead thought it self-evident that you would get a good government if you took power out of the hands of the acquisitive and gave it to the learned and the cultivated. At present, a child in kindergarten knows better than that.

It is remarkable how many outstanding persons who achieved much in life were savagely asinine at the age of twenty. "What They Said at Twenty" would make a curious collection. I just read a statement made by Dos Passos in 1916 when he was twenty: "My only hope is in revolution—in the wholesale assassination of all statesmen, capitalists, warmongers, jingoists, inventors, scientists."

January 22, 8:00 A.M.

An individual can probably thrive without illusions, but it is doubtful whether a wholly disillusioned society can be vigorous. Such a society will be awkward in dealing with internal adversaries and will not know how to impose its values on the new generation and on outsiders. The thirty million immigrants who came to America after the Civil War were quickly assimilated by a society that had extravagant illusions about the future. On the other hand, the present integration of twenty million Negroes is proceeding in a climate of disillusionment.

In the past I could carry a complex train of thought in my head, formulating and revising, without writing down a word until I had it all tied up. At present I cannot think without pen in hand. Clearly, old age has its own requirements and rules. The old must break with the past and learn anew.

To feel well, the old need the forbearance and regard usually given to people of outstanding achievements. In countries where age is revered, the old look beautiful.

The things which corrupt the young may help the old stay young.

January 23, 7:15 A.M.

I am reading Trevelyan's biography of Sir Edward Grey. On the evening before war was declared, as he looked through the window of his room in the Foreign Office and saw the lamps being lit in the summer dusk, Sir Edward said to a friend: "The lamps are going out all over Europe; we shall not see them lit again in our lifetime." Next day, in a note, he expressed his dismay: "Europe is in the most terrible trouble it has ever known in civilized times, and no one can say what will be left at the end."

Grey's passion was for bird watching, fly fishing, and hiking. But his darkened spirits enabled him to sense the fate awaiting the Occident. In a letter in 1913 he foresaw a disastrous end for industrial civilization: "This boasted civilization that has defiled beautiful country, made hideous cities, been built up and maintained by ghastly competition and pressure, makes men swarm together and multiply horribly, is so abominable that God will sweep it away."

January 24, 6:30 A.M.

Everyone expects 1975 to be a year of decision for the Occident. My fear is that it will be a year of protracted crisis. It is the lingering crisis that debilitates. An explosion would cleanse the air. I would welcome a blowing up of the oil wells in the Persian Gulf. A dramatic end of the fossil-fuel age could be the opening act in the renewal and rebirth of the Occident. The balance of the century should be devoted to the search for cheaper and cleaner fuels. In the meantime the Occident should adopt a simpler and slower mode of life and use its manpower in a concerted effort to cleanse air and water of pollution, replenish the soil, reforest the hills, and clean up the cities. The added bonus of such an undertaking would be to give our vast population of adolescents a healthy way of attaining manhood and probably accelerate racial integration.

Who in the 1950s had a premonition of the witches' sabbath that would be enacted in the 1960s? Once events have taken place, a horde of learned commentators demonstrate that the unexpected was inevitable. Actually, chance, stupidity, and cowardice were chief factors. Nothing was inevitable.

6:45 P.M. I walked along the waterfront for about three hours. It has been a long time since I was there. The walk is easy since there are many places where I can sit down and ease my right leg. I hardly saw a familiar face. Almost all the people I worked with have retired. It was a surprise to be recognized and greeted by young longshoremen who came to the waterfront after my retirement. Several of them are the sons of longshoremen.

January 25, 8:15 A.M.

Were it not for women and children the Industrial Revolution might not have got started. They were made to work twelve hours a day, seven days a week, from the word go. Adult males stubbornly refused to be harnessed to this endless grind. The masters were unbelievably ruthless and arrogant. We read that in 1830 there were still forty-two traditional holidays. Some years later there were only four. The middle class that started the Industrial Revolution lived in its own world and cared less for the people who worked in the factories than for beasts of burden. The lower orders were seen as a different species.

The working people of Britain began the Industrial Revolution with a whimper and they are now bringing it to an end with a bang. They now have the upper hand. But the reversal of roles is taking place in a Britain impoverished and dispirited.

A generation that wearies of technology is bound to turn to magic. Those who refuse to use machines that move mountains will pray for a faith that moves mountains.

January 26, 5:00 A.M.

Old age has made me common. I have the typical aches and predicaments of the old. It is true that my nose is not dripping when my head nods in drowsiness and I manage to keep the corners of my mouth clean.

It is also true that I am easy on myself. I have a right to an unstrenuous old age. But it must be free of boredom and a feeling of stagnation. This means that I must go on thinking, learning, and writing. All I can allow myself is a slower tempo.

January 27, 8:30 A.M.

Nations tend to see their great men as the expression of their quintessence and uniqueness. Great men are also assumed to embody the spirit of their age. Actually, the essential characteristic of a great man is his timelessness and universality. The great man of any age is our contemporary.

It is by their commonness that people are linked to their time. Hence, by how much a great man is of his age, by so much is he less great.

January 29, 7:00 A.M.

Do eras vary in their degree of forgetfulness? Certainly our century forgets more readily than any preceding era. It is difficult in the 1970s to remember the 1950s. So much has happened!

The tendency to forget does not originate in the need to efface unpleasant memories. Germany could not forget its humiliation after the First World War and France its humiliation during the Second World War. Forgetfulness is linked with a break in continuity. The total difference between the 1960s and the 1950s created a feeling of remoteness. The same is true of the sharp break between the 1960s and 1970s.

We somehow take it for granted that drastic changes undermine authority. In the new book I have a short chapter on change and authority in which I show that the most successful drastic changes took place in an authoritarian atmosphere. A society racked by drastic change needs a strong framework of authority and an anchor of continuity to keep it from falling apart. Yet the intellectual establishment which advocates the permissive society thinks that the new can germinate and grow only when it breaks through the integuments of authority.

January 30, 9:50 A.M.

Right now, hope has become the monopoly of the slave-masters in Russia. In the free world, desire has taken the place of hope and it looks as if soon the Occident will weary of desire.

In a free society it is necessary to spell out what people cannot do, while in an authoritarian society it is vital to spell out what people can do.

January 31, 7:10 A.M.

No one has explained the present failure of nerve of people in authority. The erosion of authority in government, family, school, factory, and even in the armed forces is the most bothersome phenomenon of our time. Many blame it on change: rapid, drastic change disintegrates values, renders skills and experience obsolete, and drains adults of confidence. Others see the cause in affluence. Well, affluence is no more. We also know that the most drastic changes of the past—the modernization of Japan and the rapid industrialization of Germany—were realized in authoritarian societies. There was no erosion of authority during England's rapid transformation in the early decades of the Industrial Revolution. So too in this country, the rapid changes after the Civil War occurred in an atmosphere of political and cultural conservatism.

My hunch is that the reason drastic change erodes authority at present is that we are without hope. Where things have not changed, authority remains intact even in the absence of hope. But when the social pot is boiling with change and no one knows what is cooking, authority seems helpless and loses its power to awe.

February 2, 7:20 A.M.

I have not found the reason why a society without illusions becomes flabby and unsure of itself. De Tocqueville has it that "Everything is feared when nothing is ardently desired." There is also the Spanish proverb: "Whoever is not called upon to struggle is forgotten by God."

How vital is experience to the creative flow? A creative person is not eaten up by his experience. Indeed, it is remarkable how the genuinely creative instinctively shy away from a full-blooded experience. They want to make much out of very little, and need but a crumb to know the taste of a loaf.

When we speak of authority at present we usually have in mind governmental authority. Actually, social order is most firm when imposed and maintained by the limited authorities of family, school, church, job, neighborhood, and so on. In 1848 the Spaniard Donoso-Cortés predicted that "when religious discipline ceases to exist there cannot be enough of government; all despotisms will not be sufficient." This holds true to some extent of the other minor authorities.

6:00 P.M. Walked leisurely through the park. Wound up at Tommy's Joynt at five and ate lustily a heap of fettuccini topped with beef burgundy.

It occurred to me that the First World War was a dividing line for emigration from Europe. The stability of nineteenth-century Europe was in no small part due to the emigration of the restless and disaffected. Had America and the British Empire welcomed emigrants from Europe after the First World War, there might have been neither a Fascist nor a Nazi revolution.

February 3, 9:30 A.M.

Despite the drastic changes all around us, it is remarkable how rare is the sense of newness. Perhaps to feel that something is truly new we have first to expect it. It is the realization of the expected that strikes us as the birth of the new.

I am haunted by Tennyson's lament in old age: "I am the greatest master of English that ever lived and I have nothing to say." He intoxicated himself by endlessly repeating his name.

February 4, 5:50 A.M.

It seems hardly credible that this country should have attempted Prohibition. What confidence, and what ignorance! It certainly is a different country now. Both Prohibition and the Great Depression had profound effects on our national character.

In any discussion of the breakdown of authority in this country the "noble experiment" should be given a prominent place.

The Communists try to eliminate the subtly interwoven appetites, inclinations, and impulses which normally keep people striving and searching. They want a society that is energized by noble motives untainted by gross promptings. It is like trying to eliminate sexual desire as a factor in procreation.

February 5, 7:00 A.M.
It was only in the late 1840s that adult Englishmen finally became steady workers. Someone clever suggested that when the children who made the Industrial Revolution possible (January 25) grew up they became steady adult workers. Today I found the following in Arthur Bryant's *English Saga:* "Many of the child workers were crippled for life; few grew to mature manhood or womanhood. . . . Every street had its company of cripples, of permanently aged and arthritic youths bent double and limping."

February 6, 6:35 A.M.
The phenomenal conformity in America is perhaps an indication of how lost people feel on this vast continent. As Whitehead suggested, when a man is lost his chief question is not where he is but where the others are.
It is also true that in a competitive society to act and be like others is a guarantee of not being left behind. My hunch is that competitive people feel alone in the world.

Somehow connected with the fact that creative periods are relatively brief is the fact that outstanding achievements do not emerge slowly but appear full-blown. The reason is probably that anything perfect is the creation of an individual and evolves in less than the span of an individual life.

February 7, 6:45 A.M.
This country was in worse shape in the 1930s than it is

today. There was more unemployment, there was hunger, and there was a greater paralysis of will. Capitalism was more bankrupt and discredited than it is in the 1970s. Yet the feeling of doom is stronger now. There is a widespread feeling that our economic system and our civilization are nearing their end. In the 1930s we still had values, ideals, hopes, illusions, certitudes. In the 1970s many people see life drained of meaning, and there is hardly a certitude left. Arthur Koestler compares the impact of the 1960s on our traditional values to the impact the European invaders had on the traditional life of the American Indian and the Pacific Islanders. The 1960s were decisive. We cannot understand what is happening in the 1970s unless we know what happened in the 1960s.

February 8, 10:10 A.M.

Old age is teaching me to take joy in the existence of beautiful and desirable things without wanting to possess or even savor them. I have not enjoyed the sight of beautiful women in the past as I do now. The same is true of the new, magnificent buildings, paved plazas, fountains, and flower beds. Life seems richer now.

February 10, 7:10 A.M.

What were the terrible 1960s (February 7) and where did they come from?

To begin with, the 1960s did not start in 1960. They started in 1957. A bell rings in my mind every time I hear the date 1957 mentioned. On October 4, 1957, the Russians placed a medicine-ball-sized satellite in orbit. It needs an effort to remember how stunned we were when we discovered that the clodhopping Russians were technologically ahead of us, and that we would have to catch up with them. We reacted hysterically. We set out to produce scientists and technologists wholesale by shoveling billions into the universities. And where the billions went there went also millions of persons who were not primarily interested in learning but wanted a piece of the action.

Thus Khrushchev's Sputnik toy brought about a change in the tilt of America's social landscape from the marketplace to the universities. After October 1957, many young people who would normally have gone into business ended up climbing academic ladders and throwing their weight around in literary and artistic cliques from Manhattan to Berkeley, California.

It was to be expected that the potential business tycoons would feel ill at ease on the campus. Where was the action? The university seemed to them a bloated, sluggish giant cut off from the stream of life. They were going to wake up the academic world and turn the university into an instrument of power. They were going to make history, which is an acceptable substitute for making and losing millions. It was these misplaced tycoons who set the tone and shaped events in the 1960s.

February 11, 9:30 A.M.

It is of interest that almost exactly a hundred years before Sputnik this country experienced another change in the tilt of its social landscape, but in the opposite direction—from the academy to the marketplace.

The first half of the nineteenth century was the age of the gentry, whose preoccupation was with education, cultural affairs, and public service. But the opening of the West in the 1850s caught the imagination of the young, and the sons of the gentry scattered in all directions. Many who would have become teachers, ministers, writers, or artists were seeking their fortunes in railroads, mining, manufacturing, and the like. Instead of potential business tycoons throwing their weight around on campuses, as we had in the 1960s, there were potential poets and philosophers washed into business careers. I have always felt that it was not conventional businessmen but misplaced poets and philosophers who gave American business its Promethean sweep and drive. To a potential philosopher turned businessman all action is of one kind. He combines mines, railroads, oil fields, factories the way a philosopher collates and generalizes ideas.

9:00 P.M. How strange that misplaced philosophers should have become grandiose builders while misplaced men of action became revolutionary wreckers. It is probably true as I suggested long ago in *The True Believer* that revolutionary intellectuals are

mostly people "whose talents and temperament equip them ideally for a life of action but are condemned by circumstances to rust
away in idleness." Most of the outstanding revolutionary leaders
of our time spent the best part of their lives talking their heads off
in cafés and meetings.

The significant fact is that men of action metamorphosed into
men of words are more readily corrupted by power than conventional men of action. Words are a potent source of self-righteousness; they serve to mask questionable motives, and justify ruthlessness. Paradoxically, the metamorphosed man of action has faith in
the magical powers of words. He becomes irrational and primitive
and is a threat to civilized life. Though we find it hard to accept
that "In the beginning was the Word," and that words created the
world, we know that words can ignite genocidal passions and
squash civilized societies. It is not hard for us to believe that words
may eventually destroy our world.

February 12, 6:45 A.M.

Some of the potential business tycoons washed by Sputnik
into academic careers became truly creative. They became outstanding sociologists, philosophers, scientists, even Nobel Prize
winners. Still, there was something that distinguished them from
regular scholars. They did not see learning as an end in itself.
They saw words, ideas, and theories as instruments of momentous
action and history making as a vital component of an intellectual
existence. They felt superior to the trivial businessmen and politicians who were running the country. They were going to create a
new society in which every act was pregnant with meaning and
destiny hovered over everyday life.

It is interesting that whereas the potential philosophers who
became businessmen were uniquely American, unlike businessmen anywhere else, the potential tycoons who became academics
were like intellectuals everywhere. They were twin brothers of
intellectuals in Latin America, Europe, Asia, and Africa.

In a previous entry (January 2) I described the effects of permissive child rearing promoted by avant-garde experts after the

Second World War. In 1964 a considerable segment of the student population was made up of eighteen-year-olds who were born in 1946 and were the products of a permissive upbringing. They were putty in the hands of any two-bit manipulator.

I happened to be in Berkeley in 1964 when the first wave of the new generation hit the campus of the University of California. President Clark Kerr had made me a professor—it was my first taste of getting paid for doing nothing—and I had a room on the eighth floor of Barrows Hall, where I held open house one afternoon a week. So I was right in the midst of the mess when the Free Speech Movement exploded in 1964.

The spark which set off the explosion was the discovery made by the students that the power structure of the university was manned by toothless lions. President Clark Kerr, one of the finest products of our culture, knew how to build a great university but did not know how to defend it. He had not an inkling of the vulnerability of institutions—that they are more vulnerable than individuals—and did not know the first thing about the nature of authority. I cannot resist the feeling that things might have turned out differently had President Kerr had a taste for theorizing. He might have known that authority is an instrument for the repression of individual willfulness and that social authority had its origin in the need to tame juveniles as they came out from underneath parental authority. Instead, President Kerr dealt with the rampaging juveniles as if they were his equals, and a punk like Mario Savio, the leader of the Free Speech Movement, ran circles around the great Clark Kerr. Much of the teaching at the University of California was done by teaching assistants not much older than the students. Monkeys with academic degrees opened all the cages and let the tigers out into the street.

I remember how one afternoon, as I stood on the eighth-floor balcony of Barrows Hall and watched swinish punks lay low the proud institution of the University of California, there flashed before my mind's eye an event of long ago. On the evening of November 16, 1532, the swineherd Francisco Pizarro pulled down the Inca Atahualpa from his proud litter and in scarcely three hours the most powerful state of pre-Columbian America was broken forever.

The people who want, and are fit, to live in a free society

cultivate patience, and make of compromise a holy cause. The militants who clamor for freedom most of the time want power power to retaliate. The means for establishing freedom are altogether different from the means for attaining power.

To William James the most crucial habit of an effective democracy is "a fierce and merciless resentment towards every man or set of men who break the public peace."

February 13, 8:00 A.M.

Psychoanalysts have a bias for deep, obscure causes. It was to be expected that the psychoanalyst Franz Alexander (*Western Mind in Transition*) should find that "a spiritual change preceded the First World War"; that the war only gave the coup de grâce to a spent cultural and political structure. He maintains that "the signs of decline presaging apocalypse were numerous and steadily growing." The main sign was a shift from a search for absolutes to an acceptance of relativity in all human endeavors. He sees an interconnection between Einsteinian physics, the new interpretation of space in cubistic painting, cultural relativism in anthropology, the war, the departure from the gold standard, and the rejection of classical rules of diplomacy. It was this pernicious relativism that prevented Europe from regaining its equilibrium when the war was over.

Actually, we have the testimony of knowledgeable observers on the stability and hopefulness of the prewar era. To Alfred North Whitehead, who was immersed in the new physics, the period 1880–1910 was "one of the happiest times that I know of in the history of mankind. . . . We often used to speak of what a wonderful world to live in our children would have." The inability to pick things up after the war was due largely to France's determination to prevent Germany's recovery as a great power, and Lenin's rejection of civilized values as bourgeois prejudices.

February 18, 6:00 A.M.

There ought to be a small book on *The Logic of Events—* its rules and regularities; and its difference from a priori logic. Here is a jumbled summary:

A priori logic assumes that poverty breeds crime, that necessity is the mother of invention, that permissive upbringing will produce self-reliant adults, that authority hampers change. The logic of events shows the opposite to be true. Rich countries have a higher crime rate than poor countries, invention is least where the pressure of necessity is greatest, permissive upbringing produces conformist adults lacking confidence, authority is crucial for the realization of drastic change.

A priori logic assumes that people will be happier when they have more. The logic of events shows that we are less dissatisfied when we lack many things than when we seem to lack but one thing. A priori logic assumes that we have less when we give part of what we have to others whereas the logic of events shows that we multiply by dividing—that we are happiest when we share our happiness with others. A priori logic says that a straight line is the shortest distance to a goal whereas in human affairs a straight line is the shortest distance to disaster.

February 19, 6:30 A.M.

It sometimes seems that I can remember every unseemly thing I have done in my life. I do not remember the fine things.

Now and then I feel that before I am done with the world, I shall be punished for past transgressions. There is not much time left, and there is no one from whom to ask forgiveness. Yet, strangely, the more unworthy I feel, the lighter seems the burden. If I am damned already, it cannot matter much what happens to me.

February 20, 9:00 A.M.

Civilized countries fell over each other to court Hitler even as he turned Germany's Jews into pariahs. The same countries are now falling over each other to court the Arabs, who are determined to destroy Israel. The world feels no shame when it betrays Jews. It is as if fate has placed the Jews outside the comity of mankind.

The twentieth century is a Jewish century (Marx, Freud, Einstein), yet this century has seen the most fearful slaughter of Jews.

February 22, 9.30 A.M.

1 have assumed that a society that cannot safeguard its young and defend its old cannot be buoyant. Yet while England was bursting with energies between 1820 and 1840 the English working people could neither protect their children nor give security to the old. The children went into mines and factories, and the old ended up in the poorhouse.

February 23, 7:30 A.M.

The legacy of the 1960s: a revulsion from work; a horde of educated nobodies who want to be somebodies and end up being busybodies; a half-submerged counterculture of drugs and drift still able to swallow juveniles (of every age) who cannot adjust to a humdrum existence.

The sickness of the twentieth century has been cowardice— the cowardice of millions allowing themselves to be liquidated by Communists and Nazis without hitting back. If every victim had done all he could to take one murderer with him, history might have been different.

Anger is the only cure for cowardice—anger strong enough to overcome fear. Right now people are afraid to get angry.

February 24, 9:15 A.M.

To learn from experience can be painful, expensive, and time-consuming. The wise learn from the experience of others, and the creative know how to make a crumb of experience go a long way. The Greeks derived their theories not from experience but from looking on. The Greek *theorein* means to look on.

I have learned more from the ancient Hebrews than from the ancient Greeks. But lately I find myself preoccupied with pre-Socratic Greeks. I have the feeling that post-industrial society will have to be Greek in spirit. Industrial society with its single-minded drive and its passion to master things has its roots in the Old

Testament. But a post-industrial society will not follow the injunction to subdue the earth.

The Greeks had no clichés, no fictions, no vital lies. They were not afraid to face the facts of life. They had nothing to hide, nothing they wanted to escape from. Conversation was their passionate pursuit. But whereas in America the passionate pursuit of business drained energies from other departments of life, in Greece conversation canalized energies into all sorts of pursuits. The Greeks were many-minded. Just as in their conversations in the agora men of every variety communed with each other, so in their minds all sorts of interests and bents intermixed. They had no specialization. The men who managed the state, fought the wars, and sailed the ships also wrote the poetry, thought the philosophy, and carved the statues.

The Greeks invented logic but were not fooled by it. They had an eye for the inner logic of events. They were close observers and based their thinking on what they observed. They had none of the clichés and platitudes mouthed by our logicians.

February 25, 9:45 A.M.

I was highfalutin when I said that a society needs a passion for excellence if it is to stay vigorous. Another way of putting it would be that a society stays vigorous so long as it can educe dedication and craftsmanship from the people it pays well to do the world's work.

In human affairs a device or a policy is most successful when rendered invisible. Changes are most successful when they are scarcely perceived. A successful manager makes management invisible, and authority is most potent when hidden in hearts and minds.

February 26, 6:30 A.M.

Both the ancient Greeks and Chinese had an exaggerated idea of the power of music. Pythagoras used music as a medicine to purge souls. To Plato, a change in music was a prelude to social change. Do we know anything about Greek music?

According to Confucius: "The spirit of a community is formed by the music it hears. Hence a government must encourage one kind of music and forbid another." When one of his disciples became the governor of a city, he instructed the people in music as a first principle of government.

February 27, 9:00 A.M.

Last night I dreamed about God—a grayhaired old man with bloodshot eyes surrounded by commissars. Something had been completed, and he came down to inspect. He looked tired. The commissars kept repeating: "They ought to love us."

No one has said worse things about the Russians than the Russians themselves. Russia's chronic despotism has its roots in the boundless contempt for the Russian people which possessed anyone who had power over them. A recurrent epithet in the expressions of contempt is "deceitful savages." Dostoevski believed that Russians are most easily won over "by an open advocacy of a right to be dishonorable."

To Eisenhower, an intellectual is "a man who takes more words than are necessary to tell more than he knows." As President, Eisenhower mastered the art of saying nothing at great length—he used more words than were necessary to say less than he knew.

February 28, 2:10 P.M.

Right now in every country not under Communist rule a high percentage of the intellectuals are contemptuous of capitalism. The fact that in capitalist countries most intellectuals are fairly well off—that they often combine anti-capitalist opinions with capitalist bank accounts—only serves to fan their hostility. Their influence has been increasing since Sputnik. They are brainwashing politicians, civil servants, judges, editors, publishers, journalists, teachers, students, broadcasters, and even "concerned" businessmen. It is obvious that a capitalist society must know how to deal effectively with its would-be destroyers if it is to survive. But it is difficult to see how a society can fight its educated classes.

March 1, 8:00 A.M.

It will need a new type of businessman to cope with the writers, artists, scholars, and so on who shape our attitude toward business. I have suggested (February 11) that potential poets and philosophers originally gave American business its Promethean sweep and drive, and it may take culture-bearing businessmen— as much at home in literary and artistic circles as in board rooms—to guide business at present.

Is underestimation of its own strength inherent in a democratic society?

Up to the First World War neither Britain nor America underestimated its strength. In France there was overestimation. The democracies lost their nerve after the war, and it was the underestimation of their strength that made possible the rise of Hitler and the coming of the Second World War.

During the Second World War Britain and America courted Stalin, who needed them more than they needed him. Even after America's superb performance in the Pacific, Roosevelt did not believe we could defeat Japan without Russian help.

Right now Israel is the only democracy that does not underestimate its strength, and it is being warned by the Western democracies that overconfidence may endanger its survival.

Logicians are baffled by the logic of events (January 2), which upsets their predictions. They tend to see it as a mysterious, even spiteful, power. Hegel spoke of "the cunning of history." René Grousset saw a mocking demiurge playing tricks behind the scenes and delighting in drawing from men's actions consequences least foreseen. Henry George remarked on the fact that the excellent mind that conceived and built the Brooklyn Bridge could not prevent a lot of condemned wire from getting into the bridge.

March 2, 6:50 A.M.

The educated classes: on the one hand a large number of educated people who want to live important lives. They cannot find fulfillment in making a good living by doing their share of the world's work. And they lack the humility and patience which might enable them to achieve distinction by realizing their capacities and talents.

On the other hand, there are a number of creative, prestigious individuals—scholars, writers, artists, scientists—who are averse to the practical, materialist temper of capitalist society. They are contemptuous of the triviality and banality of the marketplace. They want a society in which souls are stretched by grandiose tasks and noble challenges.

How is capitalist society to deal with them? I am playing with an idea that is perhaps impractical but which I find attractive: to find grandiose tasks for the educated by having them do the things capitalist society cannot do.

I have to chew on this some more.

March 3, 9:00 A.M.

The elegant way to solve problems is to put one problem to solve another. You solve the problem of adversary educated classes by giving the educated a chance to solve some of the problems capitalism cannot solve.

Capitalism is ideal for people who can take care of themselves but it cannot do much for the helpless. Capitalism cannot cure chronic poverty, cannot do much for the old, and cannot ease the passage of adolescents to adulthood. My suggestion is that the educated classes should be given a free hand and the required means to deal with the helpless, and in the process find the high drama and grandiose challenges that would quicken their spirits.

There should be an enclave wholly in the keeping of the intelligentsia—perhaps a whole state run by professors, students, writers, artists. They will probably fashion a communal society. The chronically poor will be settled in cooperative hamlets, where they will be taught to produce vegetables, fruit, eggs, and milk. Juveniles will become members of large kibbutzim engaged in both agriculture and industry. The old too will live in a communal milieu, where they will find a sense of usefulness and opportunities to learn and grow. Finally, the temporarily unemployed will be given plots of ground on which to grow vegetables, and be encouraged to hunt and fish.

The communal state will not be cut off from the rest of the country. Those who weary of the rat race will be free to transfer to the new state. It is also possible that once the chronically poor become self-reliant they may choose to return to the free-swinging capitalist society. The same might be true of the adolescents who attain manhood, and of the unemployed who are offered jobs.

4:00 P.M. Bought a shirt, cigars, and tobacco. Spent a fortune and feeling fine. Can't tell why.

10:15 P.M. The shirt is shoddy. The buttonholes are frayed and there are loose folds of cloth inside. I shall drop the thing in hot water and hope it dissolves.

March 4, 6:00 A.M.

The eighteenth century was the golden age of the intellectuals. They were feared and courted by the mighty. Frederick the Great courted Voltaire, and Catherine the Great went to great lengths to woo Diderot. Frederick and Catherine feared Voltaire's and Diderot's power to shape European opinion. One wonders whether the heads of large business corporations would take the trouble and be as skillful wooing the intellectuals who are shaping America's attitude toward business.

March 5, 8:45 A.M.

On the threshold of the twentieth century, two Jews—Theodor Herzl and the English Rabbi Moses Gaster—foresaw the coming of a dark age.

Herzl in an address to Lord Rothschild in 1897: "It is impossible to hope that the Jewish position will improve. If I am asked how I know it, I should say that I can tell you where a stone rolling down an inclined plane will go—right to the bottom. . . . I cannot foretell the forms it will take. Will it be expropriation through revolution from below or confiscation by reactionary forces from above? In some countries they will drive us out, while in others they will slay us. Is there no way out?"

Rabbi Gaster (in a symposium, *The Great Religions of the World*, Harper, 1901): "A mighty wind of reaction is blowing over all Europe. We are moving on a downward plane leading from equality, fraternity, freedom and right to radical hatred, national exclusiveness, military brutalization ... from the free and serene atmosphere of human faith to the swamps of mysticism, occultism; to the inquisition and the stake."

About the same time, the Zionist leader Max Nordau predicted that beautiful socialism would end in anti-Semitism: "If we should live to see theory become practice you'll be surprised to meet again in the new order that old acquaintance anti-Semitism, and it won't help at all that Marx and Lassalle were Jews."

March 6, 7:00 A.M.

In preceding entries I pointed out the almost total unawareness of impeding catastrophe in the decades before the First World War. The German Jewish writer Stefan Zweig, for example, said that he had never had more faith in the future than in the years before the war. Herzl, Rabbi Gaster, and Nordau were poignantly Jewish, and never recovered from the shock of the Dreyfus affair. Zweig, on the other hand, saw himself as an outstanding German writer and a European. His suicide in 1942 suggests an inability to draw strength from an identification with the Jewish people.

How is one to explain the blindness of the German Jews during the 1920s and the early 1930s? There was the widespread delusion that the Russian Revolution and Weimar Germany had created a new climate of enlightenment. The German Jews refused to take Hitler seriously until it was too late. They had not an inkling of what the average German felt and thought. They could not see, as Jung did, that Hitler "magnified the inaudible whispers of the German soul"; that he was articulating what Germans had been thinking since the defeat of the First World War.

The blindness of the German Jews strikes me as a mark of decadence. It will fare ill with Jews everywhere if they allow the memory of Hitler's holocaust to be blurred during the remainder of this terrible century.

March 9, 6:00 A.M.

Greek individual freedom was not a by-product of a stale-mate between the two coercive powers (Church and State), as it was in the West, but the result of a fortuitous break with coercive patterns of the past. The Dorian invasion, early in the first millennium B.C., washed remnants of shattered communities and tribes onto the shores of Ionia. This mixed multitude was almost without a memory of the past.

What was it that generated in the Greeks a creative tension? They were the first free men immersed in a sea of barbarism. Without the binding power of dogmatic religion and traditional patriotism, their society hovered on the brink of anarchy. They had to search for the foundations of the beliefs, customs, and attitudes indispensable for a stable social existence. Everything had to be discussed and analyzed. There were few things they could take for granted.

March 10, 7:15 A.M.

Those who rate heredity higher than environment in the shaping of a society have a lot of explaining to do. They have to account for the long periods of stagnation and the usually brief outbursts of creativity. You cannot attribute the petering out of Periclean Athens or of the fabulous era of Dutch painting to a loss of genes. Someone said that heredity proposes and environment disposes, which is a way of saying that environment is decisive.

It is startling how often an outburst of cultural creativeness is associated with economics and social decline. Great literature and great art are rarely found in countries that are expanding and growing. America after the Civil War was seething with energies yet its literature, art, and science were anemic. So too the rapid industrialization of Imperial Germany after 1870 went hand in hand with a cultural decline. Germany's greatest literary age, 1760–1830, was an age of economic and political stagnation. The greatest Russian writers, composers, and scientists made their appearance in stagnant Czarist Russia just as the phenomenal intellectual and artistic vitality of Vienna at the turn of the century was the product of a stagnant Hapsburg empire. The most striking association between creative vigor and social stagnation is of course the flowering of classical Greece at a time when Athens was in economic and political decline. We also know (December 27) that at the height of the Renaissance, Italian banking and trade were losing their paramount position in Europe and the Mediterranean countries.

Still, the relation between action and creativeness may not be as automatic as I have made it out to be. Through most of history, general stagnation was the rule—absence of action was concurrent with an absence of cultural activity. It is also conceivable that in a society bursting with energies action and creativeness may, under certain conditions, go hand in hand.

March 11, 10:00 A.M.

The century 1550 to 1650 was one of great literature in both Spain and England although economically and politically England was on the rise and Spain in accelerated decline. Could there be perhaps a difference between insular and continental patterns of energy? In Elizabethan England the rule did not hold that opportunities for impressive action draw energies away from cultural pursuits. So too in the first half of the nineteenth century the unprecedented opportunities for action opened by the Industrial Revolution did not leave English literature anemic. On the contrary, this age of economic and political expansion became one of the greatest poetical epochs in England's history. It was the age of Wordsworth, Byron, Shelley, Keats, Coleridge, Browning, Tennyson, and others. The literary output outweighed in volume and value that of any other period.

It is of interest that England's insular pattern seems to have been carried over to New England, and persisted there until the middle of the nineteenth century. With the opening of the West in the 1850s the familiar continental pattern made its appearance. The cultural flowering of New England came to an abrupt end when potential writers, artists, scholars, and philosophers went off to seek their fortunes in mining, railroading, manufacturing, and the like.

Finally, it seems that Britain's decline signals the loss of its insular uniqueness. The present economic and political crisis is due partly to the fact that Britain's finest brains and energies are going into universities and cultural pursuits. We are seeing the association of economic and political stagnation with undiminished creativeness in literature, music, and science.

March 12, 7:15 A.M.

Yesterday I received an invitation from Herman Kahn to attend a seminar on the prospects of mankind to be held at Rockefeller University in New York. The truth is that I am not interested in the prospects of mankind but in the prospects of families—few of them without tragedies.

1:30 P.M. The idea of insular and continental patterns of energy does not stand up. France, a continental country, offers the example of an even creative flow unaffected by the oscillations of the economic or political pendulum. The reason is probably that in no other country are writers and artists so admired and honored. There is the story about Clemenceau breaking up a cabinet meeting when told that Monet had become dejected and stopped painting his famous water lilies. Clemenceau rushed to cheer him up and get him painting again. One cannot see a President of the United States interrupting a cabinet meeting to call up a despairing Hemingway and perhaps save him from suicide.

Ortega y Gasset when exiled from Spain wandered alone through the streets of Paris, where he knew not a soul, only to discover that he was surrounded by old friends, the statues of writers and thinkers he had known all his life, and he could now discuss with them, face to face, the great problems of mankind. An American writer who lived in Paris tells how the neighborhood grocer and baker who knew he was writing a book treated him as they would a woman big with child. How many statues of great thinkers, writers, and artists are there in our cities?

March 13, 7:20 A.M.

Last night I spoke to an audience of common people, half

of them black. I told them, among other things, that if they believed in God they must know that he loved them since he made so many of them. He is also a just God. Hence it would be blasphemous to assume that a loving, just God showered all his gifts on a chosen few and left our minds and hearts empty and shrunken. We are actually richer than we think. God has implanted in us the seed of all greatness and it is up to us to see that the seed germinates and grows. Learning and growing should be a kind of worship. For God has given us capacities and talents and it is our sacred duty to finish God's work.

Many have remarked on the capacity of popular opinion to foretell events. The unlearned apply what they see around them to the affairs of the great world. I heard an illiterate longshoreman predict on V-J Day that America would soon be quarreling with Russia, citing the behavior of boys playing on a sandlot. It has been my impression that the unlearned can read the book of the world better than the learned.

March 14, 6:45 A.M.

According to Bergson, "the intellect is characterized by an inability to comprehend life." Kant was certain that "the origin of the cosmos will be explained sooner than the mechanism of a plant or a caterpillar." How outlandish then is the belief that the intellect can fathom man's soul?

How can science unravel the chemistry of the soul when what we have here is actually an alchemy? Good and evil, beauty and ugliness, truth and error, love and hatred, the sublime and the ridiculous continually pass into each other. And alchemy is ruled not by the intellect but by magic.

March 15, 6:20 A.M.

We need a sense of grandeur. Were I an architect I would give every public building, even a post office, a lofty ceiling, soaring columns, marble floors—and tack utility onto the grandeur. We need the frequent enactment of grandiose public ceremonies. My feeling is that it is vital for democratic societies to cultivate the grandiose the way churches and monarchies did in the past.

March 16, 7:40 A.M.

Cleansing souls is risky. Bizet declared that "if you suppress adultery, fanaticism, crime, fallacy, the supernatural, there is no more means of writing a note." Montaigne saw our being so cemented by sickly qualities that "whoever should divest men of them would destroy the fundamental conditions of human life." Sir Francis Bacon had no doubt that "if there were taken out of men's minds vain opinions, flattering hopes, false valuations and the like, it would leave the minds of men poor, shrunken things." Renan feared that we can get rid of the bad only at the sacrifice of what is excellent, remarkable, and extraordinary.

The proponents of reason who set their hearts on cleansing souls of the irrational released demonic forces beyond control of reason.

Capitalism is in trouble because of its belief that everyone can take care of himself. It does not know how to help those who cannot help themselves. On the other hand, socialism is in trouble because it believes that no one can take care of himself.

Except the love for a child, all love is flawed. All that one can say of love is that it enables us to put up wholeheartedly with imperfections. This is true also of self-love.

March 17, 8:45 A.M.

It seems to be true that all great events come unheralded. I cannot think of a war or a revolution that did not come as a surprise. The fact that the Second World War was expected marks it as a continuation of the First World War. It seems incredible that the Industrial Revolution, one of the greatest events in history, was not foreseen by anyone. No one forecast the development of a machine industry.

It was not long ago that national greatness seemed a legitimate goal for almost any country. At present, a deliberate reaching out for national greatness is not found outside Russia and China. It is curious that at a time when every two-bit intellectual in a democratic country wants to make history, the free world has become skeptical of great feelings and sacrifices. The democracies aspire not to historical greatness but to the attainment of a modicum of material prosperity. Will this retreat of the free world from greatness make the world ripe for universal Russian dominion?

March 18, 6:40 A.M.

I cannot think of anything more un-Oriental than the first chapters of Genesis. The theorizing is in the grand scientific style even though the theories are based on fictions rather than facts.

A case can be made out that the ancient Hebrews were the first Occidentals. In the Orient power has always been absolute, as implacable as a force of nature. The Hebrews invented the division of power—between kings and prophets and later between Pharisees and the secular power. Finally, it was the Hebrew influence that created the tension that stretched Occidental souls, and generated the Occident's unique dynamism. Greek-dominated Byzantium knew no separation between Church and State, and became an Oriental despotism. I remember reading somewhere that in both Byzantium and Russia the Old Testament did not enter the lives of the pious as it did in the West.

One hears a lot about the primacy of Greek influence in the shaping of the Occident. But Greek influence flowed eastward, to Antioch, Alexandria, Persia and all the way to the borders of India. Until the fall of Constantinople Greek influence reached Europe through Arab channels. On the other hand, Hebrew influence penetrated Europe directly after the birth of Christianity and the destruction of the Second Temple. The Hebrews turned their backs on the Orient.

However vital the Greek heritage has been for the Occident's science, art and literature, it did not enter the lives of the people. The Occident's temper has been not Greek but Hebrew, and much of what is good and bad in us has Hebraic roots. And when Europeans crossed the Atlantic to possess the new world they carried not the Greek but the Hebrew heritage with them. It was Jehovah's injunction to subdue the earth that sustained the pioneers in their attempt to tame a savage continent in an incredibly short time. Greek learning came later. It was brought over by scholars and remained confined to houses of learning.

Still, as I have suggested (February 24), it could well be that if the post-industrial era evolves a new style of life it may follow the Greek model.

March 19, 8:30 A.M.

Even when I force myself to appreciate what is good in Communist Russia—the spread of education and the modernization of the Central Asian states and of Siberia—I keep remembering de Custine's belief that providence created Russia not to diminish the barbarism of Asia but to chastise Europe. I cannot help feeling that Russia is destined to destroy Western civilization.

No similarity is so genuinely similar as a difference is different. Most of the time an insistence on similarities is an attempt to evade thinking, whereas a probing of differences is almost always seminal. Our understanding of Russia is not furthered by the assumption that Russians are like everybody else. It might be intellectually more profitable to go to the other extreme and assume that the Russians are a species apart. The acceptance of fundamental differences would not only make us better observers of Russian behavior but might make our dealings with the Russians less frustrating by moderating our expectations.

March 20, 7:15 A.M.

In Soviet Russia scientists, ballet dancers, musical virtuosi, and chess players often achieve excellence while writers and artists remain on the whole mediocre. The reason is not mainly that writers and artists are more under the thumb of the censor. Even without censorship literature and art will not thrive where there are no friendship, no free conversation, no shame, and no extravagant dreams. Moreover, science, ballet, and so on live each in its own world while literature and art derive their nourishment from the social milieu.

The middle class is the only revolutionary class in history—the only class that accepts and promotes ceaseless change. The middle-class revolution changes not only a country's technology but its physical appearance and its way of life. Revolutions by other classes—by aristocrats, intellectuals, soldiers—change fundamentally little and terminate in stagnation. When, as in Britain at the turn of the century, the middle class embraces aristocratic values, it loses its revolutionary ferment and tends toward stagnation.

How has middle-class domination affected the human spirit? It has brought unrest, frustration, tension, insecurity, triviality, and insatiable desire. It has also brought unimagined affluence and given rise to great literature, art, and science. Middle-class domination stretched but did not cripple the human spirit.

March 21, 10:00 A.M.

I have set out a dish of bird seed and a basin of water on the balcony. I no longer have any illusion about birdlike innocence. One bully gets into the dish and drives off all other birds. The bullies seem demented and malicious. They skip about pecking at other birds rather than eat the seed. Why don't the birds gang up on the bully? Is it because of a lack of language? Birds are capable of united action: they flock together and organize themselves into flights to the ends of the earth.

It wearies me to think that the senseless pecking is part of the energy that fueled the ascent of life—the manifestation of a tireless, blind drive that will go on forever.

It occurs to me that only birds, two-legged creatures, can simulate human speech. Nothing that crawls or walks on four legs can utter words. The snake who spoke to Adam and Eve walked erect. He became mute when made to crawl. "Upon thy belly shalt thou go."

How did the snake manage to walk erect? Probably with the aid of hummingbird wings. He must have been a proud sight. To me, the story of the fall is above all the story of the fall of the snake.

March 22, 6:25 A.M.

It is doubtful whether writers and artists will ever be worshiped as they were during the Renaissance and the 1700s. One cannot see present-day presidents, prime ministers, or bankers vying for the favor of Leonardo, Raphael, Michelangelo, Erasmus, Voltaire, and Diderot. The worship had a religious quality. Both the Renaissance and the eighteenth century were preceded by periods of intense religious devotion. The habit of adoration lingered on but was transferred to nonreligious objects. When religious intensity returned with the Reformation and Counter-Reformation the adoration of writers and artists subsided. It reappeared when religiosity was discredited by the excesses of the Thirty Years' War.

Thucydides quotes Cleon that "Ordinary men usually arrange public affairs better than their more gifted fellows." It is something I have known all along (December 23).

Why should ordinary people be better organizers than people who feel themselves above the average? Ordinary people have more trust in their fellow men, and trust is a precondition for effective organizing. It is also true that ordinary people are never certain that they know best, hence their willingness to listen and compromise. Finally, ordinary people are not likely to demand perfection and will settle for the possible.

March 24, 8:30 A.M.

According to Paul Valéry, no great power in modern times has been able to hold on to its conquests for more than fifty years. Should this be true, Russia's day of judgment will come in the 1990s. Yet the staying power of the colossus seems awesome. Russia seems large and rich enough to weather any crisis. It may well continue more or less unchanged despite the chronic inefficiency of its economy and the antihuman absurdities of its system. However, if Russia's day does come, everyone will wonder that few people foresaw the inevitable end. The final breakup of a clumsy conglomerate of a hundred nationalities situated between nine hundred million irreconcilable Chinese and millions of resentful colonial subjects in Eastern Europe will seem to have been foreordained.

March 25, 6:00 A.M.

The fundamental difference between the thinker and the artist is that the thinker looks for a universal truth that will help explain unique events while the artist endows the unique with an intimation of the universal. What they have in common is that to both the visible is mysterious.

Things I cannot understand: the passion for immortality; the delusion that there is a cure for all the world's ills; Hitler's rise to power; the morbid hatred of some intellectuals for America; the belief of many people that good things will come to pass without effort; that so many well-educated people consider Lenin a great man.

They have been doing it all the time: they raze Bastilles and raise Kremlins.

March 26, 9:15 A.M.

It would be an understatement to say that the world has treated me better than I deserve. I have been favored by chance and treated royally by circumstances. Moreover, I have been spared both envy and greed.

It never bothered me that there are people who live in fabulous opulence. And I never assumed that to be rich is to be happy. However, the present galloping inflation is darkening my view of the rich. They are getting richer while the value of the few dollars I have saved is melting away. Should I live a few more years, I may have to pinch pennies in my last days. The rich raise prices in order to maintain a steady increase of profits. The rich are not paying taxes. There is not a law the rich and their shyster lawyers cannot get around. On Friday, April 4, I have to speak to a group of lawyers. I shall speak of the sins of the rich.

I am reading Nietzsche's letters. I used to be scornful of his pathological vanity—he actually expected an earthquake every time he had a new idea. But now I am overcome with compassion. The man was losing his mind. Reading about his breakdown in Turin in 1889, I suddenly saw the soul-wrenching predicament of a great spirit who needs a state of exaltation to do his best. An addiction to ecstasy may lead to madness and self-destruction.

I have always equated individual as well as social health with the ability to perform well at room temperature.

6:00 P.M. A rare electric storm. Thunder, lightning, and an angry north wind whipping the rain across the balcony almost to the glass wall. The barely visible docks below remind me of ceaseless toil, short lives, and brooding eternity.

March 27, 8:30 A.M.

In the city of Antwerp in 1560 there were three times as many working artists as there were butchers. The butchers had an exclusive union and a strict pattern of apprenticeship. Only the few could become butchers but every mother's son could become a painter.

Sixteenth-century Antwerp was a compact neighborhood, where children could watch artists at work. Tales about the fame and fortune of great painters were known to all. Becoming a painter was no more beyond reach than becoming a baseball player is today. Appreciation of art in sixteenth-century Antwerp was probably as diffused as the appreciation of baseball is in an American city.

March 28, 11:00 A.M.

Was Christianity a factor in the release of Jewish energies? In the non-Christian world the Jews sank to the level of the natives, both intellectually and economically. It is true that during the Muslim renaissance the Jews were in the van, but they declined with the Muslims after A.D. 1200. On the other hand, the Jews preserved their intellectual prowess in the inert Christian world of the Middle Ages, and later in the stagnant atmosphere of Eastern Europe. In the eighteenth century, in dark, illiterate Lithuania, the Jews produced the great Rabbi Elijah Ben Solomon, the "Gaon" of Vilna.

With emancipation at the turn of the eighteenth century, the pent-up Jewish energies burst over central and western Europe and contributed, disproportionately, to the fabulous economic and scientific expansion initiated by the Industrial Revolution. This was particularly true in Germany. It is significant that virulent German anti-Semitism did not stifle the Jewish creative spirit.

One wonders what would have happened had Jewish energies been canalized eastward and given free play in the vast expanse of Russia. Chances are the Jews would not have performed as well in Russia's Byzantine climate.

March 29, 6:00 A.M.
When I read what Paul Valéry wrote about the Occident after the First World War, I am surprised by its contemporaneity. It is as if he were writing about the 1970s. This reminds me of de Custine's description of Russia in the 1840s, which strikes me as a description of the Stalin era. It is as if we predict the future when we exaggerate the defects of the present.

Senility consists partly in not being able to take things for granted. The old are not sure that their legs will carry them, their arms will lift, their eyes will see, their stomach will digest. Would this be true also of a society? Does a society become senile when it no longer can take familiar practices and attitudes for granted?

March 30, 7:15 A.M.
Modern manufacturers invent a product and then find a use for it. Psychoanalysis tries to induce the disease for which it offers itself as a cure. The revolutionary strives to produce the evils he denounces in order to apply the cure he prescribes. We have here three different human types resorting to a similar strategy. Do they perhaps respond to a similar need—the need for a sense of usefulness? No one in modern times can savor usefulness the way people did when going to bed on a full stomach was a triumph. We have now to invent uses in order to feel useful.

March 31, 9:40 A.M.
It seems to me that deeds do not bite deeply into the mind. I doubt whether people can become incurably damaged by what they do. I believe it is possible to do the terrible things many Germans did in Hitler's time and still lead a decent life afterward. It is possible to blur or completely wipe out the memory of evil

deeds. Remorse is not what moralist logicians make it out to be.

Actually, it is the things we have missed doing that are likely to fester in the mind.

April 2, 9:15 A.M.

Democracies are naked. Anyone can see their weaknesses and shortcomings, whereas their hidden strengths can only be guessed at. The Japanese had every right to believe that hedonistic, undisciplined Americans would be no match for the fanatically dedicated Japanese warriors. Many knowledgeable Americans thought so too. It is quite natural to underestimate democracies, and it is not a mark of decadence when a democracy underestimates its own strength.

April 3, 7:00 A.M.

Capitalism's greatest predicament is that several paradoxes of the human condition combine to turn capitalist successes into failures.

Take affluence: capitalism is the only system that can create abundance. The noncapitalist world, no matter how rich in natural resources, has been and is likely to remain a world of scarcity. But it turns out that affluence is straining capitalist society to the breaking point. We were not prepared for the disintegration of values and the weakening of social discipline caused by the elimination of scarcity.

Take efficiency: capitalist production is the most efficient the world has seen. It takes fewer workers to do a job in a capitalist society than anywhere else. But, by using as few workers as possible, capitalist society is without the wide diffusion of a sense of usefulness essential for social stability. So far, capitalism has not known how to cope with chronic unemployment.

Take change: capitalist society is the most open to change. It is the only truly revolutionary society. The self-styled revolutionaries once in power prize stability above everything else, and the societies they dominate become economically and culturally stagnant. However, as change accelerates, capitalist societies are finding themselves in deep trouble. They are discovering that even the most desirable changes are upsetting traditions, customs, and routines—all the arrangements which make everyday life predictable. And there is no telling how long a society that cannot take things for granted—a society with few axioms—can keep on an even keel.

Take mass education: it was the capitalists and not the intellectuals who initiated and promoted mass education. In capitalist America every mother's son can go to college. Most capitalist societies are being swamped with educated people who disdain the triviality and hustle of the marketplace and pray for a new social order that will enable them to live meaningful, weighty lives. The education explosion is now a more immediate threat to capitalist societies than a population explosion.

April 4, 6:40 A.M.

Small tightly knit circles are a peculiarity of creative milieus. You find them in Periclean Athens, in Renaissance Florence and Antwerp, and in Paris and late Hapsburg Vienna. Emulation, example, praise, and assistance are at their best in such circles. Nevertheless, I shudder when I imagine what my life would have been as a member of such a circle. I always wanted to be left alone—not to have anyone to vie with, and not to have an example.

April 5, 9:45 A.M.

Taking too much for granted cuts people off from reality. The generation that stumbled into the First World War took civilization for granted. There was nowhere an awareness that a civilized pattern of life is almost as easily marred as the markings on butterfly wings. Yet we are also finding out that without axioms there is no social stability or continuity—that without taking things for granted there can be no civilized living.

How good I feel when I do my duty! I ought to invent a whole chain of duties and revel in their performance. Is not this the way the pious live full lives?

April 6, 4:00 A.M.

A painful twist of the left arm woke me up. I do not feel sleepy.

I try to imagine what Prime Minister Rabin said to Secretary of State Kissinger at their last parting. America's abandonment of Vietnam was in the air. "You are an American Secretary of State, and the interests of America should be uppermost in your mind. You are also a Jew whose relatives died in gas chambers while the whole civilized world looked on and did not lift a finger. The destruction of Israel would not affect America more adversely than did the fall of South Vietnam. Can we accept a condition in which our survival would depend on America's good will and good faith? Would you accept such a condition were you the Prime Minister of Israel, which you might have become had your parents gone to Israel instead of the United States?"

It does not make sense for a non-Israeli, however knowledgeable, sensitive, and benevolent, to tell Israel what to do in order to survive. Israel is the foremost authority on national survival.

Do my dark thoughts reflect the weariness of a troubled old man rather than objective situations? Do I give voice to personal weariness when I maintain that this country cannot go on indefinitely as it has done in the past—the same squirrel cage, the same ups and downs? I am convinced that we have to stop running, stop wanting what we no longer really want.

April 8, 7:00 A.M.

I have assumed that the stagnation of the Arab world is due to the congeniality of the religion of Islam—its lack of the inner contradictions and tensions which stretch souls. But it seems that hashish is also a factor. The Mongol invasion in the thirteenth century which put an end to Arab supremacy also introduced hashish. Egyptian doctors have blamed this drug for the sluggishness of Egyptian workers. Will the use of marijuana have a similar effect on American workers?

We can never love as totally as we hate. Hitler hated the Jews more than he loved Germany, more than he loved power, and more than he loved victory.

April 9, 7:50 A.M.
Reading Hans Kohn about his youth, I am aware how hard it is for an educated young man to develop his own thoughts and shape his own attitudes. At his age I was on the run. I was not immersed in the spirit of an age. I lived in a timeless world.

One need not be profound to predict the future. On the contrary, the seed of the future is on the surface of the present and is not seen by those who look for hidden truths. During the first miners' strike in 1910 the near-sighted Sir Edward Grey, by magnifying what he saw, predicted that trade unions would ultimately supplant parliament. It is true that in this case a naïve view of history aided prediction. Sir Edward saw a chain of displacements reaching back into the past: the barons displaced the crown, the middle class displaced the barons, and the workers were destined to displace the middle class and its parliament.

April 10, 9:30 A.M.
The nineteenth century was dominated by men of action. The men of words just talked: they philosophized, theorized, prophesied, and schemed extravagantly and recklessly because they knew that their words would not lead to action.
The twentieth century became a century of words par excellence. It not only saw the extravagant words of the nineteenth century become flesh but in no other century have so many men of words become spectacular men of action. In no other century have words been so dangerous. Yet few have recognized this fact. The free world refused to take Hitler's words seriously and at present hardly anyone outside Israel is alarmed by wild Arab talk about eliminating the Jewish state.

Hans Kohn's *Living in a World Revolution* was written in the early 1960s. It is good about Europe before the First World War but anemic about contemporary affairs and the recent past. There is no mention of the world's indifference to the fate of the Jews under Hitler. He includes Lenin among "the great emancipators of modern times."

April 11, 7:50 A.M.

Hebrew fanaticism was born during the Babylonian captivity and became full-blown when the fascination with Hellenism threatened Jewish uniqueness. Fanaticism was the invention of a small, weak national entity fighting for survival. It became a scourge when appropriated by large, powerful bodies—churches, states, parties—in a struggle for supremacy. The unexampled success of organizations armed with fanaticism has led clear-sighted thinkers like Renan and Keynes to believe that "Only fanatics can found anything," that "The future lies in the hands of those who are not undeceived," and that "An age can only be great if it is bred up in believing what is preposterous."

Yet the Greeks achieved greatness without a belief in "vital lies."

April 12, 10:30 A.M.

Since Communist countries are not equally inefficient, one ought not to blame communism for Russia's incredible inefficiency in the mechanics of everyday life. Repairing a car in Russia is a nightmare of negligence, ignorance, chicanery, theft, and general bungling. There is evidence that things are different in Rumania, Hungary, and several other Communist countries. One is justified, therefore, in blaming the Russians rather than their system for the mess.

However, judging by the wonders performed by Russian peasants on their tiny private plots of land, there is reason to believe that a machine shop run by Russians as a private undertaking would be as efficient as any in the world. The present inefficiency should be attributed, therefore, to a Russian inaptitude for communism.

April 13, 7:30 A.M.

There were anarchic intervals in the history of most countries: "In those days there was no king in Israel: every man did

that which was right in his own eyes." We are told how unprece-
dentedly new our time is, but our troubles and difficulties are not
new. There is nothing new in the decay of communities, the
crumbling of authority, and the defiance of the young.

In an authoritarian regime it looks as if despotic power has
usurped the authority of family, church, unions, and so on. Actually, it was the decay of traditional authority that prepared the
ground for dictatorship. Those who try to weaken established authority in order to enlarge individual freedom unknowingly clear
the way for the coming of tyranny.

April 20, 7:00 A.M.
In his autobiography John Nef says of the philosopher
George Mead that "One thing that kept him from publishing as a
philosopher was a strong belief that anything he wrote would no
longer be true by the time it got into print." This suggests that
contemporary philosophy is a fad that sooner or later goes out of
date. The strange thing is that at present books based on facts
rather than philosophical speculation are often overtaken by a
similar fate. Facts have become as perishable as opinions. This
holds true even of scientific facts. Only the human condition has
remained timeless.

April 21, 8:50 A.M.
At present, to be practical is to expect the worst.

Machines may make people superfluous, but they cannot
make them harmless. No matter how many and how ingenious
the machines, there will always be people around to mess things
up.

I am more than ever convinced that the intellectual's hopes
and fears are not shared by the majority of common people. The
dismay which darkens our spirits has nothing to do with the sins
of government or with the threats to human survival such as population explosion, pollution, or a nuclear holocaust. No, our dark

mood stems from the inability of parents to protect their children against pitfalls and snares, and from the inflation which puts to naught our efforts to provide for a rainy day.

Lenin sprang a leak in the cesspool of Russian history and the stench has poisoned the civilized world.

In human affairs the immaterial is more weighty than anything that can be weighed and measured. The unpredictability of man has its source in the interaction between the fictitious and the real. The purely fictitious and the purely real are usually predictable.

April 22, 6:00 A.M.

I am still looking for a wholly new train of thought. Actually, at my age, the mind is better elaborating and deepening the familiar than groping for a new beginning. I find I have my own key for any problem that is brought up. Thus, although I keep looking for something totally new, there is the conviction in the back of my mind that there is nothing new under the sun.

The early Greek philosophers were fantastic creatures. They were immersed in revelations and visions. "A light," said Kant, "broke on the first man who demonstrated the properties of the isosceles triangle." The world was a fabulous goldfield—the meanest fact had in it nuggets of ideas. They expected the unexpected and found it. And there was not an idea they could not express in a sentence or two; and what they wrote sounded like inspired oracles.

After all that we have seen with our own eyes there ought not to be a grownup person who is not contemptuous of the gibberish about an ideal society and does not look for the lineaments of a commissar in the features of an idealist loudmouth.

It is disconcerting that the young who want to make history are so unbelievably ignorant of much that has happened in this terrible century. They do not know that you cannot build Utopia without terror, and that before long terror is all that is left.

April 25, 7:30 A.M.

I ought to have a good chapter on hope in the new book. The role hope plays in the life of a modern society is so taken for granted that we are unaware of its novelty. Through most of history mankind lived without the vision of a shining future around the corner. The conviction prevailed that successive generations and ages would be "as alike as drops of water." The belief that the future will be better and happier than the past was introduced by the French Encyclopedists and preached by the French revolutionaries. "Happiness," said Saint-Just, "is a new idea in Europe." America's birth almost coincided with the birth of this climate of hope.

Hope is a vital social ingredient. It is indispensable not only in the maintenance of social vigor but in the preservation of social cohesion and discipline. And nowhere in the modern world has hope been so central and natural as in America. The taming of a savage continent in an incredibly short time was powered by boundless hope. As recently as the 1950s Americans still felt themselves in the van, pioneering the future. Yet by 1970 a British correspondent in Washington could pontificate without being challenged that if America is the future, the future does not work.

Who slew America's hope? We were all there—workingmen, businessmen, politicians, soldiers, old and young, rich and poor, learned and ignorant. But the murder weapon was forged in the radical-chic salons of Manhattan and Washington, and in the word factories of our foremost universities.

April 26, 7:45 A.M.

The ancient Hebrews were precursors not only of the Occident (March 18) but of the modern age of hope. Usually, when we speak of the uniqueness of the ancient Hebrews, we have in mind their worship of one, invisible God. Actually, Hebrew monotheism went hand in hand with two other unique manifestations. The Hebrews were the first optimists. Alone among the peoples of antiquity they located a golden age not in the past but in the future. Their *tikva*, hope, envisioned a glorious future for humanity on this earth. (The Old Testament makes no mention of a heavenly kingdom. All of God's promises were to be fulfilled here on earth.)

Curiously, this faith in the future was joined with a passionate preoccupation with the past. The ancient Hebrews made history rather than cosmic events the meaningful drama of the universe. Their rites and celebrations concerned themselves not with the cycle of the seasons but with historical events.

It is my feeling that there is an interconnection between faith in one, invisible God and a vivid awareness of future and past. People without hope need tangible idols to worship. It is only when we hope "for what we see not" that we can believe in what we see not. So, too, the making of historical rather than natural events the central drama of the universe was part of the downgrading of nature which made possible the belief in a God who was not part of but the creator of nature. There can be no monotheistic faith without a belief in the uniqueness and primacy of man. The one God who created nature made man his viceroy on earth.

Strangely, a modern Occident that functions largely without faith in God has embraced the Hebrew *tikva* and the passionate preoccupation with history.

April 28, 7:50 A.M.

We usually think of youth as an age of hope. Actually, the young are immersed in the present and their hopes are so immediate as to be indistinguishable from desire. On the other hand, to the old, hope is a tonic that stimulates digestion and blood circulation and makes sleep more restful. The old are stretched by expecting something around the corner.

I have suggested (April 12) that Russia is in chronic trouble because of the incompatibility between Russian nature and communism. Yet it is by no means self-evident that an incompatibility between a doctrine and those who adopt it unavoidably spells trouble.

One cannot think of a more profound incompatibility than that between the Christian doctrine of meekness and Europe's warrior tribes who embraced it; yet this contradiction generated a tension which made Europe the most dynamic part of the world. Why, then, does the contradiction in Russia result in stagnation? The answer probably is that, whereas the warrior tribes fervently believed in a Christianity that went against their grain, the Russians do not believe in communism. There is no pull between opposites which would stretch souls.

April 29, 8:00 A.M.

I have never had absolute command of language. Words have always been to me accidental, unnatural, uninevitable. I have spent my life trying to master words, but they never became part of me. I always have to search for them, pull them in by the neck. I use as few of them as I can.

Several years ago, I gave the University of California at Berkeley a sum of money that would yield at least five hundred dollars a year to be given as a prize for an essay for five hundred words. A dollar a word! There was an outcry from students and some of the faculty: "What can one say in five hundred words?" My answer was that there is not an idea that cannot be expressed in two hundred words, and the prize allows words enough for two and a half original ideas.

April 30, 8:00 A.M.

As long as a society has an enclave of legitimate recklessness, spoiling children need not have fatal consequences. In the heyday of Britain's aristocracy, Lord Holland could propound the doctrine that "the young are always right," and indulge his son Charles when he smashed a gold watch, saying: "If you must, you must." This Charles grew up to be a reckless gambler and womanizer but also a brilliant, daring political figure—an aristocrat who toasted "Our Sovereign the People."

In this country, business is the main enclave of recklessness and it is my hunch that spoiled children have the makings of daring business operators. It was disastrous that in the 1960s the spoiled children of the rich turned their backs on business and vented their recklessness on campuses.

May 1, 7:00 A.M.

It is incredible how much pampering and bribing it needs to induce the rich to get richer. They call the bribes incentives. Clearly, it is assumed that it is the rich who keep the wheels turning. They not only avoid paying adequate taxes but are paid not to raise wheat and not to pump oil.

Despite space exploration and unprecedented discoveries in science and technology, the spirit of our age expresses itself more clearly in failures than in achievements. Our age is documented by fears rather than hopes.

7:45 A.M. Perhaps, under ideal conditions, communism might be compatible with individual freedom and even with abundance. What are the ideal conditions? A fairly advanced country with a disciplined, energetic, and highly skilled population that has wearied of competition and the lust for possessions. The aim of such a society would be an unhurried, culturally rich existence. Whatever it had of abundance would be an accidental bonus.

May 3, 8:30 A.M.

You would think that when a man had something worthwhile to say his chief concern would be to make himself understood and he would write as simply as he could. But it is not so. There are not above a score of scholars in this country at present who express themselves in lucid prose.

In Britain good writing has a long tradition, and it is practiced by scientists and scholars. Lord Rutherford used to say that he was not sure an idea had merit until he could express it in ordinary language understood by charwomen.

The French have long been masters of lucid writing. French thinkers from Descartes on believed that there is not an idea that cannot be expressed in language intelligible to everybody. In the eighteenth century Rivarol maintained that that which is not lucid is not French. Of late, however, French writers have become enamored of existentialist, Marxist, and Hegelian double talk. It is the British who now write English the way the French used to write French.

Hegel's great victory in the twentieth century has been to make Frenchmen write like Germans. Actually, it was Hitler who made Frenchmen receptive to Hegel. They needed fig leaves of obscurantism to cover the shame of the German occupation.

May 4, 6:30 A.M.

I woke up this morning thinking about old King David. I reread the opening paragraph of the first book of Kings: "Now king David was old and stricken in years; and they covered him with clothes, but he gat no heat. Wherefore his servants said unto him, Let there be sought for my lord the king a young virgin: and let her stand before the king, and let her cherish him, and let her lie in thy bosom, that my lord the king may get heat. So they sought for a fair damsel throughout all the coasts of Israel and found Abishag a Shunamite and brought her to the king. And the damsel was very fair, and cherished the king, and ministered to him: but the king knew her not." Has anyone painted David with the Shunamite maiden? David's leathery, worn face, the lost look in his brooding eyes, the white hair on his skeletal chest. I cannot see the maiden.

It is probably extremely rare for a person to feel, even for a brief moment, that what he is and does are absolutely fitting and cannot be bettered. And it is a gift from heaven for an older person to have such a moment.

May 5, 9:45 A.M.

I suspect that American obscurantist writing has German roots. German universities were the nursery of American scholarship during the nineteenth century. The Germans disdain lucidity as superficial. The least-understood philosophers have among them the greatest authority. It has been argued that the inability of the Germans to develop lucid prose has been one of the disasters of European civilization.

Strangely, two great Germans—Frederick the Great and Charles the Fifth—thought that German was good only for talking to horses.

American articles are usually longer and American books thicker than their British counterparts. When I go through a shelf of books on a subject I begin with the thin volumes. Now and then I find a thin and a thick book by the same author on the same subject. Usually, the thin book is of an earlier date; and it often turns out that in the thin book the author reveals what he knows and in the thick book he tries to conceal what he does not know.

Good historians are an exception. They may produce a thin volume toward the end of their days summarizing their ideas, and it is a treat to read them.

About David and the Shunamite maiden: "The lost look in brooding eyes" is wrong. Rather eyes like live coals glowing in a shriveled face, and the hair on his head standing on end. The maiden at his side is excited, with twinkling, mischievous eyes. Two playmates.

May 6, 8:00 A.M.

It is becoming increasingly difficult for haves and have-nots to live together in one society. As never before, it is clear that a massive attempt to end poverty must in various ways discomfort the haves, while under conditions optimal for the haves the disillusionment of the have-nots threatens social stability.

The hopeful nineteenth century took it for granted that the march of progress would turn have-nots into haves. The Bolsheviks tried to solve the problem by turning haves into have-nots. But in the last third of the twentieth century we have seen it demonstrated that money, education, and armies of dedicated social workers cannot cure chronic poverty. We also know that turning haves into have-nots results in social decline and stagnation. The only alternative left is separation—to have two different societies side by side (March 3). In one society the chronically poor will have ideal opportunities to learn new skills and become self-reliant. In the other society the haves will be free to wheel and deal, compete, run risks, build and tear down, experiment—in short, do as they please.

May 7, 7:50 A.M.

I doubt whether any book or film could do justice to the battle of Midway. The Americans did not fight for a fatherland or a holy cause. There was a job to do and they did it. They were not only outnumbered by the Japanese but also outclassed. The Japanese Zero fighter could outclimb, outrun, and outmaneuver any plane the Americans had. The American fliers were inferior in battle experience and in morale. There was nothing on the American side to match the fanatical dedication of Japanese fighting men. The Japanese had every reason to believe that taking Midway would be "as easy as twisting a baby's arm."

The American planes came in clumsily, doggedly, and recklessly. A large number of them were blown out of the sky, and most of their bombs missed the target. But they kept coming, and eventually sank all the Japanese carriers with all their planes, and most of their irreplaceable veteran crews. It was a fateful victory and a turning point in the war. Yet, throughout the battle, all that the American commanders, from Admiral Nimitz down, could tell their men was, "There is a job to do."

During the Civil War, educated people in Europe took it for granted that America's days were numbered and they were on the whole glad of it. It is startling to read what the enlightened Walter Bagehot had to say on the subject (*Historical Essays*): "Europe at large and England especially have not grieved much at the close proximity of America's fall, but perhaps rejoiced at the prospect of some marked change from a policy . . . of which the events were mean, the actors base, and the workings inexplicable. A low vulgarity has deeply displeased the cultivated mind of Europe, and the American Union will fall little regretted even by those whose race is akin, whose language is identical, whose weighted opinions are on most subjects the same as theirs. The unpleasantness of mob government has never before been exemplified so conspicuously, for it never before has worked on so large a scene."

It needs an effort to realize how offended Europe's cultivated, aristocratic minds were by the spectacle of common people eloping with history to a vast, new continent and essaying to do there all the things—build cities, found states, lead armies—which from the beginning of time were reserved for the privileged orders.

May 8, 6:40 A.M.

In any consideration of creative milieus Hungary of 1867–1914 should occupy a prominent place. The Hungarian aristocracy in its effort to hold up its end in the partnership with the Austro-Germans did all it could to stimulate the growth of Hungarian culture. There was a massive, methodical effort to realize creative potentialities. The spotting and encouragement of talent in the Budapest of that period were as effective as they were in Renaissance Florence. Most of the fabulous Hungarians who made their mark in Europe and America had their start in this creative milieu. If I remember correctly, they were all graduates of the same famous high school.

When Wycliffe translated the Bible from the Latin into "the tongue of the Angels," he was excoriated by his betters for scattering the evangelical pearls "to be trampled by the swine." The educated have equated common people with swine almost from the invention of writing. It is curious that in Russia, despite the official glorification of the masses, there is an intense loathing of common people among the intellectuals. In this country in the 1960s the SDS semester-intellectuals spoke of the majority as "honkey swine."

May 9, 8:00 A.M.

When we read what some revolutionary intellectuals wrote about the evils of the nineteenth century we are startled by how closely their words fit the realities of twentieth-century Russia. Here is Alexander Herzen's description of Western Europe in the middle of the nineteenth century: "A secular inquisition reigns supreme, civil rights have been suspended. . . . There is only one moral force that still has authority over men . . . and that is fear which is universal."

The revolutionaries made of history what Engels said it was: "the most terrible of divinities driving its triumphant chariot over piles of cadavers."

9:00 P.M. I spent four hours in the park walking leisurely. The call of the quail reminded me of the great silence of the wilderness I knew in my gold-prospecting days. I am like a man with a heart condition who has not a thought on which death is not engraved.

May 10, 6:30 A.M.

The nineteenth century was naïve because it did not know the end of the story. It did not know what happens when dedicated idealists come to power; it did not know the intimate linkage between idealists and policemen, between being your brother's keeper and being his jailkeeper. The nineteenth century was both hopeful and rational. Is naïveté a by-product of hope and logic?

Some of the hands seen in cave paintings have a finger or the joint of a finger missing. The conclusion of the scholarly experts: "Mutilation; the sign of religious practices." It did not occur to these experts that hunting and the chipping of stone tools can be hard on fingers, at least as hard as longshoring. Missing fingers or joints of fingers are common on the waterfront.

May 11, 8:45 A.M.

To maintain social discipline, an affluent society must know how to create a new kind of scarcity—a new category of vital needs that are not easily fulfilled. In an affluent society the vying and ceaseless striving which made material abundance possible will have to be directed toward new goals. Just as in a time of general scarcity societies had to implant and nurture the work ethic in order to survive, so in an era of general abundance they have to know how to induce a ceaseless striving for the realization of individual capacities and talents in order to preserve their stability and health. And by passing from an economy of matter to an economy of the spirit a society enters a world of incurable scarcity.

May 12, 6:30 A.M.

In a creative milieu the talented are not only encouraged and cultivated but are also left alone to stew in their own juice. This is something a Communist regime cannot do. It both worships and fears the creative individual. It is convinced that the field of culture is also a seedbed of dissent and subversion, and needs constant weeding.

May 13, 8:10 A.M.

Von Karman's *The Wind and Beyond* is a delight. He is one of the prodigious Hungarians I have mentioned (May 8). I am learning something and also enjoying myself. Good stories. The one I like best is about David Helbert, the great mathematician. At a party in his house, his wife asked him to change his tie. He went up to the bedroom and did not return. When his wife went up to see what had happened to him she found him fast asleep in bed. He had taken off his tie, and since this was normally the first step in undressing he simply continued and went to sleep.

This story reminded me of the predicament of the old: they have the failings and the needs of genius. They are as absent-minded as a great mathematician, and like creative people they need recognition and praise in order to function well.

Von Karman's father thought that the life span of an idea is 150 years (five generations). He predicted that nationalism, which took hold in 1800, would begin to die in 1950.

Of what do ideas die? Some die of excess. The excesses of the religious wars put an end to religiosity just as nationalist excesses are bringing nationalism to an end. Industrialism too seems likely to die of excess. The idea of hope died from expecting too much and taking too much for granted. The hopeful generation that stumbled into the First World War took civilized life for granted. The life span of the idea of hope, from the Encyclopedists to 1914, was about 150 years.

May 14, 7:30 A.M.

Social scientists dream of situations immune to interference by unpredictable human factors. But it turns out that in human affairs no situation is manproof. However high the degree of automation and however overpowering the nonhuman factors, the human elements of enterprise, courage, pride, faith, malice, stupidity, sloth, and the capacity for mischief remain decisive.

Reading von Karman, one realizes what a potent key mathematics is for the unlocking of nature's secrets. One is also aware that in aerodynamics, as in man's soul, the trivial is not trivial. A slight change in design can have momentous consequences.

I love ideas as much as I love women. I derive a sensuous pleasure from playing with ideas. Genuine ideas dance and sing. They sparkle and twinkle with mirth and mischief. They titillate the mind, kindle the imagination, and warm the heart. They have grace and promise.

May 15, 7:00 A.M.

Latin countries seem always politically on the brink. Non-Latin countries in Western Europe and North America have economic crises but are on the whole politically stable. It is of interest that Latin Quebec is introducing a brink into Canada's political life.

The greater political involvement of intellectuals in Latin countries may be a factor. The intellectuals are there at the center of the web of power. They not only organize political parties and shape public opinion but are often elected to high office. And there is clear evidence that intellectuals are too self-important and self-righteous to practice the give-and-take vital for the stability of a free society. Where there is no restraining power, intellectuals in politics are a divisive element with a natural bent for pullulating, zealous sects, cliques, and factions. If an organization dominated by intellectuals is to keep stable it has to be authoritarian and intolerant of dissent. This is true of the Catholic church and of Communist parties. De Gaulle, who sensed France's incompatibility with parliamentary democracy, did not go far enough in his innovations to ensure political stability. And it is quite fitting that the largest Communist parties in Europe outside the Soviet orbit should be found in Latin countries.

May 16, 2:30 P.M.

Czarist Russia was an inefficient, backward, and somewhat chaotic despotism. Its cultural life was dominated by a tyrannical censor. It was racked by violent dissent and police brutality. Yet, surprisingly, during the second half of the nineteenth century Czarist Russia produced writers, composers, and scientists who rank with the greatest of our time. Clearly, despite its appalling drawbacks, Czarist Russia had the elements of a potent creative milieu. What were they?

There was an appreciative reading public that welcomed a good book as a national event. The publishing establishment celebrated and rewarded excellence. The censorship was inefficient. It compressed rather than repressed the creative drive. A paucity of opportunities for impressive action in business and politics allowed a copious flow of energies into cultural pursuits. There was a passion for discussion; talk was a national pastime. Finally, Russian society in the second half of the nineteenth century was subject to the pull of opposite poles, which stretched souls: national pride and self-contempt, hope and fear, worship of freedom and a slave mentality, a pull toward and a repulsion from Western Europe, a suspension between East and West and between barbarism and civilization.

About the capacity for prophesying. The Baltic barons, suspended between Germany and Russia, and with a foreign peasantry on their land, had both the inclination and the gift for prophesying. On the eve of the French Revolution, Baron Grimm wrote to Catherine of Russia: "Two empires will divide the world between them: Russia in the East, and America, which has gained its freedom in recent years, in the West; and we the people in between shall be too degraded to know what we have been." Thus when, about fifty years later, de Tocqueville prophesied the impending domination of the world by Russia and America, he was echoing something that was floating in the air.

9:00 P.M. Though my life is meager, I have yet to meet a person with whom I would like to change places. I never wanted to be other than what I am. I have been wearing the same kind of clothes, cut my hair the same way, lived in the same style all my life.

Nor have I ever become disenchanted with America. I somehow always felt that I had no right to expect too much from this country. I know all the flaws and blemishes. But I also know that America was built largely by hordes of undesirables from Europe, and that had this country been populated by Europe's best and finest, we would now be in a worse mess.

May 17, 6:35 A.M.

In a post-industrial society it will become increasingly difficult to find work for everybody. How will the presence of millions of energetic, skilled workingmen rusting away in inaction affect social vigor?

A concerted effort to clean up the continent and renovate the large cities might offer a temporary solution. But in the long run, post-industrial society will have to accept a drastic reduction of the work week to, say, twenty-four hours or less. This will involve a change in the role of work: rather than being the main content of life, work will be seen as a ritual and drill to maintain physical and mental health.

The distribution of goods was a problem of industrial societies. The problem of post-industrial society will be the distribution of work.

May 19, 10:30 A.M.

We must never get over the fact that one of the best-educated and most-advanced countries of the Occident became a willing instrument of Hitler's holocaust. Instead of repeating the clichés about the humanizing and civilizing effects of education we ought to think and speak about the dehumanizing effects of humiliation—how easily the bruised self sheds its humanity and its veneer of civilization. The humiliation of Germany by France after the First World War was a monumental blunder. It is to America's credit that it did not humiliate its defeated enemies after the Second World War. The humiliation of France during the Second World War will go on having pernicious consequences for decades.

A war is not won if the defeated enemy has not been turned into a friend. It should be easy for a conqueror to court the conquered. The injunction to love our enemy is easy to obey when it is a defeated enemy.

May 20, 8:00 A.M.

In a Communist country there is no pornography, no violence in the streets, no unemployment, no rat race, no corrupt welfare and poverty programs, and no ceaseless din of inane, brazen advertisements. Why, then, would I never choose to live in a Communist country?

In a Communist country the individual is never left alone. He is spied upon, bullied, and paralyzed by fear and distrust. Above all, the savagely enforced prohibition of emigration makes it plain that a Communist country is basically a prison. When you go to prison in a free country you escape pornography, unemployment, the rat race, and so on. Yet no one chooses to go to prison to escape the evils of the outside world.

May 21, 7:00 A.M.

It is a general assumption that America became a great nation because of the abundance of its natural resources. The assumption is not shaken by the fact that Canada and Mexico did not become great despite their natural riches, and that a Japan that imports over ninety percent of its raw materials is catching up with the United States.

Whether Marxist or not, American historians are not hospitable to the idea that man makes history, that the human resources are more decisive than the natural—that courage, enterprise, skill, and a passion for excellence are the ingredients of national vigor and greatness. Do they see doom around the corner now that our stores of oil and natural gas are running out, and other raw materials are nearing exhaustion?

Still, I wonder whether the vastness and riches of this continent were not a precondition for the formation of our unprecedented mass society in the second half of the nineteenth century. The masses who plunged into a virgin continent and tamed it in an incredibly short time were mindlessly wasteful. The fabulous natural riches gave them the time to become skilled men of action even as they wasted, so that eventually they could turn the ravaged land into a cornucopia.

11:00 P.M. I spent almost two hours tracking a mistake in my bank book. The elation when I finally spotted the mistake is comical. I realized that since my retirement from the waterfront I have been without the frequent feeling of well-being that comes from a job well done. Happiness comes from small things.

May 22, 9:15 A.M.

Coming of short-lived stock, I have felt most of my life that my days were numbered. Yet only now, at seventy-three, do I have the feeling that there is no time left to make good what is lost or damaged—that any mistake I make is irremediable. Obviously, the sense of time is not purely a mental attitude but a function of the body.

What happens when a highly endowed person does not develop with his talents? It all depends on whether he has clear proof of his exceptional capacities. If he has, the unrealized talents will gnaw at his heart and mind. But, if a person is unaware of his talents, the buried gifts will give zest and sparkle to his everyday life.

May 23, 6:00 A.M.

The present manufactures both past and future. A good book about the present should tell how past and future are made.

It should throw a new light on the past, and provide niches into which future happenings will fit.

I am reading Yevgenia Ginzburg's *Journey into the Whirlwind*. She spent eighteen years in Stalin's camps. The Stalin-Hitler decades shaped my mind and I am still obsessed with the deliberate human degradation practiced by Russians and Germans on a vast scale. The passivity of the outside world during those terrible decades makes me scornful of the present fashionable agitation against all sorts of wrongs in non-Communist countries. A world that did not raise its voice against the enormities of Stalin and Hitler is now crying out against injustice in Chile, Rhodesia, and South Africa. Arnold Toynbee, who glowed when he shook Hitler's hand, called the displacement of Arabs by Israelis an atrocity greater than any committed by the Nazis

Soviet Russia is an empire without a history. Its true history can be written only by its enemies. To the Soviets, Lenin is almost the only historical figure. Most of the other people who played leading roles in the rise of the Soviet empire have become non-persons. It is fantastic that the Marxist worship of history should have resulted in an abolition of history and a return to mythology.

May 24, 7:45 A.M.
It has been an article of faith since the French Revolution that nothing great can be accomplished without enthusiasm. Is it not possible to achieve the momentous in an unmomentous way? Surely an enterprising, skilled population should be able to do great things in a sober, workaday spirit. It has been said of the people who built Ford's first assembly line that to them work was play and that if it had not been play it would have killed them. One might say that the vigor of a society is proportionate to its ability to dispense with enthusiasm.

We are discovering that righting wrongs does not increase social concord. Women's liberation, racial equality, and the war on poverty have not made us a more united nation. On the contrary, social justice has multiplied grievances and fueled discord. Like total freedom, total justice may become a cause of social disintegration.

Civilized life is based on an acceptance of imperfection—on not trying to enforce every right one possesses.

It is the testimony of the ages that there is little happiness—least of all when we get what we want. Many outstanding persons who reviewed their lives in old age found that all their happy moments did not add up to a full day.

The entrance of the masses onto the stage of history has not produced the anarchy forecast by many social thinkers in the nineteenth century. Yet the fear of the masses persists. The reason is that the self-assertion of the masses threatens the cultural elites. Where every mother's son feels competent to write or paint, being a writer or an artist is no longer the rare achievement it has been through all of history. To Robert Graves, "Writing has become almost meaningless as a descriptive term since popular education opened the dikes to a shallow sea." According to Marcel Duchamp, "When painting becomes so low that laymen talk about it, it doesn't interest me." Abstruseness and abstraction are probably devices to preserve a cultural monopoly.

May 25, 6:30 A.M.

Has there ever been a time when people felt, as they do now, that comes the big wind not much will be left of what is now touted as great? We see an unprecedented outdatedness overtaking cultural products. When cultural life is dominated by clowns, nothing lasts.

Modernization has everywhere weakened social cohesion by draining the traditional authorities of church and family of their effectiveness, and by discrediting long-established customs and attitudes. So far, the advanced countries have failed to evolve a durable new organizing principle of society. The mushrooming big cities characteristic of our age are a dumping ground of the debris of communal entities shattered by the march of progress. Nowhere has this human debris been integrated into new social bodies.

One can see the advantage Japan and probably other countries of the Chinese Far East have in the present social crisis. Japan's strong sense of identity and group solidarity enabled it to ward off the social disorganization which accompanied modernization elsewhere. The countries of the Chinese Far East know how to transplant ancient group values to new institutions. This is particularly true of the deeply rooted family relationships. Hence the Chinese Far East is becoming an ideal milieu for the development of esprit de corps—the formation of family ties among strangers—in neighborhoods, factories, offices, armies, and so on.

The Greeks had no holy books, no received truths, no venerated classics, and no scientific or philosophical jargon. The speech of the uneducated was also the speech of the intellectuals. The Greeks had a lot to say and little to hide. They did not need obscurantist double-talk to cover up their emptiness or shame.

The ancient Hebrews were alone in their cultivation of compassion. The Bible forbids the muzzling of an ox in his threshing whereas the Romans muzzled slaves grinding grain. To the Greeks, too, slaves were not human.

It is a paradox that the Greeks, who invented individual freedom, were the first to institutionalize slavery. In the pre-Greek world all men were servile and chattel slavery was of minor importance. To the clear-thinking Greeks freedom meant freedom from the servitude of work.

The automated machinery of a post-industrial society is more than an effective equivalent of the slave population that did much of the work in classical Greece. But could a modern society match what the Greeks did with their freedom from work?

May 26, 9:30 A.M.

The silent majority has no hopes. It has fears: fear of inflation, fear of violence in the streets, fear of having houses and cars ransacked, fear of losing its children to the drug and drift culture. A party that aspires to become a party of the majority must address itself to these fears.

The Democratic party is increasingly becoming a party of the minorities. The question is whether the Republicans can develop the sweep and drive necessary to stir the majority and convince it that there are practical ways to assuage its fears.

Modern history came to an end with Lenin's revolution. The Bolsheviks aspired to bring history to an end by eliminating classes. Instead they brought modern history to an end by eliminating individual freedom and initiative and the friendship, loyalty, and honor which can mark the intercourse between autonomous individuals.

In 1917 the Germans brought a plague-carrying rat in a sealed train to the edge of Russia and let it loose. The rat set off a ravaging pestilence that killed sixty million Russian men, women, and children. No one knows whether the pestilence has burned itself out or is merely dormant.

When the rat died its body was embalmed and placed in a glass case. It is worshiped as a god in a temple in Moscow. There are many people in other countries who have been converted to rat worship.

May 27, 6:00 A.M.
Slept fitfully. The left arm is giving me trouble. The first thought this morning was about my lack of a fruitful train of thought. The short essays I have been writing are links in a chain. I could combine several of them into larger chapters. But I hunger for a totally new train of thought.

Social automatism is at its height when a society is engaged in a struggle to master nature. It is then that impersonal factors move people to action and the need for the deliberate management of men is minimal. But once things have been mastered and want is banished much of the social automatism disappears. A triumphant technology ushers in a psychological age, and history is made not by the hidden hand of circumstances but by men. Once the social anarchy released by the elimination of scarcity is brought to an end by despotic power, it will be seen that, for the mass of people, the outcome of technological progress is a passage from servitude to things to the more demeaning servitude to men.

I used to think it self-evident that freedom means freedom from iron necessity. But it is not quite so. The moment necessity no longer regulates and disciplines there is need for imposed regimentation. On the other hand, a society living on the edge of subsistence cannot afford freedom. Thus the zone of individual freedom is midway between the extremes of scarcity and abundance.

May 28, 7:00 A.M.

Does not civilized living depend on not seeing things as they are? There can be neither order nor stability and continuity without illusions about authority, about the attainability of desired goals, about the quality of our fellow men, and about our own nature. A confrontation with naked, raw reality shreds the fiber of civilized life.

May 29, 8:30 A.M.

My faith in America is partly faith in its digestive powers—its capacity to absorb and assimilate foreign bodies. During the past 150 years, whenever there was an influx of outsiders there were knowledgeable people who wondered whether the country could preserve its identity. In 1868 Sir Charles Dilke predicted that the Irish who were packing the cities would become America's new ruling class and the squeezed-out "law-abiding Saxon" a docile peasantry.

America is the worst place for alibis. Sooner or later the most solid alibi begins to sound hollow. Even the alibi of heredity becomes irrelevant. To come to America is to be reborn, to start with a clean slate. Here you are your own creator and your own ancestor.

In America nothing is finished. The social and political chemistry is still active. Everything is still in solution, and every reaction reversible.

America is the classic land of rebirth and new beginnings. You cannot predict the performance of an American from his past.

4:15 P.M. I met Jack Lurie outside the Safeway market near

where I live. His face looked drawn. He is eighty-three years old and has been retired from the waterfront for fifteen years. His stomach is giving him trouble for the first time in his life and he is panicked. He also feels terribly alone—has no kin or close friends. All of a sudden he started to cry. I put my arms around him and tried to console him. I did not know what to say.

May 30, 7:20 A.M.

Every era has a currency that buys souls. In some the currency is pride, in others it is hope, in still others it is a holy cause. There are of course times when hard cash will buy souls, and the remarkable thing is that such times are marked by civility, tolerance, and the smooth working of everyday life.

At present, no matter how prosperous a free society might be it is still plagued by inflation, chronic unemployment, and mindless violence. There is no reason to believe that copious new sources of fossil fuels and serviceable substitutes for scarce raw materials would change the situation. There is evidence on every hand that material resources are not as decisive as they used to be. Have we entered a new era in which old axioms are no longer valid? It might well be that at present advanced countries can remain free and stable only when they realize and utilize their human resources. Intractable problems would solve themselves once there was a wide distribution of work, a participation of common people in cultural pursuits, and unlimited opportunities for the young—from the age of ten—to acquire skills and become self-reliant.

3   THE HUMAN FACTOR

WHEN I STARTED on the diary that became "Before the Sabbath," I wanted to find out whether the necessity to write something every day would revive my flagging alertness to the first, faint stirrings of new ideas. I also hoped that some new insight caught in flight might be the beginning of a train of thought that could keep me going for years.

Did it work? The diary reads well, and here and there I suggest that a new idea could be the subject of a book; but only one topic, "the role of the human factor," gives me the feeling that I have bumped against something which is, perhaps, at the core of our present crisis.

From the early days of the Industrial Revolution, intellectuals of every sort predicted that the machine would make man superfluous. Right now it would be difficult to find a social scientist who does not believe that automated machines and computers are eliminating man as a factor in the social equation. There is even an academic joke on the subject: Descartes said, "I think, therefore I am"; the computer says, "I think, therefore you are not."

The belief that the machine turns men into predictable robots is not based on experience or observation. It is an a priori assumption that blinds social scientists to what is happening under their noses. It prevents them from seeing that a triumphant technology

---

Previously unpublished; elements appeared in the Afterword of *Before the Sabbath*.

is doing the opposite of what they predicted it would do. There is evidence on every hand that the human factor has never been so central as it is now in technologically advanced countries. It is the centrality of the human factor that makes industrialized societies so unpredictable and explosive.

All through the millennia work has been the main theme of human existence. Society itself originated in the need for a concerted effort to wrest a livelihood from grudging nature. In the modern Occident work became as well the chief source of a sense of usefulness, and the means by which the young proved their manhood. You became a man by doing a man's work and getting a man's pay.

The battle against want mobilized and disciplined. It was the hidden hand of scarcity that regulated and managed men through most of history. In a world of scarcity, the innate anarchy of the human condition is kept locked in the dark cellars of the individual's psyche and is not allowed to inject its unpredictability into everyday life.

During the nineteenth century, a nation that was engaged in the Promethean effort to harness nature gave little thought to the management of men. The ruling middle class could proceed on the principle that government is best when it governs least. Everyday life had a fabulous regularity: millions went to work each morning and returned from work each evening "with a regularity akin to the moon's tide." Obedience to authority was automatic as a reflex movement. Social processes were almost as rational and predictable as the processes of nature which the scientists were then probing and elucidating. It was reasonable to believe in the possibility of a social science as exact as the natural sciences. Walter Bagehot wrote a book, *Physics and Politics*. There was also boundless hope—a belief in automatic, ceaseless progress—which infused people with patience. No one foresaw the startling consequences of a taste of limitless plenty made possible by a triumphant technology. No one foresaw the twentieth century: hectic, soaked with the blood of innocents, fearful of the future criss-crossed with frontiers that prevent free movement, stripped of certitudes, unpredictable, and absurd.

Was it logic and hope that kept most nineteenth-century thinkers from contemplating an unpleasant, let alone an apocalyptic, fulfillment to the Industrial Revolution? Few in the nineteenth century were aware of the explosive irrationality of the human condition. No one suspected that once nature had been mastered and scarcity no longer regulated and disciplined people, industrial societies would enter a psychological age in which man would become a threat to his own survival.

In the rational, hopeful climate of the nineteenth century there was little place for fearing that the paradoxes of the human condition would combine to turn the successes of an industrial society into failures. A logician like Marx could not foresee the downfall of capitalism as a result of ever-increasing affluence rather than ever-increasing misery. Hardly anyone foresaw the chronic unemployment and the loss of a sense of usefulness caused by increased efficiency. No one feared that rapid change would upset traditions, customs, routines, and other arrangements which make everyday life predictable. Finally, no one foresaw that the education explosion made possible by advanced technology would swamp societies with hordes of educated nobodies who want to be somebodies and end up being mischief-making busybodies.

In technologically advanced countries at present there is little that can be taken for granted. There is no certainty that the end result of a course of action will be what it was reasonable to expect. It often seems as if some cunning, spiteful power is playing tricks behind the scenes, delighting in drawing from men's actions consequences least foreseen. The centrality of the human factor makes it impossible for a free country to have a strong government. Everywhere we look we see the paradoxes of the human condition play havoc with the best laid plans and the best intentions. It is becoming evident that in the post-industrial world, human rather than natural resources will be the wellspring of a country's wealth and vigor.

Viewed from any vantage point the nineteenth century was a sharp historical deviation. All around us now we can see the linea-

ments of a pre-industrial pattern emerging in post-industrial societies. The explosion of the young, the dominance of the intellectuals, the savaging of the cities, the revulsion from work are
characteristics of the decades which preceded the Industrial Revolution. We are not plunging into the future but falling back into
the past. We are rejoining the ancient caravan.

The significant point is that the people who are rejoining the
caravan are not what they were in pre-industrial days. They are
more dangerous. The unspeakable atrocities of the twentieth century have demonstrated that man has become the source of a
great evil and that the central problem of the post-industrial age is
how to cope with man himself.

It is conceivable that if the exhaustion of raw materials and
sources of energy compel societies to tap the creative capacities of
their people they may, in doing so, also tap a new source, of social
discipline. For there is no invention that can take hard work out
of creation, and the creative flow is never abundant. Thus the
creative society is immersed in hard work and chronic scarcity
and is unavoidably a disciplined society. Still, the coming of the
creative society will be slow and faltering, and meanwhile we
must find other defenses against evil.